"*Inner Strengths: Contemporary Psychotherapy and Hypnosis for Ego-strengthening*
made a substantive contribution to the theory and practice of hypnosis through
providing a framework for understanding the personal strengths we have within,
and giving practitioners the tools to elicit these strengths. It is a book that
remains relevant, and I will personally return to it when engaging in research
and practice."

Professor Tharina Guse, *University of Pretoria*

"This is an outstanding book which combines thoughtful scholarship with
clinical utility. While primarily conceptualizing egomastery techniques from
a contemporary psychodynamic perspective, the book is transtheoretical with
applicability to both hypnotherapy and to more general psychotherapy.
Enhanced self-stability, self efficacy and self esteem form the heart of nearly
every psychotherapeutic encounter and process. I suspect that this book will
prove to be a central text for any psychotherapist's library. I recommend it with
enthusiasm."

Elgan L. Baker, *President Society for Clinical and*
Experiemental Hypnosis; Indiana Center for Ps

"In a book that ranges from psychoanalytic to transpersonal perspectives, and
from treating dissociative disorders to facilitating patients' self-care, Claire
Frederick and Shirley A. McNeal present a treasury of concepts, techniques, and
examples that will enrich any practitioner who explores them. *Inner Strengths*
is an inspirational commentary on the human condition, its resilience, and how
dividied, broken, and violated selves can be mended through the wise application
of psychotherapeutic procedures that are at the cutting edge of clinical practice."

Stanley Krippner, *Saybrook Graduate School; Coauthor,*
The Mythic Path; Coeditor Broken Images

"*Inner Strengths* is an important book for all clinicians working with traumatized
patients. Drs. Frederick and McNeal draw upon the major psychotherapeutic
and hypnotic traditins to present an integrative approach to ego-strengthening
treatment that is grounded in both respect and compassion for the client. In easily
read prose, important concepts are robustly defined, linked to the theoretical
literature, and clinically explained and illustrated by means of detailed case
examples. The authors' considerable scholarship and clinical acumen guide
both novice and experienced clinicans through an informative and wide-ranging
exploration of both hypnotic and non-hypnotic ego-strengthening techniques."

Francine Shapiro, *EMDR Institute*

Inner Strengths

Inner Strengths is the first book to meet the need for a comprehensive treatment of approaches to ego-strengthening in psychotherapy. It provides a historical breakthrough in the history of ego-strengthening education, and explores contemporary psychodynamic, object relations, self-psychology, ego state, and transpersonal theoretical models for understanding how and why ego-strengthening occurs.

Written by two experienced psychotherapists, who were active in developing the newer, projective-evocative ego-strengthening techniques, this book emphasizes the utilization of patients' inner resources. They survey the history of ego-strengthening efforts and show how that which has been considered intrinsically hypnotic connects with the great traditions of psychotherapy. Additionally, they offer step-by-step instructions for a diversity of ego-strengthening methods that can be used for patient self-care, internal boundary formation, and personality maturation in a wide range of clinical conditions. Their discussion of the fundamental concepts of ego-strengthening draws on their theoretical and clinical explorations of dynamic internal resources such as memory, strength, wisdom, self-soothing, and love.

Throughout the book, theory is balanced by an unusual richness of extended clinical examples and a wide variety of practical ego-strengthening scripts. This classic edition is essential reading for seasoned clinicians of hypnosis and beginners alike.

Claire Frederick, M.D., was a psychiatrist, who taught, consulted, and presented papers nationally and internationally. She was a co-author, with Maggie Phillips, Ph.D., of *Healing the Divided Self: Clinical and Ericksonian Hypnotherapy for Post-Traumatic and Dissociative Conditions.* She received multiple awards from the American Society of Clinical Hypnosis.

Shirley McNeal, Ph.D., has been a psychologist in private practice, who also presented papers, taught, and consulted nationally and internationally. She has received awards for her writing from the *American Journal of Clinical Hypnosis* and the *International Journal of Clinical and Experimental Hypnosis.*

Routledge Mental Health Classic Editions

The *Routledge Mental Health Classic Edition* series celebrates Routledge's commitment to excellence within the field of mental health. These books are recognized as timeless classics covering a range of important issues and continue to be recommended as key reading for professionals and students in the area. With a new introduction that explores what has changed since the books were first published, and why these books are as relevant now as ever, the series presents key ideas to a new generation.

Beyond Empathy
A Therapy of Contact-in-Relationship
Richard G. Erskine, Janet P. Moursund, and Rebecca L. Trautmann

Hidden Treasure
A Map to the Child's Inner Self
Violet Oaklander

Married Women Who Love Women
And More...
Carren Strock

Playing Sick? Untangling the Web of Munchausen Syndrome, Munchausen by Proxy, Malingering, and Factitious Disorder
Marc D. Feldman

Inner Strengths
Contemporary Psychotherapy and Hypnosis for Ego-Strengthening
Claire Frederick and Shirley McNeal

For more information about this series, please visit:www.routledge com/Routledge-Mental-Health-Classic-Editions/book-series/RMHCE

Inner Strengths

Contemporary Psychotherapy and Hypnosis for Ego-Strengthening
Classic Edition

Claire Frederick and Shirley McNeal

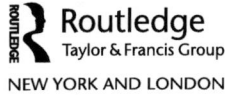
Routledge
Taylor & Francis Group

NEW YORK AND LONDON

Designed cover image: © Getty Images

Classic Edition Published 2023
by Routledge
4 Park Square, Milton Park, Abingdon, Oxon, OX14 4RN

and by Routledge
605 Third Avenue, New York, NY 10158

Routledge is an imprint of the Taylor & Francis Group, an informa business

First Edition Published by Routledge 1999

British Library Cataloguing-in-Publication Data
A catalogue record for this book is available from the British Library

ISBN: 978-1-032-58100-2 (hbk)
ISBN: 978-1-032-58086-9 (pbk)
ISBN: 978-1-003-44258-5 (ebk)

DOI: 10.4324/9781003442585

Typeset in Times New Roman
by Apex CoVantage, LLC

In loving memory of my mother, Beulah Brown McNeal:
Who taught me to love the written word.

To Claire Frederick: This book could not have been written
without her ongoing encouragement, support,
and collaboration.

Contents

Foreword to the Classic Edition

Shirley McNeal

During the years since its original publication, Claire Frederick and I had spoken about updating this book. We had discussed adding chapters based on what we thought at the time were new developments in psychiatry and psychology. Specifically, we considered material on the reemergence of the theory and treatment of attachment disorders, and on new discoveries in the area of brain functioning and hypnosis. However, because we were working on opposite sides of the country and had busy schedules, this task was not completed before Claire's death in 2015. In 2019, I was asked to be a plenary speaker at the annual meeting of the American Society of Clinical Hypnosis. On that occasion I had the opportunity to summarize Claire's and my past work on hypnotic ego-strengthening and to make some suggestions about future directions. Most of these ideas are included in a follow-up journal article published in the *American Journal of Clinical Hypnosis* (McNeal, 2020). I thought that article would be my last publication because I was planning to retire. However, when the publishers contacted me to say that they were contemplating reissuing this book as a "classic," I was willing to contribute what I could. I also wanted the opportunity to present other ideas pertaining to hypnotic ego-strengthening.

My review of this book convinced me of its continued relevance to the fields of psychiatry, medicine, nursing, dentistry, psychotherapy, and all ancillary forms of treatment within the healthcare professions. Clinicians of all theoretical orientations continue to emphasize the importance of the therapeutic alliance and of the patient's ability and motivation to change. A patient will only make changes if he or she feels strong enough to do so, so ego-strengthening is not only helpful but necessary. Also, the techniques, suggestions, and scripts presented in *Inner Strengths* can be used today, and in the future, because they are not tied to any particular historical period. Especially relevant are the projective/ evocative imagery techniques which are very client-centered, and depend on the specific aspects of the current goals of treatment, and all the resources that are available at the time. It is unfortunate that the term "ego" has a negative connotation in our popular culture. It usually implies an inflated ego. This book makes it clear that the ego is the energy of agency, that part of an individual that takes action. Thus, ego-strengthening continues to be a vital ingredient in all forms of treatment where the patient needs to take action for self-improvement. Within psychotherapy, ego-strengthening helps the patient access their internal resources, hence the book's title, "Inner Strengths." Ego-strengthening helps the individual to move from insight to action. Hypnotic ego-strengthening provides patients with tools that they can then use on their own.

Attachment theory was touched upon in my last article (McNeal, 2020). There I emphasized how the attunement between therapist and patient that mimics secure attachment between infant and caregiver can be healing and promote self-regulation of affective arousal for the patient. Ego-strengthening from an attachment perspective thus increases self-regulation, self-soothing, and self-compassion. It is possible that hypnotic suggestions and scripts, the Inner Love script in particular, can increase self-compassion.

Neuroimaging techniques have advanced to the point that hypnotic suggestions can actually stimulate specific regions of the brain (Landry & Raz, 2017). Currently, it often happens that seminars on psychotherapy will stress how knowledge of brain functioning can dictate appropriate treatment interventions. Such knowledge could be of particular relevance to ego-strengthening suggestions that address specific perceptual, cognitive, and behavioral treatment goals.

Polyvagal theory (Porges, 2011) builds on attachment theory and the involvement of the autonomic nervous system, the vagus and cranial nerves in particular, in self-regulation where the influence of the environment plays a major role. Porges describes how facial expressions and vocalization between humans can stabilize physiological arousal and shift the individual out of fight-or-flight-or freeze reactions. These findings are obviously applicable to psychotherapy and hypnosis. Maggie Phillips (2018), in her plenary address during the 2018 annual meeting of the American Society of Clinical Hypnosis, spoke about creating relational safety in the treatment of trauma and pain with reference to the polyvagal contributions to the countertransference trance. Practitioners of clinical hypnosis are very aware of the importance of vocalizations for an effective hypnosis experience along with rapport and a positive therapist–patient relationship. Establishing safety and stabilizing affect are indeed ego-strengthening during all phases of treatment. As discoveries about the neurophysiological aspects of hypnosis progress, we can expect to see more relationships between various aspects of states of consciousness and neurophysiology, providing even more material for specialized ego-strengthening suggestions and hypnotic scripts.

Another new and developing area of psychotherapy and hypnosis is the increased focus on creating states of consciousness that can be healing and ego-strengthening. The relationship between mindfulness and hypnosis has been explored to a considerable extent by a number of professionals who have been utilizing clinical hypnosis in treatment (Yapko, 2011). Alladin (2014) has described a treatment approach that he calls Mindfulness-Based Cognitive Hypnotherapy (MBCH), which includes ego-strengthening. Elkins, Roberts, and Simicich

(2018) wrote about mindful self-hypnosis for self-care, and Carolyn Daitch (2018) combined hypnosis, mindfulness, and cognitive behavior therapy for the treatment of generalized anxiety disorders. She utilized the ego-strengthening techniques of age regression and age progression as well as mindfulness and CBT techniques. These studies are described in more detail in my article about the road ahead for hypnotic ego-strengthening (McNeal, 2020).

An additional new direction in treatments that involve states of consciousness is psychedelic-assisted psychotherapy. Clinics are popping up all over the US and other countries offering the patient the opportunity to ingest a controlled substance, usually ketamine, which is legal, and then to be guided on a journey of self-discovery. During a seminar that I attended on this topic, one of the professionals who had studied to be a guide in psychedelic-assisted psychotherapy mentioned that she had training in clinical hypnosis, and that this training had been very helpful to her as she interacted with individuals while they were in the drug-induced trance state. Although we did not discuss ego-strengthening in particular, I strongly suspect that ego-strengthening would be involved in helping the patient to feel safe and to have an experience that could be deemed successful. I also would expect a successful psychedelic-assisted psychotherapy experience to increase conscious–unconscious complementarity. I believe future research should look at the similarities and differences between states of consciousness created by psychedelic substances, mindfulness meditation, certain forms of yoga, and hypnosis.

Finally, I believe it is important to take a look at hypnosis teletherapy. During the Covid-19 pandemic many psychotherapists continued to see patients using video platforms. Initially, caution was recommended for therapists using hypnosis with patients through telemedicine. However, a recent article on hypnosis teletherapy (Hasan & Vasant, 2023) indicated that in a study by Palsson et al. (2023), a world-wide survey found that approximately two-thirds of clinicians reported providing hypnotherapy over video. Over half of the clinicians reported that hypnotherapy delivered remotely is just as effective as face-to-face therapy. The majority of clinicians in the survey did not feel as positive about telephone hypnotherapy and used it much less frequently. The authors of the study feel strongly that hypnosis teletherapy is here to stay. However, the Hasan and Vasant (2023) study discussed advantages and disadvantages of delivering hypnosis via video and concluded that patient selection is very important. They also stressed the importance of training in hypnosis teletherapy and called for further research. I have used hypnosis remotely with patients whom I knew well and with whom I had a well-established therapeutic alliance. I have found hypnosis teletherapy to be quite successful, and recordings from our sessions have provided my patients with self-hypnosis recordings of ego-strengthening suggestions to use on their own.

In summary, I believe that ego-strengthening continues to be an important part of all hypnotic treatment and will continue to be included in all forms of psychotherapy and medicine. Because there appears to be a tendency toward greater integration of hypnosis with other forms of treatment, there could be even more opportunities for creating ego-strengthening techniques, especially those that are of a projective/evocative nature. As previously mentioned (McNeal, 2020), more research into ego-strengthening techniques is needed along with more precise definitions of what constitutes ego-strengthening, and what results should be expected. This book provides considerable historical context, a variety of theoretical approaches, and many tools for the clinician to utilize that are timeless and invaluable in all areas of healthcare and healing.

References

Alladin, A. (2014). Mindfulness-based hypnosis: Blending science, beliefs, and wisdom-sto catalyze healing. *American Journal of Clinical Hypnosis, 56*(3), 285–302. doi:10.1080/00029157.2013.857290

Daitch, C. (2018). Cognitive behavioral therapy, mindfulness, and hypnosis as treatment-methods for generalized anxiety disorder. *American Journal of Clinical Hypnosis, 61*(1), 57–69. doi:10.1080/00029157.2018.1458594

Elkins, G., Roberts, L. R., & Simicich, L. (2018). Mindful self-hypnosis for self-care: An integrative model and illustrative case example. *American Journal of Clinical Hypnosis, 61*(1), 45–56. doi:10.1080.00029157.2018.1456896

Hasan, S. S., & Vasant, D. H. (2023). The emerging new reality of hypnosis teletherapy: A major new mode of delivery of hypnotherapy and clinical hypnosis training. *International Journal of Clinical and Experimental Hypnosis, 71*(2), 153–162.

Landry, M. & Raz, A. (2017). Neurology of hypnosis. In G. E. Elkins (Ed.), *Handbook of medical and psychological hypnosis* (pp. 19–28). New York, NY: Springer.

McNeal, S. (2020). Hypnotic ego-strengthening: Where we've been and the road ahead. *American Journal of Clinical Hypnosis, 62*(4), 392–408.

Palsson, O. S., Kekecs, Z., De Benedittis, G., Moss, D., Elkins, G., Terhune, D. B., Varga, K., Shenefelt, P. D., & Whorwell, P. J. (2023). Current practices, experiences, and views in clinical hypnosis: Findings of an international survey. *International Journal of Clinical and Experimental Hypnosis, 71*(2), 92–114.

Phillips, M. (2018). *Relational safety as the treatment for trauma and pain: Polyvagal contributions to the countertransference trance.* Paper presented at the annual meeting of the American Society of Clinical Hypnosis, Orlando, FL.

Porges, S. W. (2011). *The polyvagal theory: Neurophysiological foundations of emotions, attachment, communication, and self-regulation.* New York: W.W. Norton.

Yapko, M. (2011). *Mindfulness and hypnosis: The power of suggestions to transform experience.* New York, NY: W.W. Norton.

Foreword

Stephen Gilligan

A letter arrived in the mail yesterday. It was from a woman who had been in therapy with me some years back. Out of the envelope fell a picture of her, so happy and proud, holding a beautiful, bright-eyed infant. A typed message formally announced that she had adopted this baby, and written underneath were simply the words, "With amazement, gratitude, and joy!!" Indeed! What an incredible sight to behold the beauty of both mother and child, reflected in their sparkling eyes. How different was the look in her eyes from when she had started therapy. Then she was depressed, suicidal, deeply pained. She felt useless, unlovable, and isolated. For my part, I felt overwhelmed by her at many points in the work, wondering if and how her healing might occur. Even when she terminated therapy after several years, coinciding with a job-related move back to the east coast, I wondered how she would fare. I was cautiously hopeful but then lost track of her. The picture was a welcome answer to my curiosities and hopes about her continued development.

Part of the difficulty was that many things I tried with her just did not work. They seemed to appropriately map into the client's patterns, but something inside her just couldn't or wouldn't positively respond. It was dismaying and frustrating to both of us that the therapeutic work progressed so slowly and haphazardly. That it was ultimately successful despite my fumblings is a testimony to her great strengths and commitment.

That therapy can succeed without the therapist being brilliant or all-knowing is one of the better-kept secrets in the clinical field. Actually, it seems that many times the therapist actually needs to fail in order for the therapy to succeed. It is only then that the patient's own resources can adequately be appreciated as the ultimate determinant of therapeutic success.

I wish that this wonderful book written by Claire Frederick and Shirley McNeal had been available to me then, for it would have helped me immensely. *Inner Strengths* is a book true to its name, and is full of extremely important ideas. For example, the authors emphasize how the ego strength of the patient is more important than the brilliance of the therapist. They describe how this ego strength is reflected in many skills, such as the capacities for self-care and self-confidence; the abilities to play, self-soothe, trust one's self and others in a healthy way, and tolerate conditional love; and the capacities to be creative, to know "safe space," and to have a positive sense of the future.

Frederick and McNeal provide excellent theoretical frameworks and multiple clinical examples of how these basic ego skills may develop and how they may be arrested or undeveloped via trauma, neglect, bad luck, biological predisposition, or poor relationships. They are especially artful in weaving different theoretical traditions into a coherent clinical description that provides a tremendous guide for helping therapists with even the most difficult cases. And they include abundant suggestions, protocols, and examples of how therapists may help clients build and use their ego strength as the basis for a happy, productive life. They impress on the reader that being a good therapist is a tremendous undertaking, but one well worth the considerable efforts.

In drawing on the work of Milton Erickson, my old mentor, they actually go beyond him in certain important respects. For example, Erickson was quite fond of emphasizing how the "unconscious mind" of the patient was very intelligent and resourceful. But he never quite explained how if a person's unconscious was so intelligent, then why on earth was the person acting so poorly before Erickson came on the scene? Frederick and McNeal address this paradox clearly by emphasizing that it is the relationship between the person's conscious and unconscious processes—between the agency of the ego and the multiple primary processes of the unconscious mind—that determines the mental health of the person. They further elucidate how the relational space created by therapist and client is a sort of a "third self" that constitutes a transitional space for the client to develop this relationship between his or her ego and unconscious. Thus, whereas one who reads Erickson is often left with a sense of Erickson's brilliance, Frederick and McNeal's writing leaves one with an appreciation of the inner strengths of patients, and how patients may learn to access and use them in their own ways.

This is what I really could have used with my old client. I was too busy trying to help the client with my brilliance, rather than appreciating how she could (or could not) help herself. I was too busy trying to connect with her unconscious, rather than helping her to connect with herself. I was too busy thinking of clever techniques, rather than wondering if and how she was able to incorporate and use these new learnings.

I still have these failings as a therapist, so I am grateful for this book by Frederick and McNeal. It is a very helpful guide for me as I continue the journey of being a therapist. I hope and trust that it will be helpful for you, too.

About the Author

Stephen Gilligan, Ph.D. is author of *Therapeutic Trances: The Cooperation Principle in Ericksonian Hypnotherapy* and *The Courage to Love*. He is coauthor of *Brief Therapy: Myths, Methods and Metaphors* and *Therapeutic Conversations*. Dr. Gilligan is in private practice in Encinitas, California.

Foreword

John G. Watkins and Helen H. Watkins

The title, *Inner Strengths: Contemporary Psychotherapy and Hypnosis for Ego-Strengthening*, is accurate in that the work is oriented around the concept of "ego strengthening." Moreover, Claire Frederick and Shirley McNeal have rightly claimed that strengthening the ego is a most significant element in all successful therapies. In this book they clearly describe many techniques for accomplishing this worthy goal.

However, the title greatly underrepresents the scope of this significant book. One cannot help being impressed by the solidness and immense breadth of scholarship here as the authors draw from basic sources throughout the entire range of psychology, empirical research, psychotherapy, philosophy, history, folklore, ethics, and religion. They paint broadly with a many-hued brush.

Furthermore, the authors are also very sensitive and innovative therapists. They offer many techniques and applications, drawn both from the contributions of others and from their own experiences in treating patients with a wide variety of disorders.

Within the field of therapy, they show how techniques and concepts from psychoanalysis, hypnosis, Ego State therapy, Jungian theory, Ericksonian psychology, object relations, self psychology, and many other psychotherapeutic systems can be effectively utilized to strengthen the ego during treatment. They demonstrate that by such ego strengthening, every approach to treatment can be made more potent and efficient. This is, therefore, a treatise on psychotherapy itself and will be a source for all who treat the emotional and behavioral ills of mankind regardless of theoretical orientation.

Specifically within the general field of psychotherapy, the orientation has been heavily influenced by the theory, research, and practice of Milton Erickson and the Ego State therapists. These have been integrated within a broad speculum of hypnotic and hypnoanalytic techniques into a highly efficient and effective approach to treatment. But while building from these approaches, the authors have added many original techniques, angles, and twists (both hypnotic and nonhypnotic) that give it its new and creative flavor.

Their general format is first, naming a particular procedure and indicating from what system or contributor it stems. The background and history of that source are then described, followed by an explanation of the technique and its theory. In most cases, after this exposition, a case example is presented illustrating the specific application of that procedure.

Because one of the authors is a physician, the physiological aspects are not neglected, and the presentations include many references to the medical diagnoses and organic factors involved.

Although written in clear, understandable language, this is not a text for the lay person. It is assumed that the reader is an experienced mental health professional.

Throughout the book, the importance of the therapeutic relationship is emphasized. Mental health professionals who digest this work carefully and apply its recommendations will find their own practices and research studies significantly improved.

About the Authors

John G. Watkins, Ph.D., is Professor Emeritus, University of Montana. He is the author of *Hypnotherapeutic Techniques* and *Hypnoanalytic Techniques*. He is also co-author of *Ego States: Theory and Therapy*. Dr. Watkins is in private practice in Missoula, Montana.

Helen A. Watkins, M.A., is retired from clinical psychology practice at the Counseling Center, University of Montana. She is coauthor of *Ego States: Theory and Therapy*. Ms. Watkins is in private practice in Missoula, Montana.

Preface

Ego-strengthening techniques are the bedrock of therapy.

—Frederick (1993a, p. 1)

Our clinical and teaching experiences, and those of our colleagues and coauthors, have led us to believe that ego-strengthening is the most important thing a therapist can do and that, when it is done successfully, it acts as "an integrating mechanism that bridges the gap between insight and the actualization of change ... in short-term and long-term therapy" (McNeal & Frederick, 1993, p. 177).

Various phrases such as ego-enhancement, increased self-efficacy, "a stronger ego," better problem-solving abilities, a greater capacity for self-soothing, increased self-confidence, and greater self-esteem are often used by clinicians to indicate capabilities that therapists hope to see emerge in their patients as therapy continues. They can all be thought of as products of ego-strengthening. Although there are numerous references to ego-strengthening in the literature, particularly the clinical hypnosis literature, there has been a dearth of explanations concerning its nature or why it can be so effective in therapy (McNeal & Frederick, 1993).

As this book proceeds, we attempt to construct explanations. We explore ego-strengthening by entering into the realms of ego psychology and other theoretical frameworks. We braid the theoretical with the historical and clinical for a better understanding of theories about the constitution of the ego that is being strengthened and how the strengthening works. We also elaborate upon and interweave the wisdom of several traditional clinical hypnosis approaches with traditional forms of nonhypnotic psychotherapy. This book is intended to serve as a practical guide to various kinds of hypnotic and nonhypnotic ego-strengthening techniques for clinicians who hold a number of theoretical orientations. We believe that all techniques become really practical only when they are understood and utilized within some theoretical framework. Otherwise they can easily become hollow, devitalized, separated from the rest of treatment, and ineffective.

Although we examine many kinds of ego-strengthening techniques (for each is potentially valuable in treatment), our emphasis is on the newer projective/evocative ego-strengthening techniques that appear to be such powerful tools in psychotherapy. These techniques are evocative because they activate the patient's deepest internal resources; they are projective because they frequently yield information about what is going on with the patient and with the therapeutic situation. This book is directed to the clinician who is working with the patient. Consequently, there are abundant case materials and a variety of detailed ego-strengthening scripts from different sources. To protect the confidentiality of our patients, the cases presented will be composite cases comprising clinical work with two or more patients.

After a great deal of consideration, we decided that no matter where we began this book, the reader would have a number of questions that would be answered later. Many explanations for the effectiveness of ego-strengthening can be found in the cognitive-behavioral tradition (Hammond, 1990d). Nevertheless, we have chosen the psychoanalytically oriented therapeutic tradition as our starting place because the ego was first emphasized there, because varieties of ego-strengthening efforts have always been important in successful psychoanalytically oriented psychotherapy, and because the roots of ego psychology theory can be found here. There is a building process within this book. Many issues that are introduced are encountered again, at a more complex level, and again at a yet higher level on which they are connected with other topics we have introduced and developed over a number of chapters.

This book is for trained and, wherever possible, licensed mental health professionals. It is designed to help them within their clinical settings. It is not intended to be used by individuals who may be certified in hypnosis as lay hypnotists, but have not received graduate and specialty training in psychotherapy in such fields as psychiatric medicine, psychology, social work, or nursing, nor had supervised clinical experience in psychotherapy. We believe that hypnosis is only an adjunct to therapy. It is axiomatic among professionals who use it that one should never attempt to do with hypnosis what one cannot do without hypnosis. We are convinced that anyone who uses hypnosis for psychotherapy has an ethical (and frequently legal) obligation to first become a trained professional psychotherapist.

Each of the authors came to a study of hypnosis after considerable clinical experience as a psychotherapist who did not use hypnosis. One of us (CF) had a longstanding prejudice against hypnosis based upon vincible ignorance about the nature of contemporary hypnosis. We have both learned how much hypnosis can add to the depth and breadth of treatment. However, we do not assume that every psychotherapist will want to use hypnotic forms of treatment. Hypnotic scripts can be modified for nonhypnotic psychotherapy and suggestive approaches can be substituted for formal trance. However, we want to caution our readers that simply calling a procedure *guided imagery* or *relaxation* does not cause it to be anything other than hypnosis in the eyes of the law. We strongly urge any therapist who desires to utilize hypnosis for treatment to get adequate hypnotic training and, when applicable, supervision. There is a list of training resources at the end of the book, and to it we have appended some of our recommendations for several paths to training in hypnosis from beginning through advanced levels.

Finally, this is not a self-help book, and we caution against any attempts to use it in that way. This does not mean that we are opposed to self-help. Indeed, self-care is an indispensable theme in this book. It does mean that the material presented here can only be understood as it is intended within the context of its being written for trained professionals.

Instead of laboriously writing he or she each time a nonsexist reference is called for, we use the pronouns he and she in such instances in alternating chapters.

Acknowledgments

We would like to begin by thanking Judi Amsel, the wonderful editor we lost to geographic relocation, for recognizing the value of this book, and Susan Milmoe, our equally splendid and most generous editor, who has encouraged and supported us every step of the way. We also wish to thank the Lawrence Erlbaum Associates staff, especially Robin Marks Weisberg for her expertise and ongoing help, and Kate Graetzer and Kathryn Houghtaling Lacey for their unstinting efforts.

Many encouraged and supported us in producing this book. Among those we wish to thank are our co-authors and co-creators of some of the projective-evocative ego-strengthening approaches presented in this book: Sung Kim, Priscilla Morton, and Maggie Phillips. We also wish to thank Jan Gregory for sharing with us her concept of the "archetypal selfobject."

This book could not have been written had we not been especially touched by these remarkable teachers: D. Corydon Hammond, John and Helen Watkins, Steven Gilligan, Elgan Baker, Joan Murray-Jobsis, and the late David Cheek.

This work did not evolve in a vacuum. Much of it has come from our work with patients who have honored us by sharing their subjective lives with us. We are grateful for their trust and efforts, and we are awed by the growth we have seen in them and in ourselves as we worked together.

Nor could this book have been written without the contributions, over the years, of our many students. Their questions and comments always animated and expanded our thinking and carried us further along the line.

We want to thank Velia Frost and Priscilla Morton for their careful and critical editing. We also extend our gratitude to Neil Young, Geri Meyer, Thomas Dickey, Jean Nunes, Connie Sheltren, Viola Nungary, and Sydney Quinn.

We are grateful to Janice Stamm, Esq. for her generous legal advice, as well as for cheerleading and moral support, and to David and Karen Tillitt for sharing the artwork of Geri Meyer that is on the cover of this book.

We offer our appreciation to those others who gave us moral support during the process: Karen Booker, Jo Ellen McNeal, Susan Unrath, Joe Palazolla, Beth St. John, Doris Munger, Alex Mitchel, and Louise Atcheson, as well as Dorann Boulian, Mai Nguyen, Daniel Peterson, and Martin Naughton.

Finally, we salute our Tahoe City canine contributors: Aurora, the wolf who is not always silent; Ginger the gentle Akita, and the late Seurat of one blue eye whose canonization is in process. It is true we often had a hard time walking around and over them, but they were always there to bolster us whenever we sat down together to work on this book.

—Claire Frederick—Shirley McNeal

Chapter 1

Ego-Strengthening
The Therapeutic Tradition

Throughout this book we present a great deal of varied material about the nature of the ego, how it develops, how it becomes strengthened or weakened, how it is similar to or different from the concept of self, and how successful psychotherapy can increase its scope and function as well as utilize its often hidden powers. This chapter focuses on some "roots" of ego theory as they have developed in the psychodynamic and psychoanalytic frameworks. In particular, we examine some aspects of the therapeutic alliance, transference-countertransference issues, and object relations concepts that are useful in thinking about ego-strengthening in psychotherapy today. Here, we begin to address some more specific questions: Are there therapeutic elements other than cognitively oriented insight or behavioral restructuring that can help strengthen the patient's ego and advance his level of psychological functioning? How much of what causes strengthening of the ego in therapy comes from the therapist, how much comes from the patient, and how much comes from the therapeutic relationship? How much do conscious interventions help to strengthen the ego, and how much appears to be totally in the hands of the unconscious? How can patient and therapist interact in ways that will strengthen the patient's ego and the effectiveness of the therapy?

Freud's (1923/1964) goal for his psychoanalytic model of therapy was "to strengthen the ego, to make it more independent of the super-ego, to widen its field of perception and enlarge its organization, so that it can appropriate fresh portions of the id. Where id was, there shall ego be" (p. 80). Although a contemporary therapist might not be a Freudian at all, he would probably agree that strengthening and expanding that organizing principle often known as the *ego* have always been important goals of psychotherapy. It is also understood that psychotherapy is aimed at helping the patient withstand and eventually ignore the primitive demands of a punitive conscience, become more aware of inner and outer realities and their possibilities in many ways, possess better organizing principles, and be able to deal with impulses more productively.

Historically, there has been an evolution in the ways therapists have viewed ego-strengthening. In both shamanic and ancient temple healings, for example, the interaction of the afflicted individual with the person of the healer priest was

DOI:10.4324/9781003442585-1

considered to be of the utmost importance (Ellenberger, 1970). The patient's ego was, presumably, so sufficiently strengthened by his encounter with this magical, powerful parental figure that it could participate in the cure. Varieties of this type of healing relationship persist today (e.g., the relationship between a reader of a popular book about healing and the medical authority who wrote it, the marvels of the cures that arise with TV evangelism, and in dramatic lifestyle changes oriented around various kinds of gurus). We might classify recoveries that spring from such activities as *transference cures*.

In the ancient Asclepian temple healings at Epidaurus, a more sophisticated level of treatment often involved dream interpretation, and memory work, and subsequent re-repression was guided by a priest. The concept of a necessary, special relationship between the patient and the therapist-healer persisted over time; eventually, it became known as *rapport*, a term still used in hypnosis today. This should not be surprising because contemporary psychodynamic psychotherapy has its historical foundations in hypnosis. Both Janet, the creator of the theory of dissociation, and Freud, the father of psychoanalysis, practiced clinical hypnosis. Janet (1897) identified rapport as a complex phenomenon observed in both hypnotic and nonhypnotic subjects. He believed that it was a necessary gateway for success in therapeutic endeavors. According to Janet, rapport was characterized by the emergence and flowering of the patient's dependency needs that became focused on the therapist. During the course of the treatment the therapist's task was to help free the patient of his symptoms and guide him to more independent functioning. Like the patient in earlier temple healings, the Janetian patient's ego became strengthened through his identification with a strong and wise parental therapist who would help guide him to greater understandings. This strengthening allowed him to uncover troublesome material and reassociate it with the rest of his mental content. Unlike the more primitive approaches to healing, this process promoted a gradual weaning of the patient from the healer. During this time the patient presumably relied more on his own ego, which had been strengthened in several ways in the therapeutic encounter. It appears that the elements of insight and reassociation were additional strengthening elements. However, the greater initiative and strength were still perceived as residing within the healer-therapist.

Early in his work with psychological difficulties, Freud, like Janet, believed that trauma caused neuroses to develop; however, he soon abandoned both the trauma theory and hypnosis (see chap. 2). His subsequent nonhypnotic theoretical framework, psychoanalysis, with its emphasis on the intrapsychic mechanisms such as repression, eventually displaced Janet's extensive theory of trauma and dissociation (Ellenberger, 1970). The concept of *transference* superseded that of rapport in psychotherapy. Transference is a complex and meaningful affective and behavioral relationship that the patient experiences within therapy. Transference is defined traditionally as a set of perceptions, affects, and behaviors that the patient directs at the therapist. These perceptions, affects, and behaviors are rooted in the patient's early life experiences with significant figures of authority and superimposed upon the therapist. It was through proper interpretation of the transference and of the patient's resistances to change that insight was able to develop in the analysis.

The Therapeutic Alliance

Historical Review

Transference is a term that comes from psychoanalysis and is used by many kinds of psychodynamic psychotherapists. Transference allows the patient's difficulties to be played out in therapy for the purpose of being understood. Eventually, the patient acquires insight as a result of the analyst's interpretations and is able to change. In psychoanalysis insight is thought of as the mechanism that leads to change. (This point of view is not universally held by psychodynamic psychotherapists. Some believe that insight actually follows change instead of causing it.) This process of analyzing or understanding the transference and other elements of therapy involves collaboration between the analyst and the patient. This idea that the patient might be some sort of partner in psychodynamic treatment has appeared periodically in the literature from the beginning of psychoanalysis. A young Viennese woman named Anna O. is credited by many with the discovery of psychoanalysis because of her frequent use of what she called "chimney sweeping" (catharsis). She was certainly a wholehearted participant in her treatment (Breuer & Freud, 1893–1895/1964). Nevertheless, emphasis on the value of the patient's most mature efforts in the therapeutic process was not a focus of a great deal of attention. Freud (1912/1961) recognized that there was a noneroticized, cooperative sort of transference to which he attached the term *effective alliance* or *rapport*. He found that this less primitive, more amiable transference could be quite helpful in the progress of therapy. With it, the patient's cooperation in achieving certain therapeutic tasks could be enlisted without a struggle. Freud spoke of the necessity of the analyst's having a "serious interest" in the patient and being able to display "sympathetic understanding." Freud also signaled his recognition of and respect for the presence of adult aspects of his patients by shaking their hands as they left their analytic sessions (Jones, 1953). Although Freud initially believed that all rapport was transferential in nature, it has been thought (Hovarth, Gaston, & Luborsky, 1993) that he may later have altered his thinking (Freud, 1940/1964b) so that he entertained the possibility of an alliance based on reality rather than transference alone. Other analysts also noted the presence of a *rational transference* (Fenichel, 1941) or a *mature transference* (Stone, 1997). The model used was always authoritarian in tone, however. The analyst maintained his position as the ultimate sage.

Sterba (1929/1940, 1934) evolved a concept of an alliance between analyst and patient called an *ego alliance*. When it was present, the patient could carry out the procedures necessary for therapy such as reporting mental content or feeling states. It also allowed the patient to examine and work with unpleasant and regressed material and accept difficult insights. According to Sterba (1934), the alliance was a manifestation of a temporary and partial identification of the patient with some of the analyst's attitudes, goals, and way of working. This alliance developed because of a split within the patient's ego which produced an observing, or reasonable, ego that could ally itself with the "analyzing ego" of the analyst (Sterba, 1934).

The term *therapeutic alliance* was coined by Zetzel (1956), who described the patient as having to move back and forth between the transference and a reality-based alliance. Greenson (1965, 1967) had a particular interest in the power of a real relationship that did not depend on transference. This relationship was called the *working alliance*. Greenson (1967) contended "that the working alliance deserves to be considered a full and equal partner to the transference neurosis [in importance] in the patient-therapist relationship" (p. 191).

Other conceptualizations of the alliance focus on object relations (Bibring, 1937; Bowlby, 1988; Gitelson, 1962; Horwitz, 1974). Luborsky (1990), in particular, pointed to the transitional qualities inherent in the therapeutic alliance. According to Hovarth, Gaston, and Luborsky (1993) there are pantheoretical models that embrace both interpersonal and intrapsychic aspects of the alliance. They believe that relevant components probably work synergistically. We refer the reader to the Hovarth et al. (1993) explication of these and other ramifications of the therapeutic alliance as well as to material on research and continuing controversies in this area.

Clinical Applications of the Therapeutic Alliance

Although the concept of the therapeutic alliance, or working alliance, was developed in psychoanalysis, it has wide applicability throughout many fields of psychotherapy today. It may well represent an evolutionary advance in contemporary psychotherapy because it exemplifies a deliberate attempt to ego-strengthen the patient and activate his inner resources for constructive participation in therapy. Until it was defined and emphasized, the patient's participation in the therapeutic process was all too frequently relegated to considerations of transference and resistances that emphasized childlike aspects of self.

There are many ego-strengthening uses of the therapeutic alliance. As is seen later in this chapter, transference may aid in the development of the alliance, or it may hinder it. In certain cases a *full* working alliance can be formed only after the patient's internal psychic structures have become more developmentally advanced as a result of the therapist–patient interaction. Frequently the alliance is a place where patients are able to advance themselves psychosocially (E. Erikson, 1959), learning to move into such landmark activities as basic trust, initiative, and cooperation.

The Elements of the Therapeutic Alliance

There are certain elements that are essential to the development of the therapeutic alliance. Some of them come from the therapist, and some from the patient. The emphasis here is on the contributions of the therapist. Although we list them separately, a number of them take place simultaneously.

Respect and Interest.   We believe that work on strengthening and expanding the therapeutic alliance must accompany every aspect and stage of therapy and that this work begins during the assessment of the patient (Phillips & Frederick, 1995). It is necessary for the therapist to openly display genuine respect for the patient during the process of history taking and assessment. Almost all patients, like those who sought the help of healer priests and shamans in the past, possess primitive transference feeling and perceive the therapist as much more powerful and knowledgeable than they. Respect on the part of the therapist can easily move into an interest in how the patient perceives his problems. The therapist must be able to look beyond the patient's defenses with respect for the human being behind the defenses and for the suffering he endures.

The therapist's awareness of the unique individuality of the patient and the existential meaning of his situation is ego-strengthening because, unless the patient is quite psychotic and/or disorganized, he no longer feels alone. He also receives important information that will affect his concept of himself: That he has value as a human being, and that his problems, fears, and defenses do not constitute *all* of who he is.

Case Example: Jake[1]

Jake called me (CF) from a remote rural area. He had been watching a TV program about schizophrenia, which he called a "split personality," and he concluded that he was a schizophrenic. For some reason we never managed to discuss at the time, he believed that hypnotherapy could help his schizophrenia. I was the closest hypnotherapist he had been able to locate.

Jake arrived at his session directly from work; he was dressed in soiled plumber's clothes. His symptom list contained many of the markers for Dissociative Identity Disorder (DID), and his early life history was one of incredible deprivation, several varieties of abuse and neglect that began at an early age, and a total lack of stability. These factors had been compounded by severe dyslexia. Beyond his dyslexia, poor education, and social impoverishment, I saw a very bright young man who was frightened and confused. I was able to give him explanations about schizophrenia

---

1 More clinical material from Jake's case will appear later in the book.

and Dissociative Identity Disorder (DID) that were meaningful to him. I then explained to him why I thought he might have Dissociative Identity Disorder (DID) and what was involved in its treatment. He was interested in acquiring this knowledge, and he appeared to feel quite relieved.

Jake appeared to have no difficulty understanding my explanations; indeed, he seemed to comprehend them very clearly. He appeared to be genuine about wanting help. He told me that he was surprised that he had been able to go to a "first session" and more surprised that he had been able to talk so freely. He told me he wanted to work with me even though he would have to travel a considerable distance and lose money for his time off from his job. His main concern was whether I would find him acceptable as a patient.

I told Jake that I had a sense that the two of us could get something done that would be helpful to him if we worked together. As the session drew to a close, Jake asked me whether people who had been abused as children became abusers. I told him that sometimes it happened, and that was understandable. I did more education with him, explaining the concept of how identification with the aggressor could cause a victim to feel more powerful and in control while seeking a solution for his own abuse through reenactment. Although he had not told me about any inappropriate behavior of his own, clearly there was a possibility that it existed, at the least, in his fantasy life.

Jake then was able to tell me that he was frightened that he might abuse someone when he was much older. When he saw again that I was not judgmental and that I was reinforcing his own perception of his need for treatment, he was able to confide that he was very frightened that he might be molesting someone now and "not even know I'm doing it." I reassured him that together we would be able to find some ways of discovering whether this was so.

Jake's initial interview illustrates how work on the alliance can be incorporated into the first session. Important elements in this interaction were:

- Respect
- Interest
- Therapist perception that allowed recognition of the patient's motivation and recognition of the patient's intelligence
- Explicit definition of therapy that included working together
- An educational model geared to the patient's intellectual and emotional levels
- Lack of judgmentalism
- Openness: The therapist did not have all the answers

There are other forces that influence the therapeutic alliance in positive ways; one of them is interpersonal safety.

Interpersonal Safety.   The fundamental inclusion of interpersonal safety is crucial to the development of the therapeutic alliance. It is within this context that the therapist is able to strengthen the patient further by providing an understanding of the conditions within which therapy can take place. The alliance grows stronger as there is comprehension and agreement about issues such as confidentiality, what kind of reporting is legally mandated, the length and frequency of sessions, the fee, cancellation policies, how emergencies will be handled, as well as any other relevant issues. These rules of therapy provide a structure within which the patient may support himself in predictable ways. They can seed "the possibility of the patient's discovering and creating a 'safe space' within" (Morton & Frederick, 1997a, p. 6). Several sessions may be needed to establish these parameters in their initial forms. However, patients may not come to appreciate some of them, such as boundaries, on a conscious level until much later in treatment.

Case Example: Jake (continued)

Although Jake and I agreed on the frequency of therapy, the length of the sessions, the fee, how cancellations were to be managed, and payment terms, the issue of confidentiality had not been broached. The introduction of the topic of his fears that he might be a current child abuser mandated my responsibility for discussing confidentiality and the limits placed on it by the reporting laws. Because the material had come up just before the end of the session, I decided not to violate the boundaries of the session time, but to bring these issues up as the first topics to be discussed in the next session.

Jake was much more sophisticated than his attire and grammar suggested. I suspected that he had felt free to bring up the doubts he entertained about his behavior because he was aware of the reporting laws and knew that he had not actually acted out sexually with a child. However, if he did not know about the laws, he could well have been planning to confess an act of current molestation of a child in the next session. In the interests of his personal safety, my putting material about confidentiality and reporting laws on the table would give him choices that would influence his sense of safety and increase his sense of trust.

Consistency.   Consistency is another aspect of structure that frequently provides the patient with ego-strengthening support. The acquisition of sameness in certain parts of our lives often provides a sense of security and releases energy that can be focused elsewhere. The therapist who is aware of this attempts to put regularity into the patient's situation. Such things include always giving the patient appointments at the same time and the same place, having the bills come out on the same day of the month, and having some sort of routine for how the sessions proceed (e.g., so much time for reporting of activities, so much time for reporting dreams, so much time for therapeutic interventions such as dealing with transference issues, so much time for processing what happened in the last session and in the current session). Therapy then begins to acquire a rhythm that can feel natural to the patient just as the tides, our revolutions around the sun, or our circadian rhythms do.

In his short novel, *The Little Prince*, Saint-Exupéry's (1943/1971) little hero, a child prince, tours a number of planets. On each one he grows wiser from his adventures. On the seventh planet, Earth, he encounters a fox, and the little prince invites him to play with him because, at the time, he is unhappy.

"I cannot play with you," the fox said. "I am not tamed."

"Ah! Please excuse me," said the little prince. But, after some thought, he added: "What does that mean (tame)?"

"You do not live here," said the fox. "What is it that you are looking for?"

(They then discuss the little prince's journey, and he continues to inquire about what the fox means by *tame*.)

"It is an act too often neglected," said the fox. "It means to establish ties."

"To establish ties?" "Just that," said the fox. "To me you are still nothing more than a little boy who is just like a hundred thousand other little boys. And I have no need of you. And you, on your part, have no need of me. To you I am nothing more than a fox like a hundred thousand other foxes. But if you tame me, we shall need each other. To me you will be unique in all the world. To you I shall be unique in all the world."

(They then discuss one another's adventures, and the fox admits that he is bored with his life.)

"but if you tame me, it will be as if the sun came to shine in my life. I shall know the sound of a step that shall be different from all the others ... (It) will call me like music from my burrow.

(The fox then explains to the little prince that, because of their connection, should it exist, he would always think of the little prince's hair whenever he looked at golden wheat in the fields.)

"Please tame me!" he said. "One only understands the things that one tames ... If you want a friend, tame me."

"What must I do, to tame you?" asked the little prince.

"You must be very patient," replied the fox. "First you will sit down at a little distance from me ... (then) you will sit a little closer to me every day."

The next day the little prince came back.

"It would have been better to come back at the same hour," said the fox. "... one must observe the proper rites."

"What is a rite?" asked the little prince.

"Those also are too often neglected," said the fox. "They are what makes one day different from other days, one hour from other hours."

So the little prince tamed the fox.

(When the little prince eventually left to continue his adventures, the fox was sad. However, he explained the great significance of their encounter to the little prince.)

"It has done me good," said the fox, "because of the color of the wheat fields."

(Saint Exupéry, 1943/1971, pp. 78–86)

To be sure, there are many therapeutic implications to the relationship of the fox and the little prince in addition to consistency. However, this vignette illustrates the importance of rite and ritual in developing a significant relationship; this can be overlooked in the therapeutic situation. Like the fox, patients in such positions, like the fox, do eventually feel unique. In this way their egos are strengthened.

Empathy. "Empathy means to share, to experience the feelings of another human being" (Greenson, 1967, p. 368). Its function in therapy is to gain and communicate a greater understanding of the subjectivity of the patient and to bridge the aloneness that he experiences when in the grips of his intense painful feelings. Without empathy there is no true understanding. There is no other quality in the therapeutic situation that can bring greater closeness and intimacy.

The therapeutic alliance has an opportunity to flourish in the presence of true empathy. Faked or pretended empathy, known at times as role-playing, is not an adequate substitute for the real thing. To experience empathy the therapist must undergo a transient identification with some of the patient's affect. When the therapist becomes empathic, he experiences regression in the service of the ego (Hartman, Kris, & Lowenstein, 1946). There are probably several reasons why empathy is necessary for a good alliance. The closeness it promotes in the relationship may well be another precursor of the development of a secure holding environment in which the patient can experience caring and nurturing. Empathy also communicates to the patient, on an emotional level, that he is understood and accepted. When this does not occur, therapy can become an occasion for the intensification of patients' sufferings instead of a source of their relief. It is not unusual for patients to leave therapy prematurely because of failures in this arena (Geller, 1987). A great deal of what is dealt with in clinical self-psychology is the healing management of empathic failures that occur during the course of therapy (Geller, 1987).

The vital roles played by empathy in psychotherapy cannot be overlooked. In addition to its necessity in the formation of therapeutic alliances, it is also an essential and irreplaceable element of the therapist's ability to make the "transmutative" (Strachey, 1934) interpretations that are so crucial in the healing process (Geller, 1987). It is within the empathic framework that the patient is able to experience interpretations with the emotional immediacy that is essential for their effectiveness. Geller (1987) has viewed therapeutic competence from the perspective and with the terminology of Piaget (1954). She believes that empathy enables therapeutic competence because through the use of empathy the competent therapist assimilates patients into his own current concepts of "… the rules, rituals, and roles of psychotherapy" (p. 466). It also allows him to simultaneously accommodate the structure of the work of therapy "to effect a better fit with the unique needs and circumstances of each patient" (p. 467). Geller (1987) perceives empathy as that which, when conveyed through understandings, is able to move patients though a succession of "more meaningful, coherent connections between disparate, and perhaps disavowed, aspects of experience. Empathic interventions so conceived serve to combine, unite, and synthesize that which has been kept apart" (p. 467).

Case Example: Jake (continued)

From the beginning of the first session, I (CF) began to experience profound empathy for Jake. I made no attempt to conceal from him that I was experiencing some part of his pain as he told me about his life and his current fears. I didn't weep (although I felt close to it at times). However, I did let Jake know, in a verbally expressive way, that I was in touch with what he was telling me.

I said, "Jake I don't know exactly how you survived all that!" I then added something else I thought might be clinically useful—an interpretation. "Probably what saved you was your ability to dissociate and to create parts that could help you."

The therapeutic balancing of empathy with the cognitive and other aspects of psychotherapy is a vital element to the art psychotherapy. It has been called resonance (J. Watkins, 1978).

Resonance.   How much empathy does an effective therapist have to have for his patients? How does he balance it with the kind of objectivity that is also necessary for him to function properly? Rogers (1961) once described the empathic immersion of the therapist in the patient's material as a cognitive endeavor that led him to "understand," but not actually experience affectively, what was going on with the patient. However, Rogers (1975) subsequently modified and elaborated his concept of empathy as a process of entering the private perceptual world of the other and becoming thoroughly at home in it.... It includes communicating your sense of his/her world as you look with fresh eyes at elements of which the individual is fearful.... To be with another in this way means that for the time being you lay aside the views and values you hold for yourself in order to enter another's world without prejudice.

(p. 4)

A valuable way of looking at empathy is embodied in Watkins' (1978) concept of resonance. Watkins became interested in Federn's (1952) concepts of ego cathexis and object cathexis; eventually, he created his own theory of resonance in psychotherapy.

Resonance is that inner experience within a therapist during which he co-feels (co-enjoys, co-suffers) and co-understands with his patient, though in a mini-form ... it is a "subject" or self-relationship, one in which he commits himself as a full fledged ally with his patient. When resonating, the therapist replicates with his own ego as close as he can a facsimile of the other's experiential world ... and identifies with that replica. Resonance, therefore is a temporary identification established for purposes of better understanding the internal motivations, feelings and attitudes of a patient.

(J. G. Watkins, 1992, pp. 281–282)

According to Watkins, there are two kinds of resonance—cognitive and affective—and there is an objective rating system for overall resonance (J. Watkins, 1978). Resonance is effective when the therapist is able to move in and out of it, resonate with the patient, and then step back into objectivity. Each time the therapist moves back into resonance and then leaves this position for objectivity, he gains a greater understanding of the patient. He may well understand the patient's psychodynamics on an objective, cognitive level, but it is his resonating with the patient that lets him know if it is the right time to give the patient an interpretation about this material. Watkins thinks that the therapist makes an "ego-loan" to the patient and gets repaid by co-enjoying the therapeutic gains the patient makes. In this economy, the experiences with the patient contribute to the therapist's own growth, "in strength and maturity as a therapist and a person" (J. Watkins, 1992, p. 287). The therapist who is willing and able to make a commitment to such a deep professional involvement with the patient is what Watkins (1978, 1992) calls a *therapeutic self*. The resonance that is produced (and worked with cognitively as well) when this therapist and his patient work together brings about a better working alliance and therapeutic outcome.

There are several necessary precautions for the therapist who approaches the development of the intense empathic relationship (resonance) with his patients. The therapist could fail to oscillate from resonance to objectivity and become lost in the patient's pathology. Lindner's (1954) depiction of the therapist who joined his patient's delusional system to effect a cure is much to the point. In his story, "The Jet Propelled Couch" (Lindner, 1954), the therapist remained involved with great interest and energy in the delusional system long after the patient had given it up.

The therapist could take on too many difficult, suffering patients, forfeit balance in his life, and literally lose himself. His temporary identification with the pathology of his patients would lead him away from his own states of health. Finally, the therapist could retreat into sheer objectivity as a defense against the painfulness of the temporary identification with the patient that resonance requires.

Somewhat related to the concept of resonance is control mastery theory (Weiss, 1993; Weiss, Sampson, & Mt. Zion Psychotherapy Research Group, 1986), which emphasizes unconscious dimensions of the patient–therapist relationship and focuses more on the patient's unconscious contributions. This theory holds that the patient has an unconscious plan for what is needed in the treatment for his own recovery. Although the patient has the plan, he has been unable to implement it. The therapist's job is to discover what the plan is and help the patient accomplish it.

Fusional Alliances

Watkins' (1978, 1992) description of what happens when the resonating therapist interacts with the patient reflects a viewpoint held by many concerning what actually happens in therapy to strengthen and change the ego. Certain patients bring extremely primitive transferences to therapy. These may reflect the earliest stages of human development beginning with the symbiotic stage.

Symbiosis in Psychotherapy

These elements play themselves out in transference-countertransference communications at the deepest levels. Searles (1965) called this deep and essential process "the symbiotic core of therapeutic interaction" (p. 539).

George Groddek (1923/1950) was one of the less inhibited minds within the early psychoanalytic movement. He called himself the wild analyst (Grotjahn, 1966) and, in his flamboyant intuitive style, generated many of the ideas and themes that have proved to be relevant in psychoanalysis. Searles (1965) reminds us of Groddek's description of the fundamental symbiotic relationship between the therapist and the patient as being one in which the patient unconsciously directed the therapist to do what was needed. Whitaker and Malone (1953) also described such a process, and in great detail, in which both therapist and patient enter into a symbiotic process from which each emerges stronger and more differentiated.

Whitaker and Malone (1953) thought that all therapy eventually entered a Core Stage in which the patient saw himself as a "Child-Self," and the therapist's self-perception was as a "Parent."

Each of them introjects the other. ... In this the greatest therapeutic depth accrues. Only at this level do the bilateral symbolic relationships converge fully. ... It is the essential therapeutic relationship in and of itself. It is the relationship which ... can be used by the patient in the attempt to work through his residual transference problems, and the problems of his emotional growth in general.

(Whitaker & Malone, 1953, pp. 108–109)

As therapy continues through subsequent stages, the therapist and patient separate emotionally in healthy ways that permit each of them to continue to grow and become stronger.

At times therapists may discover that the therapeutic relationship seems to produce or create fusional alliances between the therapist and patients with primitive and inadequate internal structures. This replay of the early mother–child relationship (or symbiosis) can be particularly noticeable in the hypnotherapeutic interaction (Diamond, 1983, 1984) when therapist and patient cue in to these patient needs in the trance situation. This important topic is addressed in chapter 7.

The Roles of Transference and Countertransference

Transference is a particular type of object relationship that has always been described as "always inappropriate" (Greenson, 1967). The reason for its inappropriateness is that it is an experience of "feelings, drives, wishes, fears, fantasies, attitudes, and ideas or defenses against them" that are derived from events with a significant figure in the past. They are now directed toward someone else in the present. "Essentially, a person in the present is reacted to as though he were a person in the past" (Greenson, 1967, p. 152).

Freud (1912/1964) considered many transferences such as negative transferences or sexual and erotic transferences to be resistances to therapy. As noted earlier, however, he distinguished from all of these a positive, nonsexual, transference reaction he called rapport or the effective alliance. Freud considered all transferences to be inherently ambivalent and believed that rapport was a reflection of the patient's identifying the analyst with positive figures in his past. Because Freud and his followers thought that transference was necessary for the psychoanalytic process, the psychoanalytic situation is designed to bring out transference reactions in patients. It is only through transference that the analyst is able to discover certain "pathogenic material that is otherwise inaccessible" (Greenson, 1967, p. 190). Ferenczi (1909/1950) believed that the patient projects transference material upon the therapist because he is seeking a different kind of response—one that would be curative.

The positive feelings and attitudes that the patient transfers upon the therapist are, without question, important forces at the heart of therapy. It is doubtful that patients without transference connections to the therapist (be they positive or negative) could really participate in therapy. The sociopath, cut off from his affective life, does not seem to develop transferences. However, a primitive transference does exist so that he sees all people, including the therapist, as objects. Lengthy and careful work must precede the development of obvious transferences in withdrawn schizophrenic patients. The "absence of transference" has been reported in borderline patients as well. Giovacchini (1996) noted that the missing transference can be a transference in and of itself for those patients who are deeply alienated from their unconscious processes and who reject the concept of psychic determinism. It would be safe to say that the apparent lack of transference only conceals the true nature of the transference which may well be pre-oedipal in nature. The absence of visible transference in borderline, schizophrenic, and sociopathic patients is always a manifestation of object relationships that are infantile and primitive. Special ego-strengthening approaches that will be discussed later are needed with such patients.

Positive transference can be ego-strengthening while also containing elements of resistance. It is the therapist's task to increase the ego-strengthening aspects of positive transference without increasing the resistance.

Case Example: Gus

Gus came into therapy because his relationship with his fourth wife was deteriorating. He believed this to be all her fault, which he was certain I (CF) would understand if I listened to his explanation of the situation. His wife had a terrible temper and would not discuss things with him. She was so touchy, he stated, that she should be the one seeking help. Gus had the symptoms of a mild to moderate depression.

Gus had one reservation about his reading of his family situation. This was what, he confessed, had truly led him to see me. He wondered if he might be doing something to contribute to the situation. His history revealed that his mother had been alcoholic and his father sadistic, overcontrolling, verbally demeaning, and physically abusive to Gus. Despite his father's behavior, he still visited him and sought his approval.

From the beginning of his therapy Gus perceived me as the "expert." He seemed to believe that if he did what I told him do and worked in his therapy sessions on material he thought I might consider important, he would grow and feel better. In the early stages of therapy Gus revealed that he partied a lot. This meant that he frequently went out with the boys, and came home drunk. He denied alcoholism. I engaged him in an experiment. I thought that because he did not believe himself to be an alcoholic, it would be enlightening to see how his relationship with his wife would be affected if he swore off all liquor for a month. He thought that might be a good idea and allowed that his drinking and absence could be alienating his wife. Should he be unable to quit the drinking, he agreed that he would consider AA.

Gus strove to be an "outstanding" therapy patient. He reported all of his dereliction, gave abundant history, and made changes in his behavior. He also utilized ego-strengthening hypnotic interventions exceptionally well. He began to get his life together. This included his business, which he had let slide. One day Gus came to a session and said, "What do we do next?"

That Gus used the word we was positive, and his willingness to do some of the difficult things I asked him to do, such as not drinking, was indicative of early positive transference and a therapeutic alliance. The positive transference had been the basis for the development of the alliance. However, Gus' transference to me had now come to reveal his deep dependency needs. Would Gus remain in therapy if he had to initiate some of its direction as well as confront his need to be cared for and directed?

I explained to Gus that often, and naturally, patients looked to their therapists for direction. However, I wondered if he might think that, like his father, I might have a road map for him. "But you're the expert!" proclaimed Gus. I explained to him that indeed that was true, but that from another perspective he also was an expert. No one knew better than he what might be his concerns, fears, wishes, and goals.

After some thought Gus decided that he would like to work on the effects on him of the relationship he has had with his father.

Gus' positive transference helped his therapy; however, it also presented a resistance and a re-living of his relationship with his controlling father. What was particularly ego-strengthening about the therapeutic intervention is that the therapist did not relinquish the role of expert (trained and able psychotherapist), but rather acknowledged it. She then invited the patient to break through his transference resistance into a positive identification with her as herself and not as his father by claiming expert status in a closely related area.

Positive transference can present an almost insuperable obstacle to treatment (Frederick, 1997), and overwhelming positive transference is invariably a manifestation of an attachment disorder. It usually carries with it tremendous unrecognized transference hatred for the therapist. Early in therapy such patients view their transference feelings and behavior in a completely ego-syntonic way. As a result of continued therapy this perspective eventually changes. Hopefully patients begin to identify with the therapist's ability to scrutinize their behavior and wonder about its meaning in a nonjudgmental, empathic, objective way. Patients who are able to do this make a role identification (Crits-Christoph, Barber, Miller, & Beebe, 1993) with the therapist, and begin to take over some of the therapeutic tasks. This turning point occurs when the inappropriate transference feelings and behaviors have become ego-dystonic to them. Patients with clinging, ego-syntonic, overwhelmingly positive transference usually require additional ego-strengthening that is centered around their disturbed object relations (Frederick, 1997).

Although negative transference is not usually thought of as ego-strengthening, it also can offer important ego-strengthening opportunities in therapy. The management of the negative transference is critical for a number of reasons. Patients may leave therapy if their negative feelings are not explored and resolved. Negative transferences can be beneficial when they permit the patient to eventually see the therapist as human and imperfect rather than godlike. This occurs when the therapist is able to heal "splits" in the patient's perceptions and facilitate the development of object constancy.

Case Example: John

John had seen a succession of different therapists on and off since childhood. As an adult he had been diagnosed as having a Borderline Personality Disorder. He was referred to me (SM) by a colleague who thought clinical hypnosis might be useful in his treatment. John's reason for entering therapy was to learn how to relate to women so that he could have a girlfriend. Forming a therapeutic alliance with John was difficult as he was generally suspicious and resentful. I knew that considerable time and effort would be needed to establish an alliance before any hypnotic interventions could be introduced.

During a session John suddenly took offense at an innocuous remark I made. He recounted in an angry fashion that the teachers of his classes for the gifted in grammar school had made remarks that indicated that his parents' pressures and indulgence created the impression of his being gifted when, in truth, the teachers believed that he was not. My remark had insulted his intelligence, he declared, and I was just like all the other teachers and therapists whom he had seen previously.

I encouraged him to elaborate on his, and as we continued to discuss his feelings about me, he broke into a wide grin and exclaimed, "I must be getting better! This is the first time I've ever said anything negative to any one." John's previous pattern had always been to drop out of therapy at such a point or abandon any relationship when he became angry.

In John's case it was apparent that addressing the negative transference in an ego-strengthening way allowed him to produce more negative material that was ego-strengthening in the sense that it enabled him to become assertive in expressing his hitherto suppressed feelings. In many instances the management of both positive and negative transferences can be ego-strengthening. There are a number of other variations on transference themes that can offer challenges to the therapist who seeks to maintain a therapeutic alliance. Among them are erotic, demeaning, psychotic, and narcissistic transferences.

The therapist must always stay in touch with the fundamental principal that the primary ego-strengthening task in psychotherapy is personal safety of both the therapist and the patient. He must be aware of the possibility of potential threats to his safety that can be connected with certain intense transferences. Among them are various potential hazards including threats to physical safety, legal and administrative dangers, and actual persecution and stalking by patients (Comstock & Vickery, 1993; Frederick, 1994d).

The Therapist as Transitional Object

The concepts of transitional object and transitional phenomena were discussed by Winnicott (1975) as an explanation for the mechanisms used by the infant to manage separation anxiety and bridge positions of omnipotence and absolute dependence on the mother to the development of an orientation to the outside world. At times the therapist must occupy the role of a transitional object for patients. To be effective in doing this, the therapist must, in some way, function like the good-enough mother and provide a holding environment that is safe. In this environment the patient learns that he can express feelings without fear of disapproval and abandonment, of harming the therapist with hostile productions, or having to continue in unending shame over his neediness and feelings of desperation over fantasied loss. By providing a facilitating environment, the therapist can adapt to unmet needs and repair developmental arrests in the maturation process.

Case Example: Kevin

Kevin was a 36-year-old man who suffered from anorexia. He was over 6 feet tall and only weighed 130 pounds. He was withdrawn and suspicious and felt he could not trust anyone. His relationships were superficial and fraught with fear. Although he badly wanted to have friends and intimate relationships, he was always fearful of being used and manipulated by others. He was aware of his tendency to want to please and therefore react to others by trying to determine their expectations and fulfill them. At the same time, he deeply resented the feeling of obligations to others and had no sense of limit setting or appropriate boundaries.

His family history revealed that he had a passive father, an intrusive, dominating mother, and two lively younger sisters. His mother identified herself as a strong feminist and had lectured him repeatedly about how men abused and took advantage of women. He was told to always be careful not to hurt women. His first girlfriend in college had also called herself a strong feminist and had been abusive to him. He had such conflicting feelings toward others, especially women, that he found social situations painful and often chose to stay at home alone. It was difficult for him to decide to seek therapy, but he ultimately felt that he did want to feel better about his relationships with others and acknowledge the need to deal with his anorexia.

The early phase of treatment was challenging for both of us because it was hard for him to trust and open up to me (SM). Kevin frequently demanded that I give him "information and knowledge" concerning social skills he felt he lacked. However, he derogated anything that he construed to be a minor piece of information in that direction. It sounded as though he viewed me as a bad mother or, at the very best, a withholding mother, at times helpful on the surface, but, like his real mother, overly intrusive and hurtful. Kevin wanted to be "a good patient," but that was problematic for him because he thought that meant he might have to provide me with information I could use against him.

I felt it was important to pace the course of treatment slowly, allowing Kevin to move at a pace that felt comfortable to him. I knew he would continually test me, and it was my task to pass the tests and provide him with an experience of a relationship with a woman that was different from those he had experienced with his mother, sisters, and former girlfriend. I knew progress was occurring when Kevin began showing up for sessions on time. Gradually, he began to trust me more and more.

As his trust increased and his therapy progressed, Kevin developed the insight that the anorexia was, in part, his attempt to avoid assuming the appearance of a male. He believed men would abuse women, and it was more ego-syntonic for him to identify himself as a victim rather than an abuser. Becoming more "manly" was associated with the fear of becoming an abuser.

I supported personality aspects that favored his eating healthily and taking care of his body. He joined a gym and began to work out in addition to becoming more conscious of when he was hungry and needed to eat. He no longer is either passively complying or resisting therapeutic interventions. He is pleased with his progress and is taking more risks in his relationships with others, experimenting with saying no, negotiating, and asking.

This case illustrates how the therapist can become a transitional object. In this case example the therapist was a consistent and constant presence. She provided a holding environment and became the focus of the patient's projections. As their work together progressed, he began to view her in a different light, not as the abuser, but as someone who could and would provide calming interpersonal experiences as well as acceptance and understanding. Within this climate, he could separate enough from his transferences so that he could begin to see himself differently. This led to his beginning to consider that he could have different and more satisfying relationships with others. The topic of transitional objects and transitional phenomena and their great ego-strengthening value in all of psychotherapy is pursued in great detail in chapter 7.

Winnicott (1962/1965) viewed the demands and acting-out characteristics of borderline patients as attempts to use others as transitional objects to rediscover a lost maternal bond. The therapeutic task is then to adapt to the patients' desires for gratification. The therapist may allow himself to be used as a transitional object (and then discarded) so that further maturation can continue. Therapists who are available as providers of transitional experiences for their patients, or who are willing to be treated as transitional objects for certain periods of time, must be able to "withstand an intense variety of feelings, be there when needed, and forgotten when not needed" (Summers, 1994).

Such a therapist strengthens the egos of these patients, whose internal structures have failed to develop, by providing the possibility of a reparative experience for the development of an adult ego. The development of self-management of affect is an ego-strengthening form of mastery that can begin when enough of the therapist has been "taken in" or internalized so that the patient has created an internal object experienced as a warm, loving, nurturing part of the self. Transitional phenomena and their role in therapy are discussed in great detail in chapter 7.

The Ego-Strengthening Spectrum

The ego-strengthening therapist's involvement in psychotherapy can be thought of as existing in a spectrum ranging from simply "being there" as the object of parental transference who offers reassurance and support, through the therapist's taking an active role in setting up and fostering a good therapeutic alliance. As the therapy becomes more complex and complete on the spectrum, it includes proper timing and interpretation of the transferences as well as recognition of and working through of counter-transference issues. Moving toward the far end of the spectrum, we find resonance, the therapist's willingness to be used as a transitional object, and even to enter into profound fusional alliances with his patient.

The Staging of Therapy

Since the time of Janet (1919/1976), psychotherapy has, traditionally, been conducted in stages that help ensure that the patient is engaged in treatment and has gained enough ego strength to be able to move forward into necessary uncovering phases of therapy and then resolve and integrate painful material. There are a number of contemporary models for maintaining safety while uncovering in psychotherapy (Courtois, 1988; Gil, 1988; Herman, 1992; Kluft, 1993; McCann & Pearlman, 1990; Phillips & Frederick, 1995). The themes that can be found in these models are similar to those in the work of Janet (1919/1976). What they all emphasize is that the patient must have consistent interpersonal and intrapersonal safety if treatment is to be successful.

We are currently using the SARI model (Phillips & Frederick, 1995), which was designed to be used in the treatment of posttraumatic and dissociative patients. We find that it can be helpful in the treatment of all kinds of difficulties and illnesses, including physical ones. This is a four-stage model that is able to focus on (a) safety and stability; (b) accessing material connected with the patient's problem (in trauma patients this would be traumatic material; in patients physically ill with cancer, this would be the neoplastic tissue being accessed by the scalpel or radiation); (c) re-working and renegotiating the troublesome material; and (d) integration of resolved pathological material as well as ego states. The SARI model is considered in detail in chapter 13.

We see a role for ego-strengthening at every stage of treatment. This book focuses on many direct, indirect, and projective/evocative ego-strengthening techniques that can greatly amplify the work with the therapy contract, with the therapeutic alliance, and with the transference.

Psychodynamic traditions offer many opportunities for ego-strengthening throughout the course of treatment. Subsequent chapters expand on some of the themes introduced here and focus in detail on relevant ego-strengthening techniques. They include the nature of the ego, how ego-strengthening techniques can advance psychological maturity and help develop internal structures whose formation has been delayed, and how continued work with the therapeutic alliance and the transference–countertransference fields act both as process and catalyst for helping patients strengthen their egos.

As we move into subsequent chapters, the reader may become increasingly aware that the psychodynamic, object relations, and self-psychology therapeutic traditions appear to lack certain elements that patients seem to need. What is usually absent in a conspicuous way from this tradition are techniques that foster self-care and self-management for internal self-soothing, affect containment, and greater self-esteem. It seems that the appearance of these elements is left to the therapeutic alliance and the transference as well as the working through process of therapy. Their focus is on what the therapist can do about it all. The next chapter begins to look at what dimensions hypnosis may be able to add to the process of ego-strengthening (especially in areas of self-calming and self-management) and personality maturation. There are, currently, two distinct hypnotic traditions: the clinical (or classical) and the Ericksonian. Beneath their avowed and apparent differences are great commonalties. The classical tradition has historical precedence.

Chapter 2

Ego-Strengthening
The Classical Hypnotic Tradition

What Hypnosis is Not: False Beliefs that Engender Therapist Disdain

What's in a name? There are two schools of thought on this matter: Shakespeare's and Gertrude Stein's. Shakespeare testified that names may not be of great significance by having one of his characters say: "A rose by any other name would smell as sweet." Gertrude Stein, on the other hand, uttered her opinion on the topic in the famous sentence: "Rose is a rose is a rose." This somewhat cryptic statement appears to have meant that names have many inherent meanings that cannot be separated from that which they designate. When we consider the effect the word *hypnosis* has on many therapists and patients, we are most inclined to agree with Ms. Stein. For therapists who integrate hypnosis into their practices, trance work seems as natural as breathing, talking, or walking. For those therapists who have had no (or worse, flawed) training in hypnosis, the term may conjure up images of the kind of master–slave relationship that any good therapist would certainly wish to avoid at all costs. This is not surprising since our literature, theater, and visual arts frequently continue to depict hypnosis as inaccurately as it was depicted 200 years ago.

The apogee of such a view of hypnosis as a sado-masochistic situation, whose aim is the control of one person by a (presumably power hungry) other, can probably be found in the old silent movie *Nosferatu*. Nosferatu, the antagonist, is Count Dracula, a vampire. In one of many notable scenes in which Nosferatu bugs out his eyes and waves his preternaturally long fingers in the direction of his prey, he is situated in an apartment across the street from the apartment of an ill-fated heroine. She is asleep when he stands at his window, pops his eyes out into a hypnotic stare and dangles his fingers in the direction of her apartment window. The sleeping victim-heroine, now under his influence, sits up in her bed, extends her arms, arises, and walks like an automaton to obey his (now her master's) will.

"There are a number of misconceptions surrounding hypnosis which cause a small percentage of patients and a high percentage of therapists to avoid using it" (Edelstien, 1981, p. 23). It is not at all unusual for therapists who are

DOI:10.4324/9781003442585-2

extremely well trained and effective to entertain a number of anachronistic and inaccurate ideas about why hypnosis should never be used as a therapeutic adjunct. For example, there is an erroneous belief that hypnosis should never be used with psychotic or borderline patients because hypnosis would supposedly weaken ego boundaries. The truth is that hypnosis offers possibilities for good boundary formation and strengthening in such patients with whom it can also offer help with affect containment. It can also be a vehicle for deep involvement in transitional and other growth-promoting experiences.

Another false belief about hypnosis is that it should not be used with dissociative patients because it will cause them to dissociate further. The truth is that well-trained therapists who use hypnosis consider it one of the premier tools for dealing with crises and emergencies in dissociative patients (Kluft, 1983). It can be used for grounding such patients, working with traumatic material safely, and integration (Frederick & Phillips, 1992; Phillips & Frederick, 1995). It has been lifesaving at times in physical emergencies such as highway accidents (Ewin, 1983; Rossi & Cheek, 1988). Another reason that psychodynamic psychotherapists may tend to avoid hypnosis has to do with both Freud's and Jung's experiences with authoritarian, suggestive hypnosis and their attitudes toward it. Edelstien (1981) has described Freud's self-reports of unusual difficulty in achieving even ordinary success with hypnosis although he had had extensive training in the technique with the world's greatest experts including Charcot, Liebault, and Bernheim (Ellenberger, 1970). He abandoned hypnosis after a female patient with whom he was using hypnosis for the control of pain awakened from her trance state and embraced him. Fortuitously, a house servant appeared at just that time, thus "relieving" Freud of the need to confront the patient with what had happened or what it meant. Freud believed that what had seemed so mysterious about hypnosis could be explained in terms of an erotic meaning:

> From being in love to hypnosis is evidently only a short step. The respects in which the two agree are obvious. There is the same humble subjection, the same compliance, the same absence of criticism, towards the hypnotist as towards the loved object.
>
> (Freud, 1921/1964, p. 114)

Freud embraced the misconceptions of his time, which his experience with the affectionate patient reinforced, and he made a decision not to use it anymore. Some (Edelstien, 1981; Schneck, 1954) regard Freud's abandonment of hypnosis as the outcome of a countertransference reaction.

Like Freud, Jung had also had training in hypnosis; like Freud, he eventually abandoned trauma oriented therapy as well as authoritarian, direct hypnosis. Jung practiced direct suggestive hypnosis and even used *mesmeric passes* on occasion (Cwick, 1989). Jung renounced formal hypnosis after he carefully considered what had happened with three cases in which he had used hypnosis.

Although the outcome of each case was successful (indeed one of the patients became the subject of his first analysis), the reactions of these patients contained strong transferential and erotic elements. Jung sought a direct encounter with the individual's unconscious content and felt that hypnosis intruded too much of the therapist's material into the situation.

> In summary Jung felt that he had to abandon hypnosis for various reasons. It had transference complications, was too authoritarian, and involved excessive direction by the therapist which circumvented the individual's ego.
>
> (Cwick, 1989, p. 19)

Instead, Jung created the technique he called *active imagination*. We believe this to be a hypnotic technique that involves an altered state of consciousness (often spontaneous trance), indirect suggestion, and the utilization of available material (Cwick, 1989; Hall, 1989; Rossi & Cheek, 1988). Jung's *active imagination* is examined in chapters 4 and 10. It is interesting that Jung's interest in the topic of hypnosis never vanished completely. He was aware that "excessive stimulation" (trauma) was capable of precipitating a hypnoid state (spontaneous trance; Jung, 1957) and that hypnosis could be valuable in integrating dissociated personalities (Jung, 1960).

It is no surprise that Freud relinquished something that afforded him experiences of success so infrequently but also appeared to him to be a Pandora's box of libidinous impulses and poor controls. Similarly, it is not surprising that Jung avoided what he perceived as a technique that provided complications and interference. However, their mistrust and abandonment of hypnosis as a therapeutic adjunct may well continue to be an important factor in the aversion of many psychodynamic psychotherapists toward it. Freud's understanding of hypnotic techniques was disappointing, and his understanding of its nature was, by today's standards, narrow and distorted. Together with his daughter, Anna, Freud believed that hypnosis generally, "obliterated the ego and made impossible the integration of unconscious material uncovered during it" (Watkins, 1987, pp. 40–41). Gill and Brenman (1959) subsequently showed that this concept is erroneous; they believed hypnosis to be "regression in the service of the ego" (Kris, 1951, 1972).

What Hypnosis is: The Nature of Hypnosis

Trance as a phenomenon that could be utilized for healing was well recognized by ancient shamans, healer-priests, and those who assumed their functions in various roles as the centuries passed (Ellenberger, 1970). The use of ritualized incantations and manual passes over the body of the patient was described by the father of Chinese medicine, Wang Tai, 4,000 years ago, in the Hindu Veda 3,500 years ago, and can be found in the 3,000-year-old Ebers papyrus as well

(Gravitz, 1991). In the 18th century Mesmer introduced hypnosis to the medical community and theorized that it was caused by a flow of an invisible fluid, animal magnetism, between the magnetizer and the subject. Formal attempts at scientific scrutiny were first applied to trance phenomena in 1784 when the Franklin Commission examined the claims of Anton Mesmer for the curative powers of what he called *animal magnetism*. The Commission rejected Mesmer's claims and declared that the effects of the observable and helpful phenomena could *only* be attributed to imagination. The tradition of dispute about the nature of hypnosis continues today (Gravitz, 1991).

Although hypnosis was named for Hypnos, the god of sleep, it is not sleep at all. Hypnosis is characterized by a state of focused attention, and there is a variety of theories about its nature. Generally, they can be divided into *state* and *non-state* theories. State theorists believe that hypnosis is an altered state of consciousness that has many characteristics unique to it. In contrast non-state theorists espouse an array of psychological and social explanations for what is observed in trance and believe that no special state is present, per se. In their penetrating book on theories of hypnosis, Lynn and Rhue (1991) suggested that another way of viewing the differences in theories is to divide them into *single-process* theories and theories that emphasize the *context of an interaction*. Early concepts of the nature of hypnosis were that is was a special state of consciousness (Watkins, 1987), possibly related to sleep (Pavlov, 1923). In spite of considerable debate between advocates of "physiological" theories of hypnosis and "psychological" theories, there is a more general agreement that it is "an altered state of awareness" (Watkins, 1987). The *state* theories include Hilgard's (1977, 1991) neo-dissociation theory, Nash's (1991) theory of psychological regression, and Edmonston's (1991) relaxation theory. Brown and Fromm (1986) are state theorists who think that hypnosis is an altered state of consciousness in which "one's perception of and interaction with the external environment are different from those in the waking state, and the individual is more deeply absorbed in internal experience" (pp. 3–4). Brown and Fromm detailed how the hypnotic experience fulfills the criteria of Ludwig (1966) and Tart (1975) for an altered state of consciousness. Watkins (1963) proposed an interpersonal theory of hypnosis that was psychodynamic in nature. He thought that the "transference needs in the hypnotic subject and counter-transference motivations in the hypnotist determined whether a hypnotic state could be induced easily, with difficulty, or not at all, and whether that state was light or deep" (Watkins, 1987, p. 41).

Critics of the state theories hold that hypnotic phenomena or behaviors can be produced in subjects with the use of suggestion and in the presence of adequate motivation. The *non-state* theories embrace Coe and Sarbin's (1966, 1991) *role theory* view of hypnosis, Spanos' (1982, 1986, 1991) *social psychological* and *socio-cognitive* theories, and a host of others. These theories explore hypnosis from the standpoint of social interactions, expectations, roles, and the psychological needs of the subject and operator.

There are many ways to consider hypnosis. A third category of thinking about hypnosis that is significant in terms of an ego-strengthening point of view is a multidimensional one. Banyai's (1985, 1991) social psychobiological model, which is highly interactive and phenomenological, takes into account multiple determinants. They include social and cognitive factors, the interpersonal relationship at many levels, the demand characteristics of the operator, and the roles that are being enacted, as well as the individuals' physiological makeup, temperament, and traits. "According to this model, a hypnotically altered state of consciousness may have a socially and biologically adaptive value by spurring meaningful cognitive and emotional experiences that enrich both the hypnotist and the subject" (Lynn & Rhue, 1991, p. 12). It is to Banyai's (1991) model that we are inclined. We view hypnosis as a complex phenomenon that is influenced by inborn, psychodynamic, interpersonal, social, cognitive, and even political factors.

The model that one selects for understanding hypnosis can be important for many reasons. Perhaps the most significant has to do with whether the trait of *hypnotizability* is thought to be a fixed one. There are several standard scales for the measurement of hypnotizability, such as the Stanford Hypnotic Clinical Scale (Hilgard & Hilgard, 1994) and the Hypnotic Induction Profile (HIP; Spiegel & Spiegel, 1978). They are attempting to measure hypnotic talents or skills. There are clinicians who attach both diagnostic and treatment import to the outcomes of these tests of hypnotizability (Frischholz, 1996; Frischholz, Lipman, Braun, & Sachs, 1992; Spiegel, 1996).

The hypnotizability scales focus on only a few hypnotic talents or abilities and fail to measure others. In our opinion they can present an incomplete picture of who the patient is and who the patient can become in terms of her ability to utilize trance in treatment. There is abundant evidence that hypnotizability can be modified as a result of the interpersonal interaction between the therapist and the patient (Banyai, 1985, 1991; Barber, 1980; Diamond, 1984). In other words, a patient who would initially be rated as a *low hypnotizable* on one of the standard measures of hypnotic capacity might well be able to develop an impressive assortment of hypnotic abilities while in therapy. This has even been shown to be true of seriously disturbed borderline and schizophrenic patients (Murray-Jobsis, 1991). Our own preference for evaluating hypnotic capacity is similar to that of Edgette and Edgette (1995): To evaluate our patients in therapy sessions, wherein they are introduced to a wide variety of hypnotic tasks, and carefully observe the manifestations of spontaneous trance that occur in most psychotherapy sessions.

Like Banyai, we believe that the adaptive value of trance cannot be ignored. It is well known that animals experience trance states when their lives are critically endangered. When the possum acts dead or the rabbit freezes in the headlights of a car, they are displaying trance phenomena thought to be related to survival (Cheek, 1959). Humans also enter trance states when they sense their survival is in jeopardy (Cheek, 1959; Rossi & Cheek, 1988), and often enter spontaneous trance states during the course of a day. Some believe that this occurs on an ultradian (or body rhythm) basis (Kripke, 1982; Rossi, 1993).

In human events, especially those related to difficulty, trauma, and survival, the body is flooded with informational substances—millions of messenger molecules (Pert, Ruff, Weber, & Herkenham, 1985) that communicate with the cells. As a result, a unique chemical outpouring of hormones such as epinephrine, norepinephrine, and endorphins occurs. Information is processed and retained within the physiological and chemical substrate of the state in which the individual is at that time. Because it is a unique portal to the *inner world*, hypnosis can allow the individual to have access to state-bound material and other inner resources (Rossi, 1993; van der Kolk, 1996a). *State-bound material* is information that is often processed and stored on a psychophysiologic level and acquired when the experiencer was in a particular state of mind–body.

For example, if George is knocked off his bicycle by a car, there is, at the time, a tremendous outpouring of hormones and informational substances into his body that is registered at the cellular level. George may not subsequently be able to get in touch with the difficulties and the resources present to him during that experience unless he is able to enter something like that physiological state again. Although George may recall little of what happened when he was knocked off his bike in his conscious waking state, he might be able to use a hypnotic state to produce memory material about what it felt like to be knocked off his bike, what his fears were, what resources he discovered to help him deal with this traumatic situation, and what decisions he may have made at that time. The triggers for this kind of happening can be various. In his book, *The Remembrances of Things Past*, Marcel Proust (1970) had his protagonist triggered into state-bound memory by the aroma of some cookies—madeleines.

Hypnotic experiences are common; we frequently have them in normal daily living. We often call them such things as *reverie, daydreaming*, or sometimes, *remembering*. We may be scarcely aware of having been in trance states when, for example, while driving we realize that we have arrived at a destination more quickly than we expected and then understand that we have temporarily lost a sense of time. We might also notice that there is similar time distortion when reading a book or watching a movie. Indeed, we might also temporarily lose our sense of place as well—when we do these things or when our minds drift, into fantasy, when we concentrate on producing a work of art, or a wonderful soup, or even when we pray. Anyone who has meditated has had a trance experience. Natural trance rhythms (Kripke, 1982; Rossi, 1993) appear to be intrinsic to human activity as are the circadian rhythms that regulate our sleeping and waking.

Normal human trance abilities can be activated in psychotherapy and used for therapeutic goals. They are always experiences in which the patient herself is in control, just as we are really in control when we are deeply absorbed in a movie. Were the theater on fire, we would get out. Were someone to whisper into our ears, "Don't go. Fire is good!", we would not regard this as anything we would need to obey. There is no master-slave relationship in clinical hypnosis, and hypnotized subjects cannot be made to do things they do not want to do, stage hypnosis to the contrary. What we see in stage hypnosis is the performance of willing extroverts who are highly hypnotizable and who are using trance states to enjoy their newfound places in the spotlight. Successful stage hypnotists are quite adept at selecting such subjects.

The Hypnotic Phenomena

The hypnotic state is characterized by many phenomena. These hypnotic phenomena are the "natural behavioral and experimental manifestations of the trance state" (Edgette & Edgette, 1995). They may not all be present with every trance. For example, in certain *awake-alert* trance states, activity rather than relaxation predominates. Among the many phenomena we can observe in the hypnotic state are:

- time distortion
- trance logic (which resembles primary process thinking)
- unusual motor responses such as catalepsy
- perceptual alteration
- dissociation
- time distortion
- amnesia
- hypermnesia
- posthypnotic suggestibility
- physiological changes such as:
- decreased pulse rate
- decreased respiration rate
- vasomotor changes
- rapid eye movement
- sensory changes
- hyperthesia
- anesthesia
- positive and negative hallucinations
- automatic writing
- transference manifestations such as:
  - more intense
  - more rapidly occurring
  - more primitive or archaic

We introduce clinical uses of these and other hypnotic phenomena for ego-strengthening throughout this book. For example, we take an in-depth look at hypnotic age regression and hypnotic age progression in chapter 5.

Rapport

It is interesting that the term rapport, historically associated with hypnosis, has its origins in the physics that was contemporary with Mesmer (Ellenberger, 1970). It referred to the transmission of an electrical current generated by a machine among people who had formed chains in which they touched one another and thereby transmitted the current. The term for this touching and transmission of electrical energy was rapport. Mesmer adopted the term from physics and conceptualized rapport as a physical process in which he, the possessor of magnetic fluid, was able to transmit it to his subjects by rapport. The psychological model this term represented already existed in countless interactions over the millennia, and the term was adopted by hypnotists in general to refer to the warm and trusting regard the person being hypnotized (traditionally called the subject) had for the hypnotist (traditionally known as the operator). As noted, Janet (1897) regarded rapport as an essential element in psychotherapy and believed it to have its roots in the individual's dependency needs. In Freudian terms rapport would be a positive transference that permitted cooperation. This positive feeling with its elements of trust can be a basis for the beginning of the therapeutic alliance.

Hypnotic Transferences and Other Psychodynamic Hallmarks of the Hypnotic State

Perhaps the most outstanding aspect of trance is that it offers the individual a possibility of entering and exploring her inner world (the internal world of subjectivity with its imagination, fantasy and imagery, hidden feelings, memories, thoughts, and creative events). Western culture is quite outer-directed, and many individuals do not get to know their imaginal, creative events. One of the inherently ego-strengthening features of hypnosis is its ability to open the door to the inner world. This inner world is well known to all manners of artists as the fertile ground of their creativity; it constitutes an accessible subjective realm of imagination and problem solving for many individuals. It is not only a place of rewarding subjectivity, but also a place that can be utilized by patients in psychotherapy for many ego-strengthening purposes such as safety, boundary formation, self-nurturing, and self-discovery.

Particular attention and a reverence of a sort needs to be paid to the deep subjective experiences of the patient in trance. For the therapist who is willing to interact with her respectfully, it becomes evident that here are certain *interpersonal features* in hypnosis that carry with them powerful possibilities for ego-strengthening as well as for the implementation of other significant aspects of therapy. Hypnotic trance is an occasion for the subject (known as the *patient* when she is in a treatment situation) to be able to explore her inner world, to expand it, and to have positive experiences of discovery, interaction, and growth with it. Much of the work that is done in individual, family, and group therapy emphasizes getting in touch with feelings. This is certainly an attempt to begin to introduce patients to their inner lives to help them get to know themselves. In the hypnotic situation, the inner life may be encountered directly and more richly as it is represented in thought, image, feeling, and, at times, bodily sensations.

Brown and Fromm (1986) have placed special emphasis on the importance of the patient's subjective experiences in her inner world. They noticed that during these experiences there tends to be a lowering of defenses, and patients often share with their therapists many feelings, facts, and fantasies with greater ease than they would in a nonhypnotic situation. When the hypnotherapist is sensitive to the patient's expanded opportunities for involvement with the resources of her own inner world in trance and facilitates this process instead of imposing authoritarian direction and heavy-handed suggestion, the development of trust is accelerated and intensified, and the therapeutic alliance is greatly strengthened (Brown & Fromm, 1986).

Some patients may avoid contact with their inner worlds because they may only find criticism or feelings of inadequacy there; others may find that looking inward causes them to feel empty or lonely. The inner world of trauma victims may not appear to be desirable; indeed it may be a place of horror that such patients try to avoid whenever possible. As is seen later, such patients need special assistance to transform their inner worlds into places of safety and beauty and to discover there their creative resources whose presence has been long obscured by the products of trauma.

Hypnosis also has a profound influence on the nature of transference. A special hypnotic transference emerges in which archaic object relationships are replayed within therapy (Brown & Fromm, 1986; Smith, 1984) and the trance induction may also foster age regression. The style of the therapist may also influence the kind of transference that emerges (Brown & Fromm, 1986). Transferences are usually more intense and archaic with hypnosis and they often develop with great rapidity. Happily, there is usually a strong *here and now* aspect to the hypnotherapeutic relationship that allows the patient to place the transference reactions in perspective (Brown & Fromm, 1986).

Hypnotic Suggestion: Direct Versus Indirect and Authoritarian Versus Permissive

Hypnosis can be used for suggestion, uncovering, the activation of untapped internal resources, and problem solving. Heightened suggestibility is frequently thought of as characteristic of hypnosis (although this may not always be the case, and considerable debate exists on this topic). Suggestion is the bedrock of "old fashioned" hypnosis, which is usually direct and *authoritarian* in style as well. This is the kind of hypnotic approach that Freud and Jung used and then renounced; it is also the hallmark of the stage hypnotist. Often patients seeking hypnosis have this model of direct suggestion in mind. It is not uncommon for therapists who use hypnosis to receive requests from prospective patients for brief direct suggestive work. We encourage therapists to carefully evaluate all patients and never to attempt to do anything with hypnosis that they are not able to do without hypnosis.

Hypnosis, often a stepchild of psychotherapy, can broaden and deepen treatment. This is not always within the awareness of many psychotherapists, although it has been carefully studied (Kirsch, Montgomery, & Sapirstein, 1995) in the case of cognitive-behavioral therapy. Kirsch et al. (1995) examined 18 studies in which cognitive-behavioral therapy had been used with and without hypnosis and performed a meta-analysis on them. They reported that clients who had received cognitive-behavioral hypnotherapy showed a 70% greater improvement than clients who had received nonhypnotic cognitive-behavioral therapy. In general hypnosis can be regarded as effective; however, it is only an adjunctive technique and always needs to be integrated with other aspects of therapy. *Hypnosis is not a substitute for therapy.*

Contemporary hypnosis is often characterized by indirect approaches and an emphasis on permissiveness that allows the patient to set the pace and select what is useful to her in the experience. It honors the inner world and seeks only to complement it. We believe that a great deal of "nonhypnotic psychotherapy" is an exercise of indirect trance work. It is ironic that Freud and Jung thought that they had repudiated hypnosis as a therapeutic tool. What Freud replaced them with—free association—is an exemplar of indirect trance work in which the patient enters her timeless inner world and approaches her primary process thinking in a noncritical way. We think that Freud adopted an indirect hypnotic approach without realizing it. Jung (1960) specifically referred to a need for an *abaissement*, or altered state of consciousness for his analytic technique, *active imagination*. The condition of the field of hypnosis at the time was of no help to either analytic pioneer in understanding what kind of trance work he was using or in allowing him to understand how the altered state of consciousness that appears in the psychoanalytic situation could be worked with in other ways that would complement and expedite psychoanalysis. Much of the "nonhypnotic" psychotherapy done today contains strong elements of spontaneous trance states and indirect hypnosis. We believe that every psychotherapist could benefit from a study of contemporary hypnosis theory and practice.

In clinical practice both direct and indirect hypnotic techniques can be useful. There is no experimental evidence that indirect techniques are superior in their results to the direct. To the contrary. There are several studies that show that each is equally as effective as the other (Alman & Carney, 1980; McConkey, 1984). Another study by Matthews and Mosher (1988) has actually shown that indirect suggestions produced more resistance in subjects than direct suggestions. The question is still the subject of continued investigation. For an excellent discussion of it, the reader is referred to Hammond (1990a).

Direct suggestions do not have to be authoritarian. The authoritarianism of Freud's and Jung's time would be a turn-off to most patients today. It is rare for authoritarian approaches to be particularly helpful as they usually tend to alienate the patient and detract from the spirit and message of the therapeutic alliance. A notable exception exists in the field of emergency medicine. Here victims of physical trauma may need authoritarian approaches to capture and direct their attention in the presence of pain and shock.

Hartland's Ego-Strengthening

Every time an ego function is improved, the ego is strengthened. This happens in nonhypnotic as well as hypnotic psychotherapy. Every therapeutic encounter has the potential for ego-strengthening, and these opportunities appear to be increased when the altered state of consciousness is added to the picture. When the subject embraces her inner world, she is automatically strengthened by it; just as strengthening also occurs when hypnosis produces hypermnesia, and the subject is able to recall something previously forgotten.

However, the field of hypnosis has offered specific interventions for ego-strengthening that have been shown to be quite helpful. Although Freud and Jung rejected direct, authoritarian, hypnotic techniques (Cwick, 1989; Hall, 1989; Rossi & Cheek, 1988) as ineffective, there is a definite role for the use of direct hypnotic suggestion for ego-strengthening. Healing arts professionals who used hypnosis began to focus on the topic of ego-strengthening with the appearance of Hartland's (1965, 1971) work. John Hartland (1965, 1971) discovered the efficacy of direct hypnotic ego-strengthening suggestions in an interesting way that he has described (Hartland, 1971). Hartland was a physician in general practice in Wales who saw many patients with psychosomatic disorders. His time with these patients was quite limited, and he realized that it would be impossible, given the system within which he was working, to discover the source and meaning of their difficulties. Although he felt his emphasis needed to be on symptom removal and he used hypnosis to help him with this, the problem he encountered was that he "found direct symptom removal to be both difficult and unsatisfactory in many cases" (Hartland, 1971, p. 1). He decided to "evolve a series of standard psychotherapeutic suggestions" that he could use in every session with his psychosomatic patients before he focused on the main symptoms. His successes were indifferent and were frequently followed by relapses into the same symptoms or the appearance of a new set of symptoms. Nevertheless, Hartland felt he had few other alternatives, and he continued to experiment with the meaning, wording, and sequencing of his suggestions. Eventually, as a result of what Hartland openly described as a trial and error approach that went on for a considerable period of time, he found a combination of general hypnotic suggestions that appeared to help his patients recover more quickly and without relapses. The other significant feature of these recoveries was that they were not followed by symptom substitution or by anxiety.

Then destiny brought Hartland an appointment as Consulting Psychiatrist to the Hallam Hospital in West Bromwich where he worked for 6 halfdays each week in the outpatient department. Of these 6 halfday sessions, he was able to devote four entirely to psychotherapy and hypnotherapy. For the first time in his professional life he had the opportunity to use hypnoanalytic methods to treat patients with psychoneuroses. As he conducted this work, Hartland discovered that when he preceded hypnoanalytic work with the same hypnotic ego-strengthening suggestions that he had originated in his general practice, "the average length of treatment was substantially shortened," and "the need for more involved analytical techniques was also greatly reduced" (Hartland, 1971, p. 2).

When Hartland wondered how and why these suggestions worked, he concluded that they strengthened the ego and the ego defenses. This theory also helped explain why symptom removal, usually thought to be dangerous by psychodynamic therapists of his time, was not dangerous at all because patients would not relinquish their symptoms until they "felt strong enough to do without them." Patients who had great needs to use their symptoms as defenses would hold onto them so strongly that they would prove to be intractable to any kind of psychotherapy.

Hartland believed that his hypnotic suggestions were effective because they were designed to relieve tension, anxiety, and fear as well as to restore the patient's confidence in herself and in her coping abilities. He decided that they were *ego-strengthening*. The strengthened ego could relinquish the symptoms and not have to replace them. Hartland recommended that ego-strengthening be done before and after uncovering with hypnosis.

> Not only will the patient obtain more rapid relief from his symptoms, but he will obviously display marked improvement in other ways. You will notice that he gradually appears to be more confident and self-reliant, and that he is beginning to find it easier to adjust to his environment. This, in itself, will render him much less likely to relapse.
>
> (Hartland, 1971, p. 3)

Hartland thought that repetition of important ideas was necessary. He expressed them several times in different ways, stressed certain key words, and, through the insertion of pauses, developed a general rhythm of delivery. Although he believed his technique worked better and faster when the patient was in deep trance, he did not believe that deep trance was necessary in all instances. He felt that his script (which is given later) could readily be adapted, shortened, or lengthened with specialized suggestions. At times Hartland discussed the technique with his patients beforehand and explained to them why it worked. According to Hartland it was a learning process in which material was learned by the unconscious. Trance facilitated this, Hartland explained to his patients, because hypnosis improves both memory and concentration. Hartland claimed that within his practice 70% of his patients improved with ego-strengthening alone and that these patients were seen on a short-term basis (20 sessions or less).

Hartland had relied on his clinical impression to arrive at his estimate of improvement in 70% of his patients. However, Calnan (1977) did a clinical evaluation of Hartland's suggestions and was impressed that many of the patients he studied used the same words to describe the changes they experienced that were present in the ego-strengthening suggestions of Hartland. Stanton (1977) discovered that patients preferred Hartland's suggestions to positive suggestions of rational-emotive therapy. Later, Stanton (1979) conducted an experiment using the Rotter I-E Scale to evaluate the efficacy of ego-strengthening suggestions in increasing internal control. His results were positive.

Hartland's Ego-Strengthening Suggestions

Once the patient is in a trance-state and is as fully relaxed as possible, I proceed as follows:

> You have now become SO deeply relaxed ... So deeply asleep ... that your mind has become SO sensitive ... SO receptive to what I say ... that EVERY-THING that I put into your mind ... will sink SO deeply into the unconscious part of your mind ... and I will make SO deep and lasting impression there ... that NOTHING will eradicate it.
>
> Consequently ... these things that I put into your unconscious ... WILL begin to exercise a greater and greater influence over the way you THINK ... over the way you FEEL ... over the way you BEHAVE.
>
> And ... because these things will remain ... these things that I put into the unconscious part of your mind ... after you have left here ... when you are no longer with me ... they will continue to exercise that same great influence ... over your THOUGHTS ... your ... FEELINGS ... and your ACTIONS ... JUST as strongly ... JUST as surely ... JUST as powerfully ... when you are back home ... or at work ... as when you are actually with me in this room.
>
> You are now so VERY DEEPLY ASLEEP ... that EVERYTHING that I tell you ... that is going to happen to you ... FOR YOUR OWN GOOD ... WILL happen ... EXACTLY as I tell you. And EVERY FEELING ... that I tell you that you will experience ... you WILL experience ... EXACTLY as I tell you. And these same things WILL CONTINUE TO HAPPEN to you ... EVERY DAY ... and you WILL CONTINUE TO EXPERIENCE these same feelings ... EVERYDAY ... JUST as strongly ... JUST as surely ... JUST as powerfully ... when you are back home ... or at work ... as when you are with me in this room.

As a result of this deep sleep ... YOU are going to feel physically STRONGER and FITTER in every way. You will feel MORE alert ... MORE wide-awake ... MORE energetic ... You will become MUCH less easily tired ... MUCH less easily fatigued ... MUCH less easily discouraged ... MUCH less easily depressed. EVERY DAY ... you will become SO DEEPLY INTER-ESTED in whatever You are doing ... in whatever is going on around you ... that your mind will become COMPLETELY DISTRACTED AWAY FROM YOURSELF ... you will no longer THINK NEARLY SO MUCH ABOUT YOURSELF ... you will no longer DWELL NEARLY SO MUCH UPON YOURSELF AND YOUR DIFFICULTIES ... and you will become MUCH LESS CONSCIOUS OF YOURSELF ... MUCH LESS PRE-OCCUPIED WITH YOURSELF ... AND WITH YOUR OWN FEELINGS. EVERY DAY ... your nerves will become STRONGER AND STEADIER ... your mind CALMER AND CLEARER ... MORE COMPOSED ... MORE PLACID ... MORE TRANQUIL. You will become MUCH LESS EASILY WORRIED ... MUCH LESS EASILY AGITATED ... MUCH LESS FEAR-FUL AND APPREHENSIVE ... MUCH LESS EASILY UPSET.

You will be able to THINK MORE CLEARLY ... you will be able to CON-CENTRATE MORE EASILY. You will be able to GIVE UP YOUR WHOLE UNDIVIDED ATTENTION TO WHATEVER YOU ARE DOING ... TO THE COMPLETE EXCLUSION OF EVERYTHING ELSE. Consequently ... YOUR MEMORY WILL RAPIDLY IMPROVE ... and you will be able to SEE THINGS IN THEIR TRUE PERSPECTIVE ... WITHOUT MAGNI-FYING THEM ... WITHOUT EVER ALLOWING THEM TO GET OUT OF PROPORTION. EVERY DAY ... you will become EMOTIONALLY MUCH CALMER ... MUCH MORE SETTLED ... MUCH LESS EASILY DISTURBED. EVERY DAY ... YOU will become ... and YOU will remain ... MORE AND MORE COMPLETELY RELAXED ... and LESS TENSE each day ... both MENTALLY AND PHYSICALLY ... even when you are no longer with me. And AS you become ... and AS you remain ... MORE RE-LAXED AND LESS TENSE each day ... SO ... you will develop MUCH MORE CONFIDENCE IN YOURSELF ... more confidence in your ability to DO ... not only what you HAVE to do each day ... but more confidence in your ability to do whatever you OUGHT to be able to do ... WITHOUT FEAR OF FAILURE ... WITHOUT FEAR OF CONSEQUENCES ... WITH-OUT UNNECESSARY ANXIETY ... WITHOUT UNEASINESS. Because of this ... EVERY DAY ... you will feel MORE AND MORE INDEPENDENT MORE ABLE TO "STICK UP FOR YOURSELF" ... TO "STAND UPON YOUR OWN FEET'... TO "HOLD YOUR OWN" ... no matter how difficult or trying things may be.

EVERY DAY ... you will feel a GREATER FEELING OF PERSONAL WELL-BEING ... A GREATER FEELING OF PERSONAL SAFETY ... AND SECURITY ... than you have felt for a long, long time. And because all these things WILL begin to happen ... EXACTLY as I tell you they will happen ... more and more RAPIDLY ... POWERFULLY ... and COMPLETELY ... with every treatment I give you ... you will feel MUCH HAPPIER ... MUCH MORE CONTENTED ... MUCH MORE OPTIMISTIC in every way. You will consequently become much more able to ... RELY UPON and DEPEND UPON ... YOURSELF ... YOUR OWN EFFORTS ... YOUR OWN JUDGEMENT ... YOUR OWN OPINIONS. You will feel ... MUCH LESS NEED ... to have to RELY ... or to DEPEND UPON ... OTHER PEOPLE.

(Hartland, 1971, pp. 4–7)

Although Hartland's script is best adopted for use with formal hypnosis, the principle of ego-strengthening as an integral part of all psychotherapy remains a significant contribution that can be appreciated by all therapists. The use of repetition of ideas expressed in different ways, the stressing of certain words, and the interjection of pauses to increase receptiveness can be employed by therapists who are not involved in formal hypnosis as a way of making ego-strengthening suggestions to their patients. The next chapter illustrates how the repetition, pacing, interspersal, and embedding of suggestions and suggestive words can be effective although they are not done within the framework of formal trance.

The Addition of Imagery

Today we would wonder what kind of patient would be best suited for Hartland's technique. Within the short passage of time that the idea of ego-strengthening became popular in hypnosis, imagery approaches experienced their own enthusiastic reception. Imagery, always a part of hypnosis, became an integral part of ego-strengthening, and imagery techniques eclipsed Hartland's direct suggestive method completely. It is our opinion that Hartland's script can still be particularly useful with a category of patients who are more auditory than visual and more inclined to respond well to authority, influence, or pedagogy. There is another category of patients—some victims of severe trauma—who do not appear to have the usual plenum of internal resources that can be mobilized for ego-strengthening. With such patients Hartland's direct suggestions may need to precede imagery or other ego-strengthening techniques (Phillips & Frederick, 1995).

Imagery is a universal language that is older than the spoken language. It is usually thought of as being connected with the right side of the brain—the side of the brain that is more involved with our survival. Although imagery was relegated to an insignificant role by the early behaviorists, old and radical concepts such as *imageless thinking* (Woodworth, 1906) waned as laboratory evidence pointed in other directions. Investigators developed growing interests in subjects such as brainwashing, LSD trips, and endangering hallucinations or mirages such as those that appear in highway hypnosis (Richardson, 1983). Richardson (1969) thought that there was adequate evidence that self-initiated imagery can deepen understanding in a way that is different from the perceptual or sensory counterparts of the images (i.e., experiences in the "outer" world). The consequences of this for psychotherapy are manifold (Sheikh, 1983), and the role of imagery has continued to assume greater and greater proportions, especially in the field of mind–body healing (Achterberg, 1985; Brigham, 1994; Dossey, 1982; Simonton, Matthews-Simonton, & Creighton, 1978).

Imagery is an important feature of trance. Trance subjects experience more imagery than they do in the waking state, and it is often more intense. They may encounter spontaneous imagery, and, although they are readily inclined to adopt the images offered them by the hypnotist, they may also create their own imagery at the same time (Brown & Fromm, 1986). "The hypnotist may also, move back and forth between the patient's imagery and his own, leading the patient into deeper trance along pathways some of which the patient is creating and therefore is more willing to follow" (Brown & Fromm, 1986, p. 92). Other sensory channels such as touch, smell, taste, and sound are frequently evoked as part of the visualizing, and the greater the patient's involvement in her inner world, the deeper she is in trance.

Visualization in trance is frequently accompanied by affect. Brown & Fromm (1986) recommend the use of imagery such as *safe place* imagery for soothing and transitional experiences, especially with the suicidal patient. McNeal and Frederick (1994) have expanded on their concept and included other reasons why *safe place* imagery is soothing and ego-strengthening (see chap. 7). Morton and Frederick (1996) have observed how internally visualized transitional space can be a vehicle for personality integration.

It is not surprising that many patients enjoy imagery in their trance experiences (Brown & Fromm, 1986; McNeal & Frederick, 1994). Ego-strengthening can be more easily accepted and expanded upon when it occurs within the patient's inner world as she already knows it or in a newly introduced internal visual locus. There are many advantages to purposely adding imagery to ego-strengthening procedures or utilizing what the patient may already be producing. One is that patients tend to respond well to *developmental* or to *archetypal* and other symbolic input that often bypasses the critical faculty. A second advantage is that dynamic visual imagery is often a display of *active imagination* in which the conscious and unconscious minds interact, often with profound problem solving (Jung, 1965; the topic of active imagination is explored in chaps. 6 and 10).

A third reason for the helpfulness of imagery is that positive associations can be expanded through imagery. Concern during the trance experience over performance anxiety ("Am I taking in what the doctor is saying correctly? Am I doing this right?") is lessened. Imagery as it appears in projective/evocative ego-strengthening is also a rich source of information about the patient's internal processes and what they might mean, as is clarified later in this chapter.

It has been thought that qualities such as self-efficacy (Bandura, 1977; Hammond, 1990d; Marlatt & Gordon, 1985) and self-confidence might give patients a greater sense of internal control. Harry Stanton (1979, 1989, 1993a) is one of the significant clinicians who uses imagery as an integral part of his ego-strengthening scripts. Stanton (1979) used Rotter's I-E Scale as a measure of internal control and discovered that generalized ego-enhancing hypnotic suggestions increased subjects' sense of internal control as measured by that instrument. In his subsequent five-step ego enhancement procedure, Stanton (1989) made several modifications of Hartland's technique that appeared to be improvements in the light of what is known about imagery. Stanton's five-step ego-strengthening approach can be quite useful for self hypnosis homework. In this procedure Stanton uses a hypnotic induction to produce relaxation. Internal calmness is promoted by the patient's being asked to gaze at the still surface of a pond. As the patient remains focused on the internal pond, she becomes more deeply involved in her trance experience. Stanton views the lake as representing the unconscious mind. The patient is asked to stand in a corridor before a rubbish chute. She then allows herself to recall negative experiences which she is able to dispose of into the chute. Unwanted habits can be disposed of in this way as well.

Next, the patient (in a large room, like a gymnasium) is instructed to walk through a fabric wall. The fabric is composed of every negative event in the patient's life. The patient accomplishes the fifth step by enjoying a special place of internal tranquillity where she is able to turn off the outside world. Here she is encouraged to have positive visualizations of herself in future activities, achieving goals and enjoying success.

McNeal and Frederick (1993) noted that Stanton had modified Hartland's direct ego-strengthening approach in several ways. We currently believe that his modifications were:

1. He added imagery to the spoken word. This deepened the trance and expanded its possible meanings. Some of his imagery was archetypal, some-involved "getting rid of the negative," while some was symbolic of the patient's having been successful in enduring the worst that life had thrown at her.
2. He was not authoritarian; the procedure acts as a guide that encourages the patient to add her own images to those supplied by the therapist. In this sense it is interactive.
3. He encouraged the patient to develop specific imagery that was related to her problem, thereby making the trance *her* trance. The therapeutic alliance is strengthened by such a trance interaction.
4. Stanton emphasized the importance of self-hypnosis and homework for on-going ego-strengthening.

Stanton managed, simultaneously, to broaden ego-strengthening and place more control into the patient's hands, allowing a therapeutic interplay between the patient and the therapist.

Chapter 5 contains a treasure chest of many excellent scripts for ego-strengthening (ego-strengthening, enhancing esteem, self-efficacy, and confidence): the encyclopedic and invaluable *Handbook of Hypnotic Suggestions and Metaphors* (Hammond, 1990b). Many of them employ the creative use of visual imagery as a way of enhancing self-esteem by addressing developmental and other intrapersonal as well as interpersonal problems. We would like to emphasize that there is nothing at all wrong with using a script, especially when one is new in hypnosis. The patient's experience will be completely unique and helpful whether the therapist uses a script, or whether she is someone who does not use scripts because she is possessed of a vivid imagination, formidable training, and an excellent command of the language.

We also refer the reader to Hunter's (1994) excellent collection of creative ego-strengthening scripts to be used with hypnosis. The following is a brief ego-strengthening script of Hunter's that can be used with many kinds of patients. It helps patients identify their strengths, take a noncritical look at their frailties, acknowledge their past successes, and form an awareness of their own priorities. Some of the themes in this script (mastery, the use of time) are expanded on later in this chapter as well as in chapter 5. Hunter (1994) has parenthetically called this script, "The Hunter Quartet" (p. 144).

Gathering Strengths and Resources

At times, it is important for us to be aware of our own talents and attributes. A person may feel that his or her self-esteem is at a low ebb. That person needs to recognize his or her own worth as a person.

There are many ways to improve our feelings about ourselves. Here are four basic steps that we can take.

First, IDENTIFY STRENGTHS. Everyone has some strengths in his/her life. Look at yourself more objectively, but at the same time from within using your own hypnosis to identify your own strengths: the things that you do well; the achievements that you may have had. Did you always come first in spelling? That is an achievement—one of your strengths.

Are you the one whom everyone can count on? Do you always remember to take the paper plates to the picnic? Will you baby-sit at very short notice for a needy neighbour? Or are you a staunch friend through thick and thin? Perhaps, for you, these are new ways of looking at "strengths." But they are valid. Everything that we have done, throughout our lives, is important in shaping what we are. When we can recognize the good things—at whatever age they occurred—we are recognizing our own self-worth. So take a little reconnaissance trip through your life, and find your own strengths. They are an important part of your resource storehouse.

Secondly, ACKNOWLEDGE FRAILTIES. Just take a look at those areas where you know you could use some strengthening, and accept them for what they are. Acknowledging our frailties is very different from berating or demeaning ourselves because of them. It just gives one a chance to put things in perspective—"Yes, these are areas that I can work on, to strengthen and improve."

Thirdly, REVIEW PAST SUCCESSES. In some ways, this overlaps Identifying Strengths but the two may be quite different in many respects. Strengths, for instance, include skills that we have learned, awarenesses that we recognize about our own talents. Past successes means just that—situations where you have been a winner. And they are valid at whatever time of your life they occurred. Give yourself the pleasure, now and several times over the next few days, of *reexperiencing* some of those past successes. Take yourself back to that time; see, hear, FEEL yourself there. Tune in especially to the feelings, and enjoy them yet again.

Fourthly, CLARIFY THE "SHOULDS." We have already talked about the "Shoulds" in earlier sessions, so let me just remind you that there are two types of "Shoulds"—those that come from outside, and those that come from inside.

Those that come from outside are very important because they provide information and an opportunity to review your thoughts, but they belong to the people who bring them. Inner Shoulds, those that come from your own deep inner knowledge of what is right for YOU, must always be given attention and priority. Whenever you hear yourself saying, "Yes, I should ...," be sure which type of "should" you are expressing, and place it in its proper priority.

Following these four steps at regular intervals will help you to understand yourself better and improve your sense of self-worth.

(Hunter, 1994, p. 144)

There is one caveat that we must place on the use of imagery. We often see patients who tell us that they have never experienced hypnosis, but that the previous therapist used imagery and relaxation. Certainly, therapists retain the right to suggest to patients that they imagine, or let their minds picture while in the waking state, but the days when therapists could call trance work *guided imagery* as opposed to *hypnosis* appear to have been swept away in the sands of time. In our litigious society relaxation and "guided imagery" are frequently identified as hypnosis because they produce the trance phenomena of hypnosis, such as increased suggestibility, time distortion, and trance logic. We believe that imagery techniques are forms of hypnosis, and we advise anyone using hypnosis today to get a written informed consent before beginning any trance work. It is also important to understand that a lack of training in hypnosis leaves the practitioner, not to mention the patient, at a disadvantage. Should she encounter negative or abreactive material during an imagery exercise, she might not be able to contain or to utilize it in a way that would be clinically helpful to the patient. Understandably, the failure to get appropriate professional training in hypnosis would make a practitioner of hypnosis vulnerable to legal attack and ethical questions. We recommend that any therapist who wishes to do trance work obtain hypnosis training for professional psychotherapists. There are many opportunities for such training today.

Hypnotic Mastery and Rehearsal

The kind of ego-strengthening that comes from a sense of self-efficacy can probably be best appreciated during experiences of mastery. Gardner (1976) has suggested that there are two basic questions that can be asked if one is interested in exploring possible connections between hypnotherapy and mastery. The first question asks if a sense of mastery enhances the effectiveness of hypnosis itself. Gardner believes that enhanced effectiveness, if it exists, can be seen in the hypnotic induction—by strengthening hypnotic suggestions—or by the patient's being able to maintain hypnotherapeutic gains. Gardner believes that there is a category of patients who fear losing control and that these patients do not respond well to many standard hypnotic induction hypnotic techniques that favor or promote passivity. Patients who present complaining of "passivity, dependence, and helplessness" (Gardner, 1976, p. 203) may not even be able to enter hypnosis when such techniques are used. However, these patients can easily enter trance when imagery techniques that emphasize mastery are used. In her classic paper on mastery and hypnosis Gardner (1976) offered two clinical vignettes of patients who had previously resisted entering hypnosis in other treatment situations. Both patients entered the trance state with great ease when she used imagery experiences of mastery with them. One patient, a man whose domineering wife belittled him, used the experience of piloting his boat during a bad storm. The other patient was a young woman with severe headaches. Her trance induction consisted of her mentally replaying the opening of a performance of the *St. Matthew Passion*, which she had recently sung with her choral group.

Both these patients improved, and Gardner (1976) believed that their inductions had been therapeutic. She cited Milton Erickson's (1959) belief that if the hypnotic induction truly utilizes behaviors that allow patients to meet their needs, it is not necessary, nor even desirable, to concentrate on completion or resolution of the problem (see chap. 3). This sophisticated approach, claims Gardner (1976), is one in which "the induction is itself therapeutic (or counter therapeutic) as the case may be" (Gardner, 1976, p. 204). Her thinking is based on Erickson's belief that it is the unconscious mind, once activated in the proper direction, not the conscious mind, that is the agent of change (see chap. 3).

In her consideration of what allows patients to maintain their improvements, Gardner (1976) felt that patients who believed they were actively involved in their treatment did better than those who simply accepted or received what the hypnotherapist suggested to them. Gardner (1976) thought such involvements were transferable to the environment outside the therapy room. Like many other therapists she emphasized the importance of the therapeutic alliance, which she perceived as a way of helping patients see their own activities as helpful, even crucial to their therapy. The good therapist ego-strengthens the patient who has mastery needs by insisting that the patient participate in her therapy. Gardner also advocated the use of self-hypnosis as another mastery tool. Gardener's article on mastery and hypnosis is a beautiful illustration of the integration of hypnotic technique within a sensitive and intelligent psychotherapy framework.

Gardner's (1976) second question was whether "hypnotherapy, as compared with other psychotherapeutic approaches, better facilitates the development of a sense of mastery" (p. 203). In other words Gardner wondered whether hypnosis could enhance mastery. The critical issue here is how one defines *hypnosis*—the same issue encountered whenever we consider "nonhypnotic" techniques such as Freudian psychoanalysis or Jung's active imagination. Gardner perceived Hartland's (1965, 1971) ego-strengthening suggestions as failing to take into account the different needs patients have (and, parenthetically, to avail himself of many different kinds of trance experiences). His suggestions, designed to promote passivity in the patient, would probably not have been helpful with the cases mentioned by Gardner. Gardner's (1976) recommendation for further investigation of the relationship between hypnosis and mastery is clear: "... the criterion for determining hypnosis vs. non-hypnosis should be based on some aspect of the experience or the behavior of the patient and not that of the *therapist*" (Gardner, 1976, p. 211).

Another classic testimonial to the power of mastery as an ego-strengthener that can dramatically transform a personality is Dimond's (1981) report of his work with a patient who was on kidney dialysis. In his review of the literature Dimond discovered that kidney dialysis patients may be prone to "feelings of helplessness, loss of independence, and anxiety concerning the future" (p. 284). He reported the case of Ms. B. J., a dialysis patient who had needle phobia and a very low pain threshold. Ms. B. J. did not have optimal dialysis because her hysterical behavior interfered with adequate blood flow. It also greatly disturbed the staff and other patients. Dimond (1981) believed Ms. B. J. was having a behavioral reaction to the loss of her own independent lifestyle which had been replaced by the forced dependence of dialysis.

Accordingly, Dimond introduced hypnosis to Ms. B. J. as a way for her to achieve control and mastery. The first hypnotic task was to help her deal with her pain. A hypnotic technique called the black box was used. The black box employed imagery of a circuit box with fuses and switches that she could manipulate to obtain physical comfort in self-hypnosis. When pain management had been established, Dimond turned to the serious problem of her reactions to dialysis. Her behavior was seriously interfering with the dialysis and was life threatening. The problem had "remained refractory to direct hypnotic suggestions" (Dimond, 1981, p. 286). Through the use of imagery Ms. B. J. was able to explore the dialysis equipment at the pace that was comfortable to her. Eventually she conceived of the dialysis equipment as an extension of herself that was sustaining her life in much the same fashion as a future kidney transplant would.

As a result of this mastery approach, Ms. B. J. became comfortable during dialysis. Her blood flow increased by 60%, and her relationship with the staff improved dramatically. A technician informed Dimond that Ms. B. J. "was like a new woman." Like Stanton and Gardner, Dimond encouraged his patient "to experience these changes *in her own way* and at *her own pace* thus emphasizing self control" (Dimond, 1981, p. 287). Eventually Ms. B. J. became a counselor for other dialysis patients.

The Ego-Strengthening Spectrum

Ego-strengthening can be thought of as existing on a spectrum. At one end of the spectrum are direct, structured ego-strengthening interventions such as Hartland's. The introduction of imagery and mastery techniques stand somewhere in the center of the spectrum. The therapist offers structure to the patient but does not bind or chain her to it. She is free and encouraged to add her own imagery, focus on what is important to her, and go at her own pace.

Hartland's ego-strengthening techniques give the unconscious mind a definite and specific program to follow. When ego-strengthening procedures rely heavily on the therapist's conscious input, the therapist and the patient work to give the unconscious mind an agenda and an assortment of resources, views, and/or techniques. They contribute to the creation, within the patient, of senses of mastery and internal control. They also desensitize her against fearful situations, give her a greater sense of familiarity and habit about the task or situation that she will confront in the future, help her work cognitively with the material, and offer her a structure she can utilize when moving into new experiences.

At the other end of the spectrum are the projective/evocative techniques that we believe are a natural evolution that has occurred within the framework of a convergence of several orientations. These techniques achieve two things: First they activate powerful ego-strengthening internal resources. Second, they may provide valuable information about what is going on with the patient. Some of the projective/evocative techniques such as Torem's (1992) Back to the Future technique, or McNeal and Frederick's (1993) Inner Strength technique are presented in a very structured way in order to lead the patient to the place where projective and evocative material may emerge. Others of this type may be deliberately unstructured, such as unstructured hypnotic age progressions (Frederick & Phillips, 1992; Phillips & Frederick, 1992) to achieve the same purposes.

The Projective/Evocative Evolution

Projective techniques for uncovering trauma and other difficulties are well known in hypnosis, especially in hypnoanalysis (Brown & Fromm, 1986;

Watkins, 1992). However, within this framework, the range of their applicability to the field of ego-strengthening has only been partially realized. Patients added material to their inner worlds, and this material was projective in nature. Further, patients in trance seem at times to get hooked up with vast reserves as a result of their hypnotic experiences.

We emphasize the projective/evocative evolution in this book for several reasons. One is that many of the projective/evocative ego-strengthening approaches activate the patient's internal resources (see chap. 3); the other is that the therapist can learn so much about the patient from them. In this light trance productions become significant the way Thematic Apperception Test results are significant. Certain ego-strengthening trance material can be diagnostic and prognostic, informing us of the status of the patient's defenses, the nature of her internal boundaries, her capacity for internal self-soothing, and the ability of the individual to experience her own strength as well as the reservoirs of love that may reside within her.

We also favor projective/evocative ego-strengthening because we place strong value on therapy that honors the healing powers that exist within the patient and techniques that endeavor to activate these healing powers whenever possible. Projective/evocative ego-strengthening is probably as powerful as it is because it increases conscious–unconscious complementarity (this topic is discussed in detail in chap. 13). That is to say that it helps the patient's ego to extend its realm by developing a better working relationship with her unconscious mind. We believe that this is the true embodiment of the concept *client centered therapy* (Rogers, 1961).

The next chapter introduces the reader to the Ericksonian approach to hypnosis and the concepts of inner resources and utilization. From a blend of the classical and the Ericksonian traditions has emerged an expanded style of ego-strengthening that evokes unconscious inner resources and that is often projective in nature as well.

Chapter 3

Ego-Strengthening
The Ericksonian Tradition

Milton Erickson has had a profound influence on human endeavors such as anthropology, medicine, psychotherapy, family psychotherapy, and clinical hypnosis. Many clinicians traveled to his home in Phoenix, Arizona to observe his work and learn from the master with the same kind of reverence as that held by ancient nobility, generals, and sages who traveled to the oracle at Delphi.

It is interesting that a man who had to confront so many personal difficulties throughout the course of his life should have become associated with mastery. Erickson was severely dyslexic, suffered from progressive color-blindness (at the end of his life he could only see the color purple), and was tone deaf. He had polio twice (at ages 17 and 51), and in his later years he had very severe, crippling, and painful arthritis that confined him to a wheelchair. His old age was plagued with the indignity of his never being able to find a set of false teeth that fit.

Erickson was a champion of the individual human being who resisted all notions that therapy could be standardized or managed (Zeig, 1982). "Each person is a unique individual. Hence psychotherapy should be formulated to meet the uniqueness of the individual's needs, rather than tailoring the person to fit the Procrustean Bed of a hypothetical human behavior" (Erickson, 1979).

Principles of Ericksonian Hypnosis

In many ways Erickson was in the mainstream of clinical and research psychiatry during his lifetime. He worked and did research with psychoanalytic scholars such as Kubie and Rapaport. However, Erickson was a founder of the American Society of Clinical Hypnosis because of his reaction to research scientists who undervalued clinical material and who did not want to admit clinicians to their ranks. He was also the founding editor of the *American Journal of Clinical Hypnosis*.

There are certain features about the way he understood hypnosis that characterized what is known today as Ericksonian hypnosis. Because he was atheoretical and did not systematize his approaches, it has been left to others to interpret his work. There exist many versions of the underlying principles of Ericksonian

DOI:10.4324/9781003442585-3

hypnosis. Among them are those of Gilligan (1987), Rossi (1980), Beahrs (1982a), Bandler and Grinder (1975), O'Hanlon and Weiner-Davis (1989), Yapko (1986, 1990), and Zeig (1980).

Despite different emphases by Erickson scholars, there are some fundamental agreements about general principles that are present in the body of his work. We believe the foundation of what is uniquely Ericksonian can be expressed in the following principles.

Every Human Is Unique

In our conforming society our uniqueness is often lost. Patients frequently feel that they should be, behave, and feel like others, and unfortunately current managed care approaches favor cookbook therapy with strict timelines for "improvement" in therapy (whatever that might mean to them). Many of our professional organizations have become deeply invested in creating "practice guidelines" that prescribe accepted treatment interventions that are based on the patient's diagnosis or a particular body of empirical research findings.

What does it mean for the therapist to regard the patient as unique? It means that each one of us is the dynamic expression of a particular combination of objective and subjective influences that cannot be duplicated. Each has his own fingerprint, his own DNA code, each has his own psychological strengths and weakness, his own sensitivities, his own character traits; each possesses his own array of psychological defenses; and each has his own position in a family that has specific dynamics. It also means that within each of us there are aspects that are singularly important and cannot be measured. Each has his own compelling goals in the passage of his life; each has his individual spiritual sensibilities.

The singular specialness of each of us has been the subject of many myths (Hillman, 1996). Plato's myth of Er, Plotinus' story of the descent of the soul, the Kabbalah, and the Native American belief that the soul originates with a divine image are all expressions of an understanding that each of us must realize that there is only one of us in the entire universe. It is probable that Erickson developed his early appreciation for the "principle" of uniqueness through his own realization of how completely singular he himself was. He appreciated how all the things that went into his makeup, even the problems, ultimately contributed to his special enjoyment of life and to his masterful development as a therapist. These points of reference apparently gave Erickson a framework upon which to stand firmly as he observed that everyone was unique. A good example of how Erickson reflected this in his formal clinical hypnosis work can be found in a comment he made about age regression:

> … its application must remain individualistic, since the varying degrees of development among different personalities and among the various aspects of the same personality may render precisely the same mode of expression

regressive for one individual, progressive (in the sense of being the opposite of regressive) for another, or regressive in relation to certain aspects of the personality and not regressive in relation to certain other aspects.

(Erickson, 1980a, p. 104)

A major implication of this principle for therapists is that there needs to be a great emphasis upon observing the patient *without preconceptions* or attempts to place him within a theoretical framework. "This is a truly radical proposition in that it requires therapists to begin each therapy in a state of experiential ignorance" (Gilligan, 1987, p. 14). Erickson and his followers are, in this respect, closely allied with the Jungians (Hillman, 1976, 1996), for whom the uniqueness of the individual is also sacred.

The implication of the Ericksonian principle that everyone is unique, and, like the Quakers we would add irreplaceable, for ego-strengthening cannot be ignored. What may be strengthening for one person has the possibility of insignificant or negative effect on another. Further, the therapist's appreciation of the unique opportunity that is challenged to meet with each patient is another factor in strengthening the therapeutic alliance. "Sarah" is not a *case*. Instead, she is one of a kind, special, never to be duplicated. Gilligan (1987) reminds us that we must learn to set our old models aside and be receptive to our patients. Each patient is a new reality, not an average, or an example of some principle.

Indeed, therapists may discover that they need to relinquish preconceived ideas about themselves as well. Although it is certainly important to learn much about theory and technique to be a *good-enough* therapist, many of us find that we are comparing ourselves favorably or unfavorably with other therapists. We recommend the use of consultation and education groups that meet on a regular basis for the discussion of case material. The group facilitator must be oriented to accentuating group perceptions of the special uniqueness of each group member. Such a group can facilitate each therapist-member in learning to become comfortable with his uniqueness and use it to enhance the quality of his therapy.

The individuality of the patient and the individuality of the therapist ultimately affect what can be called *match*. An adequate "match" is essential for good therapy; in its absence, therapy may go *on the rocks* (Phillips & Frederick, 1995). The Ericksonian principle of *uniqueness* is a lesson in life that every good therapist must learn. Those who do will probably extend the range of patients with whom they can work successfully.

Each Human Being Has Generative Resources

Ericksonians frequently refer to *resources* which reside in and about the patient and are available for the patient's use in problem solving, living, and healing. Although we believe that resources can be thought of as either external (support systems, adequate income, necessary medications, etc.) or internal, the resources to which Erickson referred were internal. Erickson believed that individuals have resources that come from their past experiences, their present situations, and even their futures (Yapko, 1990). Chapter Five presents a number of ways to use both resources from the past and visions of the future for ego-strengthening.

Resources are both conscious and unconscious processes that reside within each human being and can be accessed in many ways. Some of these resources are instinctual or innate; others are learned through normal development or in response to stress. Among the body of resources are natural endowments (such as talents, intelligence, and abilities), training and education, the quality of rearing, and life successes. Other resources include life failures such as divorce or job loss, separations caused by death, illness, inborn difficulties, and even the symptoms that plague the patient. It is usually more challenging for the therapist and patient to learn how to utilize negative qualities and events as resources. Nevertheless, such resources, when properly utilized, can become sources of strength and confirmation of the patient's special uniqueness.

A difficulty for many people is that they are frequently dissociated from their resources (Gilligan, 1987). They need help locating and recognizing them. At times they need help activating them so that they can become truly useful energies in their lives. Individuals may have inadequate resources for a number of reasons. Among them are inadequate parenting, trauma, developmental disabilities or lags, physical illness, and impoverished physical and cultural environments. For example, we think of the person who has been neglected or abused as running a greater risk of being impoverished, just as someone who was reared as a famine victim in a third world country would also lack physical integrity as well as external resources.

Many of the patients whom we see come into therapy without adequacy in quantity or diversity of resources. Although the therapist must always attempt to discover whatever resources are present and make every attempt to activate them, it would appear that Erickson did not deal with a population of the severely impoverished. With such patients the emphasis must be in "filling the glass" (Phillips & Frederick, 1995), that is, using direct ego-strengthening and other techniques in order to help the patient develop resources. (The problem of how to help patients develop or strengthen internal resources and achieve greater psychological maturity is addressed throughout this book.)

We cannot overemphasize that the resources include even the resistances the patient may bring to therapy. The therapist uses the information he gathers to create interventions that facilitate the patient's growth and healing. Thus, whatever the patient presents can be perceived as valuable and helpful in the therapeutic process. At times the therapist's function is to activate hitherto unknown resources that reside within the patient's unconscious mind. The knowledge that there are significant resources within people lies at the heart of projective/evocative ego-strengthening. The purpose of these techniques is to activate the internal resources

Case Example: Brie

Brie was 22 when her college roommates telephoned her parents. They were concerned because Brie appeared to be depressed. She was nearing the end of her third year at a large impersonal university, and she had stopped going to classes and had withdrawn into her room. Brie's parents, both physicians, helped her move back to the family home for the summer. Her mother called me (CF), seeking psychiatric help for her (now adult) daughter. She told me that she and her husband were quite concerned about Brie, that she was an only child, and that they thought her college experience was overwhelming her.

I told her I would be happy to meet with Brie so that we could see if our working together would be useful to her. However, Brie would have to get in touch with me herself to set up the appointment. Her mother's response to this was "Just a minute," and before I even realized what was happening, Brie was on the phone.

In the first session Brie told me that she had been a good high school student, but that when she went away to college, the most important things for her were joining a sorority and charging into the abundant social life of the university. They became her priorities. She went to many parties, turned night into day, cut many classes, did not study, and ended up on academic probation at the end of her first year. Along the way she had picked up a boyfriend who was insensitive and immature.

Brie managed to do some studying in her second year. She got off academic probation, but she was not enjoying her studies. She got rid of her boyfriend and changed her major from chemistry to biology. Her real major was still partying and meeting new people.

In her third year Brie met an interesting man who was engaged to another woman. When he had to stop spending time with Brie, she became depressed. She could not bring herself to attend classes and was placed back on academic probation. Her only solaces were heavy partying, sorority projects, and hanging out with her female roommates. Brie was able to tell me that she really did not enjoy classes or studying. She knew she had blown her chances for medical school, but she felt that if she could just hang in, she could get some kind of job in the health field. Perhaps she could become a physician's assistant.

Brie was working a high-pressure job in one of the casinos for the summer. She had had a series of summer jobs over the years, and she had always done well with them. She had always been on time and had always produced what was expected. In her current job she was quickly given extra responsibilities.

Her job record was a resource we could work with I thought, but was I overlooking other resources that Brie was revealing to me? I realized that her major problems at school had been her preference for extroverted social activities. I wondered if she might be telling the world that she had resources in that area.

Therapists who are faced with behaviors that are not generally considered popular in society, such as not attending classes and failing at school, may not realize that these problems can be resources of great value in therapy. We shall return to this case.

The Unconscious Mind Is on the Side of Progress and Healing, Is Positive, and Contains All the Resources the Patient Needs for Problem Resolution

Although Erickson was generally atheoretical, he did have a concept of an unconscious mind. This formulation differed from the psychoanalytic theory that emphasized uncontrolled libidinous impulses and super-ego demands. Instead it was a belief that the unconscious mind was positive and generative in nature and that it contained a plenum of resources.

Erickson was not impressed with the abilities of the conscious mind to provide solutions in the realms of human emotions and problem behaviors. He believed that the conscious mind, a fairly recent evolutionary development, could only focus on one thing at a time and could not view complex situations in a comprehensive way. The limitations of the conscious mind make it essential that it develop an adequate relationship with the unconscious mind. Erickson felt that the unconscious was so adequate that one of the best things the conscious mind could do for it was to get out of its way. He considered therapeutic trance to present a setting in which the limitations of the conscious mind could be allowed to fall away. Once the work was done, the conscious mind could hopefully bring its focus to bear upon it and integrate it into daily life. "The unconscious is a manufacturer and the conscious is a consumer; trance is the mediator between them" (Erickson, Rossi, & Rossi, 1976, p. 234).

Thus, an important role that the unconscious mind plays in healing is that of "… learning without the intervention of conscious purpose and design" (Erickson, Rossi, & Rossi, 1976, p. 147). According to Erickson it was necessary to determine whether what appeared to be unconscious learning was really just that, or whether the unconscious mind was simply responding to certain interactions with some form of automatic behavior. For him the true test was whether the patient's hypnotic experience could actually cause him to display new response capacities. He believed that trance was the optimal place for unconscious learning to occur because, in trance, preconceptions, biases, distractions, and the pull of many demands are less important and intrusive.

Early hypnotists such as Liebeault, Bernheim, and Braid were apparently aware of this, as much of their trance work contained no instructions for the patient whatsoever. They created what Erickson, Rossi, and Rossi (1976) called a healing atmosphere. They used short trances with no specific instructions as to how recovery would occur. Yet they managed to convey to their patients their beliefs that this would be sufficient for them. This atmosphere and the patients' belief systems seemed to function "as indirect and non-verbal suggestions to set in motion creative, autonomous processes within their patients that could effect a 'cure'" (Erickson, Rossi, & Rossi, 1976, p. 147). Chapter 2 describes Gardner's (1976) mastery approach to ego-strengthening. She has often espoused the principle that the therapist using hypnosis should not try to tell the unconscious mind how to do its job.

Erickson, Rossi, and Rossi (1976) have remarked how consistent Erickson's theory of unconscious learning is with what is believed to be involved in the creative process (Rossi, 1968, 1972). As most therapists realize, creativity usually plays in the fields of the unconscious mind and often reveals itself in dreams and other automatic activities. Unconscious learning and conscious–unconscious complementarity are vital elements of therapy. They are further addressed in chapter 13. Ericksonian therapy, then, aims at the activation of internal healing activities at an unconscious level. One thing that this means is that insight becomes insufficient as the agent for internal change. Healing takes place at a different level and in more comprehensive ways.

The Task of the Therapist Is to Join the Patient's Frame of Reference

The Cooperation Principle. This principle means that the therapist always seeks to adapt to the patient. He neither employs standardized, preconceived methods, nor does he demand that the patient make any great show of cooperation. The Ericksonian therapist communicates acceptance of the validity of the patient's reality. This accepting attitude aligns the therapist with the patient and promotes both the patient's self-acceptance and the therapeutic alliance. It is an element in ego-strengthening.

It is the role of the therapist to cooperate with the patient rather than vice versa. The therapist may accept and utilize the patient's history, speech, and motor patterns to create opportunities and new situations that promote more adequate functioning on the part of the patient. This adaptation to and cooperation with the patient is the basis of the cooperation principle (Gilligan, 1987). The therapist accomplishes his part of the cooperation by pacing and leading the patient's experiences in the therapy session.

Pacing is a process in which the therapist feeds back the patient's verbal and nonverbal communications to him. No new content is added. This allows the therapeutic alliance to develop and enhances the therapist's understanding of the patient as well as his empathy for the patient. There is increasing rapprochement of the rhythm of the therapist to that of the patient, and much of this reflects the internal (unconscious) resources of the therapist at work. Pacing is closely related to attunement (Brown & Fromm, 1986) and resonance (Watkins, 1978, 1992). The Ericksonian therapist also *leads* in the sense that he introduces new ideas that are different, yet consistent with the patient's goals. Thus, they help lead the patient in the direction of the desired goals. Successful leading depends on successful pacing. To be effective this must be done in a naturalistic and nonmanipulative fashion (Gilligan, 1987). Resistance within this schema does not mean that the patient is bad or is not cooperating. Rather, it means that the patient's defenses do not as yet permit him to conform to the therapist's expectations and that more pacing of other aspects of the patient's experience needs to be done until he feels safer.

Case Example: Brie (continued)

In the next session I (CF) explored with Brie how much fun she had at parties as well as how interesting it was for her to meet new people. She enjoyed her casino job very much because it gave her the opportunity to meet new people.

I also commiserated with her about having to sit in classes that were both difficult and boring for her. It seemed to me that it was unfortunate that she had chosen a field that did not seem like fun at all for her. On top of that, I told Brie it must have been a terrible shock to exchange the comfortable cocoon of the Lake Tahoe area, where everyone knew everyone else, for the large, alien university where no one cared whether you went to class. Brie was relieved that I understood this. One of the problems appeared to be that she had become depressed in her first year of college, not as depressed as she had become in her third year, but still depressed enough not to be able to use her skills for studying and learning.

I told Brie that I suspected as well, from many things that she had said, that another shock must have been to move away from parents who were so vitally interested in her that they had made their own lives secondary to her own. Brie breathed sighs of relief. The problem about it all was that she felt she was letting them down. They were paying good money for her to have a future, and she was not holding up her end of things. They had not insisted that she go to medical school; they just wanted her to get a good education so that she could have a responsible and secure career.

In the next session I learned that Brie's mother did everything for her. Brie had never done her own laundry in her own home. Her mother even registered her into her college classes each year. When Brie had been in high school, her mother had told her when to study and had reviewed all of her course material and homework with her. Brie did none of the heavy housework, and she had never learned to cook. She had been raised in a fashion that had felt very comfortable in many ways.

"It must be hard," I mused, "To give all that up."

"Yes," said Brie, "But don't you see. I have to." I had joined Brie's frame of reference, and now, it seemed to me, she was beginning to join mine.

What a Patient Experiences Is Valid for Him and Can Be Utilized

Yapko (1986) has summed up Ericksonian hypnosis in the statement "Accept and utilize." He believes that all Ericksonian therapy is based on the utilization approach (Erickson & Rossi, 1979). Erickson's use of the term *utilization* refers to the notion that the therapist works with the myriad of verbal and nonverbal self-expressions that the patient presents in therapy.

The therapist has a great deal to utilize because each patient brings much to each therapy session. In addition to his symptoms he brings his background, language, personality, frame of reference, anticipations and goals, wishes, and fears. He also brings his transferences, resistances, and state of health. If he has had too much to drink the night before, he might bring his hangover to a session. Symptoms can be viewed as resources and thus be utilized.

The therapist finds himself in the position of no longer seeing resistances as problems to be erased or corrected, but rather as expressions of the patient's need to limit his self-revelation at the time and in the current situation. The Ericksonian therapist will perceive that resistances can be treated as valuable expressions of the patient and can be utilized. The utilization principle has wide applicability. The emphasis on utilization places the focus on the relationship between the therapist and the patient. This relationship is greatly enhanced in such a way as to promote utilization by interactive trance, which is discussed later in this chapter.

Case Example: Brie (continued)

I (CF) decided it was time to begin to utilize Brie's symptoms in a way that would be meaningful to her. I called her attention to the depression as a signal that she had not been paying attention to who she really was. Her fondness for meeting people and her love of social events were good qualities. Many careers were founded on such wonderful characteristics. Further, the work that she had done for her sorority, like the employment she held at the casino, demonstrated that she had excellent organizational abilities.

Brie's eyes opened wide and her jaw became slack as I told her about jobs that allowed people to use such wonderful abilities with enjoyment.

For example, I told her about a young woman I knew who traveled around the country setting up events for a computer company at trade shows and another who set up conferences at one of the facilities of a major hotel chain and got to meet people from many fascinating organizations and businesses.

After her initial shock, Brie told me that she had never thought she could have fun in a real job. She realized that these kinds of jobs could eventually lead her to the same kind of security her parents had wanted for her. We agreed that she had been a success at being a failure so that she could solve her problem of being a square peg in a round (chemistry and biology) hole. Now the next issue would be for Brie to find the energy and direction to make her own way in the world in a way her parents had not selected for her. "Maybe I could be a flight attendant!" Brie exclaimed. "I love to travel!"

Activation of Internal Resources

Ericksonian therapy can be both subtle and complex because it emphasizes the use of multilevel communications (Erickson & Rossi, 1976) that are capable of activating a variety of resources. Therapeutic communications may be indirect and direct, nonverbal as well as verbal, and they tend to embody the notion that unconscious communication is constantly occurring.

Mutual Trance

As noted earlier, several theoreticians have been interested in how the processes of unconscious communication and unconscious learning contribute to therapy. Gilligan (1987) has observed that Freud (1912/1964, 1923/1964) believed that unconscious communication between the analysand and the analyst was necessary for analysis to take place.

> To put it in a formula: He must turn his own unconscious like a receptive organ toward the transmitting unconscious of the patient. He must adjust himself to the patient as a telephone receiver is adjusted to the transmitting microphone.
>
> (Freud, 1912/1964, p. 115)

Erickson shared this orientation: "the unconscious of one individual is better equipped to understand the unconscious of another than the conscious personality aspect of either" (Erickson & Kubie, 1940, p. 62). Erickson believed that unconscious communication and learning were more effective and reactive in an altered state of consciousness (Erickson, Rossi, & Rossi, 1976).

Gilligan (1987) advocates that the therapist adopt an *externally oriented interpersonal trance*. This allows the therapist's unconscious mind to tune in to the patient's unconscious messages, feelings, and needs. The therapist who becomes involved in this kind of trance activity "is better able to resonate" (Watkins,

1978) empathetically with the patient and to meet the patient's unconscious needs. When the therapist enters his own receptive trance while the patient is also experiencing trance, an interactive, interpersonal state of high resonance is present. In this interactive state the internal resources of the therapist are available to the patient. This open field of resources can be perceived by the patient consciously. Although technique can enhance the therapist's abilities to meet the patient's needs, technique alone is not sufficient. The body of literature on intersubjectivity (Atwood & Stolerow, 1992; Stolorow, Brandchaft, & Atwood, 1983) describes similar phenomena without addressing the specific contributions of the trance state.

From the ego-state perspective, mutual interactive trance can be thought of as a situation in which the ego-state resources of the therapist interact with the ego states of the patient in a discerning and healing way. The therapist's ego states may feel called upon to respond in a variety of ways. For example, at various times, the therapist may feel called upon to be receptive and listen, to be active in therapy by telling a story or making an interpretation, or to introduce transitional phenomena.

It is paradoxical that when therapists are willing to set aside their conscious processes and allow themselves to vibrate with the unspoken rhythms of the patient's unconscious needs, they are frequently able to supply healing experiences, although they may not consciously or specifically intend to do so.

Indirection: Metaphor, Seeding, and Interspersal

Metaphor

Erickson's indirect approach included a variety of methods for communicating messages: storytelling, metaphors, jokes, and other unusual means of communication. The use of metaphor, commonly associated with Erickson, is a way of delivering a message to the patient in a less than direct way (a message that could not be useful were it to be delivered directly). The patient's defenses and the status of his ego strength might not allow the patient to accept the therapist's message or interpretation were it to be given directly. "A metaphor provides a content to convey a therapeutic learning" (Lankton, 1986, p. 261). Metaphors are intended to give the patient new information in a way that will bypass the usual defenses. This information may be designed to help change or structure the patient's attitude, challenge a tightly held belief, to acknowledge new behavior whose import the patient does not as yet apprehend, evoke emotions, assist in the development of greater affect and emotional flexibility, and help create a behavior change (Lankton, 1986).

Although there are abundant recommendations and directions for metaphor construction (Lankton, 1980, 1986; Yapko 1990), the most effective metaphors may well be those that emerge spontaneously when the therapist and patient are in mutual trance. We share Gilligan's view that the power of metaphors lies in the fact that they speak in the more primary process language of the unconscious mind. Thus, metaphors "encourage unconscious processing" (Gilligan, 1987, p. 204).

According to Gilligan metaphors work for an assortment of reasons: "(1) the content of the story does *not* refer to the subject but (2) some major aspects of the story (e.g., the characters, events, themes, goals) are relevant to the subject's experience" (Gilligan, 1987, p. 204). Patients who hear metaphors about others, Gilligan (1987) reminds us, usually refer the story to themselves. If someone were to tell the reader a story about getting an income tax refund, most likely the reader would find himself thinking and feeling what it would be like for him to be getting one, or actually recalling such an incident. Bower and Gilligan (1979) have reported on the usefulness of self-referencing. When subjects attached personal associations to items learned, these items could be remembered much better than those that had been subject to other major learning strategies.

Gilligan (1987) also believed that another reason metaphors are effective is because they bypass potential difficulties the patient may experience in the therapeutic relationship, such as self-consciousness, inhibition, or defensiveness. They do so by attributing the conveyed wisdom to someone or something other than the therapist. With the basic interest in what the patient needs, Gilligan recommends that the therapist pay attention to the images and associations that enter his mind when he shifts into "interpersonal trance" with the patient. From the unconscious mind of the therapist comes the metaphor that can be helpful. Often therapists discover that they are doing this without realizing it. Often the best metaphors are those that are constructed from real or fantasy topics that the patient brings to therapy, although this is not always the case.

Case Example: Brie (continued)

Brie and I (CF) were able to discuss what steps she needed to take to pursue her curiosity about becoming a flight attendant. I asked her if she would be willing to call several airlines before her next session to get information on flight attendant positions. When I next saw Brie, she appeared to be guilty and ashamed because she had not called any airlines. Instead, she had phoned a cousin of a friend of hers who was a flight attendant. The purpose of her call was to find out more about this kind of job. Clearly Brie was seeing me as she must often see her parents. She seemed to feel she had let me down. As she went on, she described some successful behavior on her part. As she did, she appeared to enter spontaneous trance. Her respiration rate changed, she looked more relaxed, and her speech was slower. I also entered a light trance in which I perceived the image of a crab in shallow waters. I told Brie that I was impressed by how many constructive actions she had taken. Then, with her apparent upset about not calling airlines in mind, I told Brie this story: "Where I grew up the waters contain many wonderful blue crabs. It's interesting how the crab grows. When the crab gets a new and larger shell, that shell is very soft. The crab is quite vulnerable. She needs to spend several days in the water and the sun so that the shell can pick up what elements it needs from the water and become stronger and tougher. But that's exactly what happens to the crab. And the next time the crab grows, you know Brie, that might happen all over again."

When Brie returned for her next session, she said, "Do I have a lot to tell you!" She had called three airlines, been to one interview, and had another scheduled. She had taken charge of getting her paperwork for withdrawing from college straightened out and, in a very kind and adult way, had told her mother that she needed her to back off if she, Brie, was going to grow. Her mother told Brie she realized that this was so. Brie displayed an air of healthy pride as she told me about all this, and we were then able to discuss the value of vocational counseling about her long-term plans.

Up to this point formal trance has not been used with Brie. She had assumed a passive position in many areas of her life. There existed a strong possibility that Brie could hide in formal trance as well as in self-hypnosis by assuming passive modes of ego functioning (Fromm & Kahn, 1990) there as well.

Seeding

It has been said that, "*The more resistant the client, the more the need for indirection*" (Tilton, 1986, p. 256). The therapeutic technique of *seeding* is one that is used by many therapists, sometimes unwittingly or unconsciously. It is based on the simple principle of growth in nature: a gigantic tree can spring from one tiny seed. Seeding has been described as "the subtle introduction of ideas in a minor key before they are faced in a major way" (Phillips & Frederick, 1995, p. 97). In seeding the therapist presents an idea to the patient's unconscious mind by making statements that point to the idea. These statements are usually interjected into the session conversationally or casually.

Dolan (1991) has emphasized how important it is for therapists to engage in the "seeding of hope" with their patients from the beginning of therapy. We like to seed hope early in treatment with certain phrases such as:

* "When you are better …"
* "You will be amazed at how your understanding will grow."
* "And as you look back at today, you may find it difficult to realize how bad you felt."

- "Won't it be interesting to see what the 'new you' will be like?"
- "I wonder how your interests will develop once you are no longer using so much energy on this problem."

Dolan uses future orientations to seed hope (see chap. 5) as well as create safety and mastery (see chap. 13) in ways that are both creative and uniquely helpful.

Interspersal

Erickson (1966) reported on the therapeutic effectiveness of the interspersal technique, in which words and phrases that carry therapeutic suggestions are interlaced with the therapist's other verbal productions. Erickson thought that interspersal could be used with a variety of difficulties. In this technique therapeutic suggestions are made in such a way that they are hidden within other, more general suggestions. In Erickson's original paper (1966) he described how he concealed therapeutic suggestions among general hypnotic trance-maintenance suggestions. According to Erickson, these suggestions, both heard and understood by the patient, could not become the subject of disagreement because the trance-maintenance suggestions would come so swiftly on their heels and capture the patient's attention. Indeed, the efficacy of the technique is its ability to communicate suggestions to the patient's unconscious mind. Erickson believed that repetition added to the power of the interspersed suggestions. The best known of Erickson's cases that features interspersal as the critical hypnotic technique is the "tomato plant case." The following case example has been summarized from Erickson (1966).

Case Example: Joe

At the request of a relative Milton Erickson (1966) visited a man, Joe, who was terminally ill with cancer and was experiencing severe pain for which he could receive little relief from narcotics. He had had a tracheotomy and could not communicate with speech; he depended on the paper and pencil he kept with him. Joe had a known antipathy for hypnosis, and his son, a psychiatric resident who was present when Erickson visited his father, did not believe in hypnosis at all. Joe was a florist who had created a wonderful business. He could not understand why his physicians had not been able to control his pain. Joe wondered why Erickson was visiting him, and he asked him this in writing.

Erickson used this open state of Joe's mind to begin an indirect trance induction. He embarked on this venture although he was concerned that the drugs Joe had received were producing toxic side effects and that he might not succeed in helping Joe. Erickson reported that he kept his doubts to himself; he conveyed his genuine interest in Joe as a person both verbally and nonverbally to Joe. He spoke to Joe about how a tomato plant grows. As he spoke, he interspersed many suggestions that Joe could listen to him comfortably, and feel ... good ... comfortable ... peaceful ... restful ... happy, and so forth.

Erickson reported Joe's wife asked him when the hypnosis would begin; at the time of her question, Joe had already entered a somnambulistic trance. This had occurred as a result of the indirect hypnosis that had been generated in the story of the growing tomato plant. Erickson felt that Joe had wanted to discover something valuable in their encounter. He thought that the tomato plant story presented it to Joe in such a way that he "could literally receive it without realizing it" (Erickson, 1966/1989, p. 272). Erickson revisited Joe after Joe's lunch. He had several more sessions with Joe that afternoon. As he departed that afternoon, Joe appeared to be comfortable and shook his hand.

A month later Erickson was called to visit Joe at his home. In the interval Joe had been the subject of ineffective and heavyhanded "hypnosis" conducted by various members of the hospital house staff, and he had angrily left the hospital. His month at home had brought both comfort and weight gain to Joe. Episodes of severe discomfort were easily controlled with a standard dose of Demerol. During his home visit with Joe Erickson resumed his conversation about the tomato plant, had lunch with Joe, and visited some of Joe's very interesting plants. In his continuing monologue Erickson again interspersed many suggestions about "continued ease, comfort, freedom from pain, enjoyment of family, good appetite, and a continuing pleased interest in all surroundings" (Erickson, 1966/1989, p. 274).

Joe even made a long-distance call to Erickson to exhale a difficult "hello" through his tracheotomy tube just before Erickson left for a lecture trip. Within a month Joe died "quietly." The use of the interspersal technique had been successful in that Joe had lived longer than expected, was comfortable and free from uncontrollable pain, and had lived his remaining days with pleasure.

Multilevel communication, repetition, and unconscious communication are the principles that lie at the heart of the interspersal technique. In describing *multilevel communication* Erickson and Rossi (1976) pointed to Jenkins' (1974) contextual theory of verbal associations. Such therapeutic material as metaphors and stories present the recipient with a general context that exists on the surface—the conscious level. The exact words that are used have other contexts that are made clear by their "individual and literal associations" (Erickson, Rossi, & Rossi, 1976, p. 225). They do not completely fit with the surface, conscious contexts of the story or metaphor. These highly individual and literal associations are suppressed by the unconscious mind as it strives to focus on the general, surface context. The more literal and specific material now unavailable to consciousness does remain in the unconscious mind, where it may engender new associations. Both literalness and dissociation are trance phenomena that facilitate the influence of these unconscious and suppressed suggestions upon the unconscious mind. The story of the blue crab in the case of Brie has interspersed suggestions that have been emphasized by underlining. Although the story is about a crab and its vulnerability, the interspersed suggestions are about growth, newness, wonder, and the expectation of more of this to come within the life cycle.

Erickson felt the interspersal was best received by patients who knew and wanted what they needed and were ready to get it from therapy. Such patients are geared to respond to the first opportunity that presents itself. Erickson believed that such patients desired therapeutic assistance both consciously and unconsciously. The unconscious mind of the patient hears these suggestions well because "it is listening and understanding much better than is possible for his conscious mind" (Erickson, 1966/1989, p. 277). For this reason the patient could have a conscious appreciation of what is occurring, but it is really not relevant (Erickson, 1966).

Tilton (1986) has observed that interspersal is most effective when aimed at secondary symptoms that arise from interpersonal conflict, or external stresses, or are connected with secondary gain. They do not work well when structural intrapsychic changes are needed. We utilize interspersal for ego-strengthening in many ways. We employ metaphor with interspersed suggestions, and we also embed and intersperse suggestions within ordinary therapeutic conversations. *Embedding* can be defined as marking (Yapko, 1986, 1990) of indirect suggestions with some external, physical change over and above the literal verbal production. This can be done with tone of voice, posture, breathing and pausing, and so forth. In practice, interspersed suggestions are often embedded as well.

Case Example: Dolores

Dolores said that she had come to therapy because she was anticipating a trip to Borneo with her husband in a scholarly group and wanted to be at her best for it. She was 75 years old, and she had had a number of depressive episodes over her lifetime. She thought that perhaps some antidepressant medication might be in order. She had taken Elavil (amitriptyline) in the past. Although it had helped her, the side effects had been unfortunate. Further questioning revealed that she had never had any genuine psychotherapy; she had simply seen biologically oriented psychiatrists who had medicated her. She had lived a sheltered life before her marriage, and her second husband, Anton, had taken care of her during the many years of their marriage and her intermittent depressions.

Dolores was quite worried about her youngest son, Clarence. He had been in prison, had a history of drug and alcohol abuse, and had fathered two children out of wedlock. Dolores' nonjudgmental approach to him angered the rest of the family. At the time of her initial session Dolores was already describing symptoms of depression and displayed marked problems with her memory. I (CF) wondered whether some organic brain problem might also be present.

As I sat with Dolores in her first session, I felt nearly overwhelmed by her helpless presentation of her self. This I interpreted as a countertransference reaction that was able to inform me of how the patient must feel: Helpless to take care of herself, dependent on her husband, incapable of helping her troubled son, misunderstood by her family, and now, further compromised by her unreliable memory.

I thought it would be helpful if Dolores were to take an antidepressant agent of a newer type that would not carry the side effects of Elavil (amitriptyline). I also knew that I could only do this if the patient agreed to psychotherapy as well, because I see no patients for medication only. I began to explain to Dolores the treatment plan: "Now, Dolores, you certainly allowed yourself to make a wise choice when you decided to seek therapy. I think it is really good for you just to be able to sit here and talk. Of course there are medications that you can take that will be able to help with the depressive symptoms. The one I have in mind should not produce side effects. You do need to know, however, that it is always better when you can take it with therapy. To make doubly sure that you will be comfortable with it, we will start slowly. As a safeguard for you, you need to know that I have open telephone hours every morning in my home before 9. So if you have side effects, you can call me, and we can take care of it. I know that you have been very worried about Clarence, any good parent would be concerned. It's so important now for you to have a chance to share those difficulties by talking about them, especially when many people in your family don't understand how good your judgment can be."

Dolores was nodding her head up and down as we talked, her facial expression changing from one of worry and depression to one of smiles and relief. She had never been able to talk to a psychiatrist about her feelings before. Yes, she wanted to come in on a regular basis. And, oh yes, she wanted to try the medicine.

A week later, Dolores beamed at me. Although her antidepressant medication dosage was quite low, she was feeling much, much better. She displayed no difficulties with her memory whatsoever, and she wanted to talk about Clarence some more.

Dolores had responded well to a number of suggestions that were interspersed into a discussion of antidepressant medications. They focused on her being able to make wise choices, her wisdom in trying to find solutions to problems, and the knowledge, somewhere within her, that the talking would take care of things. Her therapy's taking care of her distress was in juxtaposition to Anton's taking care of her (i.e., keeping her dependent). Dolores found her first therapy session both validating and ego-strengthening. Although she had come about medication, she greatly preferred the expanded menu.

The interactions between Dolores and the therapist were not the outcome of the therapist deliberately planning to program Dolores with interspersed suggestions, nor did they occur within any formal trance. They occurred in an ordinary therapy intake session, and they were the spontaneous productions of a therapist who was resonating with the patient and presenting to the patient a reasonable treatment plan. Such material illustrates the fact that indirect hypnotic communication tends to occur when psychodynamic psychotherapy is practiced.

The "Corrective Emotional Experience"

The concept of the *corrective emotional experience* is one that appears periodically in psychodynamic literature (Stone, 1997). For those who seek it for their patients it is of the greatest importance. Corrective emotional experiences frequently occur in psychotherapy. Usually they are building processes that "correct" for a number of reasons. They may help the patient develop more adequate psychic structure or they may help him release energy that had been bound up in suppressing strong affect such as rage. The corrective experience may come out of identifications with the therapist; it may result from abreaction (Watkins & Watkins, 1997) or it may come from some symbolic interaction with the therapist or other reasons (see chaps. 8 and 14).

The subject fascinated Erickson (1965b). He believed that corrective emotional experiences occurred in therapy in which hypnosis was not used. However, he believed that corrective emotional experiences occurred more frequently with hypnosis. Erickson held that the corrective emotional experience was the result of a complex restructuring of the individual's subjective orientation toward, or understanding of, his own subjective experience. In short, a new identity was facilitated (Rossi, 1989). His generally atheoretical stance led him to avoid elaborate psychodynamic explanations for what may have taken place.

One of Erickson's most famous pieces of corrective work occurred in his work with what has come to be known as *The February Man case* (Erickson & Rossi, 1989). The case of the February Man was so complex that Erickson wrote a number of manuscripts about it that he never completed. Together with Rossi (Erickson & Rossi, 1979), he synthesized several of them. The question that this case report attempts to answer is one that challenges the utilization process:

What happens, however, when the patient has been severely deprived in some life experience? Can the therapist supply them vicariously in some way?

Sensitive therapists have long recognized their role as surrogate parents who do, in fact, help their patients experience life patterns and relationships that have been missed.

(Erickson & Rossi, 1989, p. 525)

Erickson was not the first to use hypnosis to create and insert new memories hypnotically in order to strengthen the ego of a patient. As Hammond (1990d) reminds us, Janet used a technique that was similar to Erickson's with his patient, Marie (Ellenberger, 1970). However, the hypnotic procedures used by Erickson were painstaking, detailed, and complex. A very simplified version of the material from the case report is briefly summarized next. The detailed and complex case report is worth a careful reading by anyone who has a technical interest in exactly how Erickson accomplished his goal.

Case Example: The February Man

Milton Erickson was asked for help by a woman who was married to a physician on his hospital's house staff. She was pregnant for the first time, and she was concerned that she might not know how to be an adequate mother to her child, because she herself had had such an unhappy childhood. She had been unwanted. Her mother repeated to her many times that her pregnancy with the patient had worked devastation on her figure, and her mother had had little time for her. The patient spent much of her early years alone in her nursery. Later she was sent away to various private schools and special camps. She seldom saw her mother, who led a very active social life and traveled quite a bit. She had a warm relationship with her father, and he made time in his busy schedule to have outings with her.

Eventually the patient rebelled against her mother's social plans for her and married a physician still in training. Now that her baby was on the way, she wondered if hypnosis could be an instrument that would help her in some way to relieve her anxieties from the past and make up for its deficiencies.

In her next session, described by Erickson as cathartic, she was quite distraught. She let Erickson know that memories and feelings concerning her childhood experiences were causing her to develop symptoms, and she wondered if he could really help her. He told her that he would have worked out a plan by the next time they met.

In the following session the patient was informed that there was now a plan for her and that it would involve hypnosis. She would not consciously have to know about it. Then Erickson spent 5 hours with the patient to train her in hypnosis. Erickson took the patient through a series of hypnotic age regressions. He began with having her recall their previous session. He gave her "many positive supportive suggestions" (Erickson & Rossi, 1979/1989, p. 529). In subsequent sessions, he continued to age regress her farther and farther back in time, and he offered her "rapport protection," a cue that would allow her to feel comfortable with Erickson no matter what kind of material they encountered. Her repertoire of regressions expanded, and they would be able to serve as a matrix or background into which new, positive material could be interpolated.

Eventually the patient was regressed to the age of 4. Then Erickson introduced himself to her as a friend of her father's. She was then allowed to have a period of hypnotic sleep. This was followed by another visit from her father's friend, and so forth. Erickson gave the patient a series of hypnotic experiences in which he interpolated himself into her life periodically as a friend of her father's who visited her every February. During each visit he built on the previous visits, constructing for them a history of their relationship that had never existed in the real world. The patient began to experience Erickson as a regular, reliable, supportive visitor "and a trusted confidant to whom she could tell all her secrets, woes, and joys, and with whom she could share her hopes, fears, doubts, wishes, and plans" (Erickson & Rossi, 1979/1989, p. 536).

As the process continued, the patient was able to do a considerable amount of uncovering work in trance and obtain many insights. The February Man had become a significant parenting figure to her, and she was able to leave her bitter experiences with her mother behind her. Erickson produced amnesia in the patient for the hypnotic work.

The patient terminated with Erickson after he gave her training in obstetrical anaesthesia. Subsequently she had her baby naturally and without pain. Two years later she visited him for a brief "refresher" course. She was once more pregnant.

In chapters 8 and 9 another useful approach to renurturing that was developed with psychotic and borderline patients will be presented.

Erickson has become an icon over the years, and a great deal of emphasis has been placed on his indirect techniques. Hammond (1984) lists certain myths about Erickson that bear little relationship to how he really worked. Although many characterize his work as swift and indirect, he frequently used deep trance with his patients and often spent many hours working out their treatment plans in great detail. He was experienced by his patients as genuine and extremely interested in them, and he usually took the time to work with his failures. He often spent hours with his patients, trying new approaches when the old ones had failed. "He did not give up" (Hammond, 1986, p. 235). He has left his impression on all of contemporary hypnosis.

There are those who believe that Ericksonian techniques are overrated. As mentioned in chapter 2, the superiority of indirect suggestion has been shown to be a myth (Hammond, 1990c). More recently, the evidence weighing against other purported mechanisms for the success of Ericksonian techniques has been reviewed (Matthews, 1998). We believe that Erickson's success with his patients was a function of his ability to discern their uniqueness and to use it as a pathway to form successful therapeutic alliances, build expectations, and tap the patient's resources. A question that can be asked legitimately is whether such highly personalized therapeutic interventions are susceptible to the usual research tools. We do not believe that most standardized research approaches could possibly measure the efficacy of this kind of highly personalized approach.

The personhood of the therapist is an important key to the degree he may be able to succeed in his endeavors. Diamond (1984) entertained the question of "Why certain hypnotists can produce deeper and more meaningful trance experiences with their subjects than can other hypnotists who may employ the very same operational procedures" (p. 3). He concluded that the hypnotherapy occurs within the context of an interactional hypnotherapeutic relationship, and that the skill of the therapist is a critical factor. He believes this skill to arise from several factors:

- The therapist must have attained a mature level of object relations development and relating and must be comfortable with deep levels of human interaction.
- He must have a capacity for empathy.
- He must have both personal and therapeutic trance skills.
- He must have healthy levels of integration of his own functions such as the receptive and passive as well as the active and cognitive.
- He must have adequate self-supervisory ability, that is, he must be able to identify and deal on some effective level with transference and countertransference issues.

According to Diamond (1984), such a hypnotherapist creates a special holding environment for the patient. Erickson undoubtedly fulfilled all these criteria and more, hence his special successfulness.

Matthews (1998) believes that Erickson's enlistment of the patient as an active participant allowed the patient to "construct a more useful life narrative" (p. 13). He has emphasized Erickson's ability to motivate patients and create belief and expectation (Matthews, 1998). We believe that Erickson's work is a sort of monument—not to techniques, but to the significance and power of the therapeutic alliance. His great contributions to therapy have as their centerpiece his emphases on the uniqueness of the individual. His interventions occurred within intersubjective relationships that could not possibly be duplicated by other therapists in any precise manner.

Matthews (1998) noted that Erickson appeared to be intuitive. Perhaps his intuitive grasp of what was needed in specific situations could never be susceptible to cognitive analysis, even his own. From what we agree appears to have been Erickson's formidable intuition came for him incredible respect for the roles of unconscious sensing, unconscious communication, and unconscious learning. His abiding respect for the resources, wisdom, and healing powers of the unconscious mind and his profound esteem for the vital role of the therapist's conscious–unconscious complementarity in the treatment process spoke to his knowledge that intuitive, feeling, and sensing functions (Jung, 1990) can inform the intuitive, feeling, or sensate therapist. His connections with Jung in these regards as well as others cannot go unnoticed. Erickson's popularity in hypnotic and nonhypnotic circles continues to grow. Perhaps he was an embodiment of archetypal healer: patient, caring, nurturing, involved, capable of looking into one's soul, and extremely powerful.

The next chapter explores several energy models of the human personality and introduces the reader to Ego State Therapy (Watkins & Watkins, 1997)—a form of therapy that offers an incredible number of opportunities for ego-strengthening and the possibilities of many new ways to accomplish that.

Chapter 4

The Ego-State Model in Hypnotic and Nonhypnotic Psychotherapy

The complexity of the universe and its components, the nature of being itself, and of the human mind have been persistent themes in Western culture. Many of the pre-Socratic Greek philosophers were preoccupied with concepts of unity and diversity, or as they often termed this *The one and the many*. In the Judeo-Christian Tradition the God of the Old Testament manifested himself in many different aspects (the God of Abraham, the God of Jacob, etc.), whereas the God of the New Testament was thought to be tripartite. It has been suggested that Judeo-Christian God is multiple by nature (Miles, 1995).

The intricacy of the self has been a factor in most attempts to understand human behavior. This has been particularly true when the behavior has been aberrant or disturbed. Unitary concepts of the human mind are unworkable. Although Freud's model of the id, the ego, and the superego added some degree of diversity and the notion of a dynamic mind, the question remained whether these particular energy concepts adequately reflected the mental state of affairs. Since the topic of ego-strengthening is intricately enmeshed with how we conceptualize the ego (see chap. 6), we now explore a model that emphasizes the complexity of the ego in terms of internal parts or subselves (the Ego State Therapy model). Although it was created as a direct hypnoanalytic therapeutic approach, there are many useful nonhypnotic applications of Ego State Therapy.

The "view of personality as unitary leads to all manner of unnecessary despair" (Schwartz, 1995, p. 11). Poor self-esteem or negative views of the self can be associated with certain thoughts, feelings, and behaviors that are only part of what the individual thinks, feels, or does. For example, an exemplary student who is appropriate in all of his behavior with his fellow human beings, is devoted to the practices of his religion, and donates a great deal of time to community projects may have a poor concept of himself that is connected with his spending a great deal of time with "twisted" pornographic material on the Internet. When he enters a state of mind that reviews some of these experiences, he may find himself thinking and feeling that *all* he is, is "some kind of pervert." When the mind is viewed as inherently multiple, a more balanced view of the self appears, and a greater hope for the possibility of resolving problems can emerge.

DOI:10.4324/9781003442585-4

Over the millennia different kinds of parts models have been proposed. Primitive healing offers several schema that implicate parts for dealing with pathology. They often focus either on losses of parts of the self or upon an intrusion into the self of unwanted parts (Ellenberger, 1970). In the former case it is thought that the soul—an essential part of the self—has fled or been stolen from the self. The cure occurs when the soul is retrieved. When parts have been thought of as alien, such as a disease object or as foreign spirits that have intruded into the individual, the cure is effected when they are expelled (Clements, 1932). Thus, physical illnesses within primitive frameworks often are thought of as manifestations of disease objects, physical in nature or of a spirit constitution, such as a devil who could produce a demonic possession. Exorcism to cast out undesired elements of the self that are viewed as alien and nonhuman has been a persistent treatment for emotional ailments over the millennia, and, unfortunately, continues to be recommended by certain therapists today (Friesen, 1991).

Although the primitives may have viewed their parts models in a concrete fashion, this is far from how the behavioral scientist of today would regard any theory. The elements of theories are not things. Just as we cannot justify the reification of the id into a monster, the superego into a contemporary version of Jiminy Cricket, or the ego into a model adult, neither can we justify turning ego states into little people. The ego-state model is an energy model (Frederick, 1994a; Phillips & Frederick, 1995; Watkins & Watkins, 1991, 1997). When we speak of ego states in anthropomorphic or other personified ways ("the Little One," "the Hedgehog," "Annie"), it is simply because we are dealing with the limits of joining our language with our clinical experience in a way that will allow us to communicate.

The belief that the human personality is composed of parts or subselves has been held by many eminent practitioners and theoreticians. Clinicians such as Janet (1919/1976), William James (1890/1983), Morton Prince (1905/1978), Franz Alexander (1950), and Milton Erickson (1948/1980) thought the mind was composed of multiple parts. Jung (1969) had a version of this orientation; he divided the parts into the complexes and the archetypes. Assagioli's (1965) psychosynthesis embraces the concept as does transactional analysis (Berne, 1961).

There is also research evidence along several lines that suggests that the mind is not unitary, but rather, multiple in its composition. Hilgard (1977, 1984) conducted a series of experiments with hypnosis that revealed the presence of a hidden observer, and Watkins and Watkins (1979–1980) found similar evidence. Gazzaniga (1989, 1995) has focused attention on neurobiological studies of the brain that suggest a substrate for such mental organization. Ornstein's (1987) interpretations of neurobiological evidence have led him to believe that we all have *multiminds*. We refer the reader to *Internal Family Systems Therapy* (Schwartz, 1995) and *The Mosaic Mind: Empowering the Tormented Selves of Child Abuse Survivors* (Goulding & Schwartz, 1995) for comprehensive views of the extent to which science, literature, and art have wholeheartedly embraced the concepts of the normal multiplicity of the mind.

Personification and Parts Models

When the theory and practice of models that work with parts or aspects of human personality are discussed, it is inevitable that personification enters the picture. Therapists begin to speak about parts as if they were indeed little people, although they may well believe that they are personality energies. Hillman (1976) has traced the historical introduction of the personification of personality energies by both Freud and Jung as a result of their contact with clinical material "in the consulting room and the insane asylum" (p. 17). Jung was comfortable with the language of myth and freely utilized personification as the best way to present his formulations and terminology. He believed that the unconscious mind spontaneously personified and that this was an inevitable human trait.

Hillman (1976) has noted that Freud constantly struggled between conceptual modes and mythic modes of expressing his ideas. Many of his terms, such as *eros, thanatos*, and *Oedipus complex*, are derived from mythology. "Others of his terms—projection, sublimation, condensation—once belonged to the poetics of alchemy" (Hillman, 1976, p. 19). The tension between our scientific formulations and our need to describe their clinical interactions in personified ways is part and parcel of all work with various parts models of personality. It can also be commonly observed in other kinds of formulations such as the psychodynamic, objects relations, self psychology, and cognitive-behavioral models.

According to Hillman (1976) personification in the depth psychologies is not a path of regression to old demonologies. It is simply an expression of a fundamental human way of formulation. He insists "that *psychology so needs mythology that it creates one as it proceeds*" (p. 20). As we proceed to a discussion of Ego State Therapy, the kind of tension Freud experienced between the conceptual and the mythic becomes evident.

Federn's Energy Theory of Ego States

One of the most balanced traditional psychodynamic approaches to the understanding of the mind as multiple was that of Paul Federn (1952). Federn was a colleague of Freud who always thought of himself as Freud's student (Weiss, 1966). He professed great admiration and loyalty to Freud, and it is probable that he may not have realized how far his ego-state psychology actually diverged from Freud's positions (Watkins, 1992).

Federn (1952) proposed a theory of ego states. These ego states were formed in early childhood, according to Federn, and they existed together in a dynamic balance. Psychic energy could be cathected (harnessed) to objects, or to the ego itself. Federn maintained that each of these ego states had its own unique combination of history, thoughts, perceptions, affects, and bodily involvement and that they existed together in a dynamic balance. Federn's theory was further elaborated by Weiss (1960), who published some of Federn's papers in English and wrote the introduction to his book, *Ego Psychology and the Psychoses* (Federn, 1952).

Freud had propounded that there was a life energy, the libido, that propelled psychic activity. Later in his career he expanded this theory to include a second kind of energy, *thanatos*, the death instinct. This energy was postulated by Freud as the explanation for the presence of aggression in the human organism. One goal of Freudian therapy was to neutralize this aggressive drive with *eros*, the positive, libidinous, life-preserving energy within the personality.

Federn's energy theory, also a two-drive theory, was unlike Freud's. Indeed, Federn eventually dispensed with the term *libido* and substituted the word *cathexis*, which means energizing or harnessing energy. Federn believed that psychic energy could be cathected (harnessed) to the ego (ego cathexis) or to the object (object cathexis) and that these two cathexes were quite different. Ego cathexis can be thought of as being synonymous with the self (Watkins, 1992); anything that is experienced by the individual as belonging to her is "by definition, invested with ego cathexis. Ego cathexis has one basic quality, the feeling of selfness" (Watkins, 1992, p. 194). When an object (the other) is invested with object cathexis, it is experienced as outside of the self. Both ego cathexis and object cathexis are held together in a dynamic interplay to accommodate the formation of the defenses and the experience of the self and the other. Federn defined *ego states* as having ego cathexis only.

Ego State Therapy

There are many psychotherapeutic elaborations of parts or multimind theories. Psychosynthesis (Assagioli, 1965) and Transactional Analysis (Berne, 1961) are among the better known. Ego State Therapy was created by John and Helen Watkins (H. H. Watkins, 1993; J. G. Watkins, 1992; Watkins & Watkins, 1990) as a hypnoanalytic form of treatment based on the integration of individual, group, and family therapy techniques with theory that is a creative outgrowth of the work of Federn and Weiss. Much of the hypnotherapy done with Dissociative Identity Disorder (DID) patients is wittingly or unwittingly related to Ego State Therapy. A knowledge of the underlying principles of Ego State Therapy makes it a practical form of ego-strengthening and uncovering psychotherapy. Although Ego State Therapy was created as a hypnotic form of therapy, many Ego State Therapy interventions can be made when the patient is not in trance.

The Nature of Ego States

In the ordinary course of events most of us show some degree of variation in our personalities. At times they can appear to be quite dramatic, but remain well within the normal range. For example, Dr. Jenkins is a renowned psychoanalytic theoretician. When she lectures, she wears well styled business suits or attire of a similar fashion. Her hair is contained in a carefully coifed French roll, and she usually adorns her blouse or sweater with a single strand of pearls. Her vocabulary is sophisticated and superb, and her bearing is dignified. It would come as quite a shock to her students to behold her behavior at most faculty parties. There she literally lets down her abundant hair, wears gypsy earrings and short skirts, and is known for her outrageous jokes and pranks as well as her frank and earthy speech. When the party is over for Dr. Jenkins it is over, just as the class is over when it is over. Both her lecture persona and her party persona are aspects of a self who is quite aware of them and actually has quite a bit of choice about her behavior. When she sings the classics with her choral group, as she sometimes does, another persona—the soprano who exults in this type of activity—becomes visible. Were Dr. Jenkins to sing arias in her classrooms, lecture at parties, or party in the middle of a choral performance, we would be concerned about her. As it is, we can know simply that she is a complex person with several well-functioning ego states.

According to Federn (1952) each ego state is particular and unique. It has its own history, thoughts, feelings, and behaviors. The particularity of ego states makes it impossible for them to be reduced to general categories such as the *inner child*, or *parent, adult, child* (Berne, 1961). Ego states are not Jungian archetypes either. They are components of an internal grouping of energies that exist in dynamic interplay.

A simple way of viewing the distribution of energy among ego states involves the concept of the *executive ego state*. The ego state that, at any given time, contains the most energy in the internal system is said to be *executive*. Anytime an ego state is executive, it experiences itself as an *I*, and experiences the other ego state as *its*, or *things*. The party ego state and the soprano ego states of Dr. Jenkins are aware of the lecturer ego state while Dr. Jenkins is lecturing, but they have relatively little energy. Most of the energy has gone to the lecturer aspect of personality, which is, at that time, executive. When it is time to sing, the soprano ego state gathers the preponderance of the personality energy, and becomes executive.

The Formation of Ego States

All ego states are adaptational. Any understanding of ego-state theory must be based on the concept that every ego state has come to help. According to Federn (1952) ego states are formed in early childhood. However, the subsequent clinical experience of many clinicians who work with ego states indicates that ego states may be formed at any time of life, although their formation is much more common in childhood.

Ego states are formed in three ways:

- *Ego states are created to meet the needs of the culture.* The various tasks that need to be accomplished within each cultural milieu are managed by various ego states. For example, a child prodigy violinist will probably have one ego state for playing a Bach violin concerto and a completely different ego state for watching Saturday morning cartoons. A child in a primitive fishing culture might need ego states of a kind that were quite different from those of the child prodigy. Such activities as social skills, creative activities, and recreational activities are negotiated by individual ego states. The reason we are seldom aware that there is a shifting of ego-state energies as we move from task to task lies in the nature of integration of ego states, which is discussed later in this chapter.
- *Ego states may be introjects of parents or other significant adults or of significant events.* In their constant roles of helping the greater personality, ego states may come into existence as childlike imitations of significant adults in a child's life. This is their way of assisting with the process of identification. At times, although less commonly, it is events, rather than people, that cannot be completely digested into the personality and are held internally as ego states that may then exercise great influence over the greater personality.
- *Ego states are created to deal with overwhelming trauma.* The Watkins (H. H. Watkins, 1993; J. G. Watkins, 1992; Watkins & Watkins, 1990) have theorized that many ego states come into existence to help children deal with overwhelming trauma. They believe that there is a limited number of responses any child can make to trauma that is overpowering. One is that the child could retreat from reality by becoming psychotic. Another, equally hopeless response is that the child could actually commit suicide. The third possibility for the child is to form a creative expression of self, an ego state, that could contain the trauma or deal with it in some other way for the greater personality.

The Ego State Spectrum

Ego states can be thought of as being separated from one another by something like a semipermeable membrane. The ideal separating membrane is thick enough to provide separation, and thin enough to allow communication. Not everyone is as complex as Dr. Jenkins. There are many people who seem to have thin barriers among their ego states and who display a sameness no matter what they are doing.

There may be some degree of variation as to separateness and accessibility to communication among normal ego states. However, as they begin to wall off from one another, pathology appears. At the far left end of the spectrum is extreme walling off or separation of ego states. When ego states become so walled off from other ego states that they come out on their own and assume control of the personality, a condition known as Dissociative Identity Disorder (DID), formerly known as Multiple Personality Disorder (MPD), is said to exist. Most ego states require hypnotic activation for their full manifestation. In Dissociative Identity Disorder (DID) the ego states do not require hypnotic activation. The ego states in Dissociative Identity Disorder (DID) patients are given a special name, *alters*.

More to the center of the ego-state spectrum are ego states that are associated with conditions not usually thought of as dissociative, such as eating disorders (Frederick, 1994g; Torem, 1987a), depression (Frederick, 1993b; Newey, 1986), obsessive-compulsive disorder (Frederick, 1990, 1996c), posttraumatic stress disorder (Phillips, 1993a, 1993b), and panic disorder (Frederick, 1993c).

Thus, ego states, depending on their level of connection with other ego states, may give color and variation to the personality, may be associated with psychopathology within the range usually thought of as neurotic, or may be associated with the kind of gross personality disorganization that Dissociative Identity Disorder (DID) can produce.

The Goals of Ego State Therapy

When pathology is present, it is a sign that ego states are not in harmony. Often something like a civil war is going on as separated or walled off ego states carry out their own agendas without concern for the needs of the other ego states or of the greater personality. The endgoal of Ego State Therapy is integration. In Ego State Therapy *integration* is defined as a condition in which ego states are in full communication with one another, share mental content, and exist in harmonious and cooperative relationships with one another (Phillips & Frederick, 1995; H. H. Watkins, 1993; J. G. Watkins, 1992). They relate to one another like members of a healthy and functional family.

In Ego State Therapy ego states are activated and worked with individually and as an internal family. Any technique that can be used with an individual patient can be used with an individual ego state. This means that ego-strengthening is an important element in Ego State Therapy.

The Activation of Ego States

It should be assumed that all ego states are aware of what is going on in therapy; although they are not executive, they are all listening in. All ego states must be considered as potential candidates for the therapeutic alliance. It is well to assume that, although there may be some exceptions, any time the therapist speaks with an ego state, all the other states are listening to everything that is said. There are many ways to activate ego states, but there is no therapeutic way to activate a state in isolation from its internal family of selves because the internal energy relationships persist.

It is important to pay careful attention to ego-state transferences during the activation process (Watkins & Watkins, 1990). Many ego states initially fear the therapist whom they may see as another potential abuser or betrayer or as someone who wants to eliminate certain personality parts. Childlike ego states cannot be blamed for fearing that the therapist will favor certain parts and consider others expendable; this misconceived version of working with personality parts can be commonly found in literature, cinema, and TV. Ego states can be activated in a number of ways.

The Talking Through Method.   Although Ego State Therapy was created as a hypnotic form of psychotherapy, activation of ego states can be done in nonhypnotic psychotherapy as well. In the talking through method, the therapist speaks to the ego state through the greater personality. Although this can also be done in formal trance, it is commonly done directly and indirectly when the patient is not in trance. The nonhypnotic activation of ego states in therapy sessions does not mean that the patient has Dissociative Identity Disorder. The heightened focus of attention to certain aspects of self appears to be sufficient for the ego state to acquire enough energy to become executive. In a reasonably integrated neurotic the ego state will not take over the personality, but rather will share the executive position with the observing patient. The patient is then aware of the images, thoughts, and feelings (perhaps memories and body sensations as well) that are manifestations of the ego state. This is a situation much like that of the ego split and the development of an observing ego described by Greenson (1967) as occurring in the psychoanalytic situation. Talking through is a great opportunity for letting ego states know that the therapist wishes them no harm and, more importantly, that she is there to understand and to help. We recommend talking through as a thoroughly ego-strengthening way of beginning Ego State Therapy. It often resolves fears and clarifies misapprehensions early in the game, thus clearing the way for the development of therapeutic alliances.

Case Example: Farley

Farley came into treatment for bulimia nervosa. A 26-year-old college student from the midwest, he had had to drop out of school and return to his parental home because his physical condition had become so compromised. At 6'3" Farley weighed only 131 pounds when he was first seen. He had initially gone to college on a football scholarship. Farley reported an interesting sequence of events. He had been obese as a child, and the other children had teased him. He took off the excess weight when he was 11 and decided to attend a boarding school in Arizona. There he rode horses and began to become involved in other athletic pursuits. It was discovered that he had an incredible ability in football. He was a high school football star, and he was offered a football scholarship to a prestigious Ivy League college. There, Farley's football scholarship became somewhat disappointing to him. As part of his effort to be the perfect, lean and mean player, he became obsessed with low-fat dieting. This required much effort on his part because he had a great interest in good food, loved to roam grocery stores, and had a mother who loved to cook and bake for and feed her family. Farley also became obsessed with weight training and aerobic exercise. Somehow Farley did not fulfill his promise as a football player. With the passage of time he played less and less, and he began to experience difficulty in eating.

When I (CF) first saw Farley, he had developed an eating pattern of prolonged and voluminous food intake that was periodically interrupted by involuntary regurgitation of food caused, he told me, by a stomach spasm. He had ended up in therapy after three outstanding medical centers had worked him up in an effort to discover some organic causation of his difficulties. It was noted that he had some hormonal deficiencies. The last medical center had diagnosed bulimia nervosa and recommended hospitalization for Farley as they were concerned that his condition could worsen quickly and result in his death.

Farley's internist and I agreed that he would examine Farley medically on a weekly basis while I saw him twice weekly as an outpatient. Hospitalization then could occur within context if his medical situation became more unfavorable or if he did not show signs of adequate motivation or response to therapy.

The eating pattern Farley described to me sounded dissociative and ego-state driven. He would be compelled to eat, would enter a somewhat dreamy state, and (in spite of negative stomach X-rays and other medical studies) would begin to automatically regurgitate. So predictable and out of his control was the regurgitation, that Farley ate in the kitchen where he had immediate access to the garbage disposal. He had a sense of not-me about his eating. However, Farley was not initially psychologically minded. He perceived the rest of his life as normal in the face of evidence of social withdrawal and gross maternal overprotection. He used a great deal of denial and rationalization about these and other symptoms: "I'm just shy like my Father," "My mother just cares about her children, and she'll do anything to help them," and "I really like it when my mother UPS'ed her casseroles to me at school because she's such a good cook."

I met with Farley and his parents, explained his treatment, and referred Farley's parents to another therapist who could work with certain family aspects of the problem such as Farley's mother sending him freshly cooked food by overnight UPS when he was in school. I worked with Farley to develop a therapeutic alliance and stabilize his situation. I also placed

Farley on an antidepressant agent although he claimed he was not depressed. Eventually I introduced hypnosis and formal direct ego-strengthening procedures. I made tapes for him, and he used them at home. His motivation for recovery appeared to be excellent. Within 3 weeks Farley began, to his complete surprise, to gain weight and experience hope. Early in Farley's treatment I had begun to talk through to the ego states:

"You know, Farley, it sounds to me ... I could be wrong, but it does sound as if perhaps your eating problem does not belong to all of you ... it's an interesting situation, and we really aren't able to understand it all yet.. but somehow I have the feeling that a part of your personality may be causing the eating problem in order to try to help you in some way ... You know, the regurgitation is so automatic ... and it will be so interesting to be able to understand just how that part is trying to help you." (Farley's response was to stare at me with a puzzled look).

"You see, Farley, each one of us has a personality that is made up of many parts. It's one of the things that makes us interesting. For example, there's probably a special part of me that energizes me when I am in the kitchen cooking and creating recipes. And there's probably another part of my personality that puts the information I need right at my fingertips when I am lecturing ... just as I bet there's a special part of you that takes over when you are playing football (Farley smiled and gave a look of recognition) ... and another part of you that has a ball when you are cruising a grocery store (Farley nodded vigorously). "Everyone of us has an entire family of parts inside, and the wonderful thing is that every part has come to help us in some way or another."

Farley indicated that he failed to see how an eating disorder could be helpful to him.

"I know that it may be difficult for us to understand now, but part of our work might be trying to understand just how a part or some parts of you could be trying to help you with these symptoms that are causing you so much discomfort."

The therapist's approach to Farley's ego state was an indirect talking through (Phillips & Frederick, 1995). If she had chosen to do so, she could have talked directly through Farley to the ego state by saying something like: "And I think that you are there listening to us right now, part, and I wonder if you are curious about how we could share our helping and problem solving energies to help Farley in a way that wasn't harmful to him." There are other ways of talking through to ego states that employ metaphor and storytelling, embedding, and seeding (see chap. 3). In the dialogue noted earlier the following idea was being seeded: that the therapist perceived the ego state producing the symptom as fundamentally benevolent and that she sought an alliance of understanding with it. Later an ego state who expressed fear of the therapist was quickly reassured, probably because of earlier embedding and seeding.

Calling Out of Ego States.   The calling out, or directly inviting, ego states to open communication in the therapy session is a traditional form of ego-state activation (Edelstien, 1981; J. G. Watkins, 1992). It is effective in nonhypnotic situations only with certain Dissociative Identity Disorder patients. Otherwise, hypnosis is necessary for this method of activation. A therapist might call out an ego state in this fashion: "I wonder if there is a part of Josh that knows something about why he is cheating in class even though he knows the material. If there is such a part, would you come forth and communicate with me ... it's alright if there is not such a part, but if there is, I would like very much to get to know you."

It is often quite helpful to use ideomotor signals to prepare the part for this approach. For example, the therapist could ask if there were a part that helped the mythical Josh by causing him to cheat and indicate that she would like the reply to come as a finger signal. Then if there is a "yes" signal, the therapist could inquire whether the part would be willing to communicate with her. Another "yes" signal could lead to the request for direct activation. In such instances the use of ideomotor signals is sufficient induction for the light trance in which most ego-state work is done; the signals offer the therapist protection from barging into direct ego-state work prematurely. A "no" signal really means not to proceed at that time.

Activation Through Imagery.   The calling out method is not for everyone (patient or therapist). Imagery activation of ego states is a gentle, no-intrusive method that allows ego state activation and also permits the patient and therapist to get an ego-state perspective on what is going on inside of the patient. Fraser (1991, 1993) uses an imagery approach called the *Dissociative Table Technique* in which all of the parts of the patient's personality are invited to sit around a table. We have modified this technique by first helping the patient establish a *safe place* and then inviting the parts to enter this region, sitting, standing, or reclining wherever they wish. Curtis (1996) has aptly demonstrated how the initial appearance of ego-state patterns (when the Dissociative Table Technique is used) may serve as metaphors for the patient's current being-in-the-world as well as for what is needed in healing.

Ideomotor Activation.   Ego states can frequently be activated through ideomotor signals as indicated earlier. This kind of activation is of special relevance with silent nonverbal or preverbal ego states (Frederick, 1994e) with whom ideomotor signals are the only way to activate and initiate communication. In the continuation of the case of Farley we show how ideomotor and imagery activations can be combined.

Case Example: Farley (continued)

As Farley's therapy progressed, he continued to gain weight. His self-esteem was visibly increasing, and he was beginning to show some signs of emancipating himself from his mother's well-meaning but crippling overprotection. From the view point of the SARI model (see chap. 1) he was stable and ready to enter the next phase of therapy (the accessing of troublesome material.

I established Farley's ideomotor signals and activated an ego state. This ego state gave a "yes" answer when I asked if it feared me. Through a variety of 20 questions, I discovered that this part of Farley's personality was quite worried that I might wish to kill off some personality parts should I discover they were causing the eating disorder. I reassured the part that I had never tried to destroy or eliminate a part of anyone's personality and that I did not think that sort of thing worked or was useful anyway. When the part appeared to be reassured on this matter, I asked it to stay around while I invited Farley to go to his safe place and construct a safe area there where he could meet parts of his personality. Farley was able to see four ego states in his mind's eye. One was a fat kid, another an emaciated version of Farley (as I had first seen him), a third part was a muscle-bound weight lifter, and a fourth a nicely proportioned, muscular version of the patient who sent the name Lightbulb into Farley's mind. "They're all me!" Farley said with some degree of surprise. The case of Farley is continued in chapters 8 and 10.

Communication With Mysterious, Malevolent, and Resistant Ego States

Not all ego states present themselves in textbook fashion, and frequently ego states communicate in what have been called *mysterious* ways. They may be easily overlooked by therapists (Frederick & Phillips, 1996). These ego states may present as visual images that are abstract or seemingly irrelevant ("I see the color green, and it has little zigzags in it") or may manifest themselves in a somatosensory manner ("I don't know why, but I keep getting a cold, heavy feeling in my right arm and shoulder"). Certain silent ego states make themselves known only with ideomotor signals in response to questioning (Frederick, 1994e). Persistent and consistent work that features attention to the therapeutic alliance and the transferences with both silent ego states and elusive and mysterious ego states can be most fruitful (Frederick, 1994e; Frederick & Phillips, 1996).

There is a variety of reasons why ego states may be resistant either to communication or to change. However, most of them can be subsumed under the categories of *fear* and *immaturity*. Mysterious ego states are shy ego states, as are many silent ones. Their resistance is a manifestation of their fears of betrayal and/or retraumatization. Some of the nonverbal states are simply too immature to be able to verbalize. Ego states may also be resistant because they experience a need for power, are frightened of extinction, or have various unresolved, narcissistic wishes and preoccupations.

One of the most daunting kinds of ego states with which therapists find themselves engaged are malevolent or hostile ego states (Beahrs, 1982b; Frederick, 1996a; Watkins & Watkins, 1988). These personality parts may prompt a variety of destructive manifestations including such things as self-mutilation, suicide and homicide attempts, physical symptoms, and antisocial behavior. They need validation (Beahrs, 1982b) of their protective functions, and an important key to working with them is the attempt of the therapist to discover what the ego state needs. It is always necessary to assure the patient and the other ego states of the value and adaptive natures of malevolent states.

Ego-Strengthening and the Ego-State Model

The first report of the formal use of an ego-strengthening technique with ego states was made by Frederick and McNeal (1993). They stressed the importance of integrating ego-strengthening with the rest of therapy and emphasized the necessity of the therapeutic alliance. Ego-strengthening has always been an essential element in all Ego State Therapy. The use of the ego-strengthening technique, Inner Strength, with immature ego states as well as with the greater personality is elaborated on in chapter 6. However, ego-strengthening with ego states is not limited to special techniques.

As with the greater personality, ego-strengthening must begin with the formation of the therapeutic alliance and often involves the resolution of transferences. These therapeutic activities must take place with every ego state with which the therapist works (Phillips & Frederick, 1995; Watkins & Watkins, 1990, 1997). For example, the presenting patient may have generally positive transferences for the therapist, whereas ego state A may be terrified of the therapist and fear that the therapist wishes to annihilate her as part of the therapeutic process. Ego state B may hate the therapist because she perceives the therapist as being like an abusive parent.

Ego states can benefit, at times, from involvement in fusional transferences (Diamond, 1983, 1984), re-nurturing techniques (Murray-Jobsis, 1990a, 1990b; Erickson & Rossi, 1989), maturational techniques used with psychotic and borderline patients (Baker, 1981, 1983a, 1983b, 1985; Baker & McColley, 1982; Brown & Fromm, 1986; McNeal & Frederick, 1994, 1997; Scagnelli, 1976), and every kind of direct and indirect ego-strengthening technique that the therapist would use with the greater personality. Integration of ego states is, per se, always ego-strengthening. We present case material that will reflect many of these techniques in an ongoing fashion and within a number of clinical contexts as this book proceeds.

Ego States as Internal Resources

The Activation of Helpful Ego States

The activation of helpful ego states can be pursued by therapists who do not use hypnosis in their practices. However, it may be a more difficult and less predictable enterprise than the hypnotic activation of positive ego states. Nonhypnotic activation is a variation of talking through to a positive or helpful part of the personality. This can be done directly or indirectly. An indirect intervention could be phrased like this:

> I wonder if there is a part of you, Sally, that would be willing to help you with the problem we've been discussing? And I wonder how this part, if it is willing to help, will let you know that it is energizing you with its help.... Perhaps you will have a dream ... perhaps you will notice some images in your mind ... perhaps, somehow, your body or some part of it will feel different.

Ideomotor activation of positive or helpful ego states is a helpful ego-strengthening technique that can be used before uncovering ego-state work is done. It also stands alone as a moving and efficient ego-strengthener. A projective/evocative hypnotic technique, it evokes or activates inner resources, it produces an experience whose specifics are unknown to both patient and therapist beforehand, and are consequently projective, and it gives the patient dramatic evidence of the presence of a benign, possibly loving, personality part within the unconscious mind. The steps for this procedure are simple:

1.) Ask the subject/patient (subsequently referred to here as "N") to think of an issue or problem he/she would like some help with. If you are doing this in a class practicum it is recommended that you use a generic issue such as "Becoming a better therapist."
2.) Establish ideomotor signals.
3.) Ask if there is a part of N's personality that would be willing, at this time, to be helpful to N in the successful resolution of this issue.
4.) If there is a "yes" signal, ask the part to go ahead and produce the experience of helpfulness and to signal with the "yes" finger when that experience is completed.
5.) Although it is not a necessary part of the technique, it is often useful to have the patient complete this experience with an unstructured age progression. While the subject/patient is still in trance, ask the helpful personality part or ego state if it would be willing to go forward in time to allow N to see how things will be in the future when the issue has been resolved.
6.) If, after (3), you get a "No" signal, ask if the ego state if it is willing to give some information about what has to be done before it will be able to provide a helpful experience.

7.) Invite the ego state to continue to be helpful to N concerning the area N sought help with over the following hours and days. Re-alert the subject/ patient and ask for feedback.

(Frederick, 1996g, p. 1)

A clinically useful variation of this technique involves asking the ego state to produce helpful positive age regressions (see chap. 5). More is said about the activation and even the possible creation of helpful ego states in chapter 11 when the topic of performance anxiety is considered.

Conflict-Free Ego States as Internal Resources

In recent years considerable attention has been focused on conflict-free ego states observed to exist within the internal system. The phenomenon of the Internal Self Helper (ISH) was first reported by Allison (1974) and has been widely observed and utilized therapeutically (Comstock, 1987).

In their pursuit of further availability of conflict-free spheres of the ego (Hartmann, 1961) as internal resources, McNeal (1986, 1989) and McNeal and Frederick (1993) developed the concept of Inner Strength which is completely explored in chapter 6. Inner Strength is "something like an ego state" (McNeal & Frederick, 1993). It is a powerful conflict-free aspect of the personality that is somehow connected with the individual's deepest survival instincts. When Inner Strength is activated hypnotically and experienced by the greater personality, there are profound ego-strengthening effects. It has also been noted that Inner Strength can be activated and utilized as an ego-strengthener and growth promoter with immature ego states (Frederick & McNeal, 1993; Phillips & Frederick, 1995). Gregory (1997) has proposed a category of archetypal selfobjects (Gregory, 1997) to which Inner Strength belongs. According to Gregory (1997), archetypes— Jungian internal resources that reside within the collective unconscious—can be activated hypnotically and function as selfobjects (Kohut, 1977) that provide ego-strengthening. Other kinds of hypnotic interventions appear to have the power of mobilizing conflict-free inner resources such as the safe place (Brown & Fromm, 1986; Gregory, 1997; McNeal & Frederick, 1994; Morton & Frederick, 1996), Inner Love (Frederick, 1994g; McNeal & Frederick, 1996), positive age regressions (McNeal & Frederick, 1993), and unstructured positive age progressions (Frederick & Phillips, 1992; Phillips & Frederick, 1992).

Conflict-Laden Ego States as Inner Resources

Although ego states born of trauma are not usually thought of as resources for ego-strengthening, ego-state therapists are aware that they are veritable cornucopias of resources at every stage of therapy (Frederick, 1996i). One source of their strength is that ego states formed at the time of trauma not only hold the negative traumatic material, but also frequently contain resources that were available before, during, and after the trauma.

Many ego states of this nature are like an ego state of Milton Erickson's patient, Miss Damon (Erickson & Kubie, 1939/1980; see also chap. 12). They are in touch with the developmental resources that are available in the patient's life. They are also actively involved in the process of continued growth and maturation. It is possible that it is these parts of the personality that may hold the key resource to the success of therapy: the ability to form therapeutic alliances. It is intriguing that, although developmental arrests that result from trauma may hamper the ability of the total personality to form trusting relationships, certain ego states whose genesis was in the trauma may have the ability to form therapeutic alliances.

One and One Are Two: Integration as Ego-Strengthening

Additional ego-strengthening can occur when individual ego states that had their origins in problem material begin to communicate and cooperate as they move along the road to integration. The power of joint efforts by ego states is frequently reported by patients who may say such things as, "I really feel stronger now!" or "Suddenly I have more confidence, more hope." Other internal resources appear to spring from work that resolves ego-state conflicts as well as from work that raises the developmental level of individual ego states. Often, the help of more mature ego states can be enlisted in these processes that provide ego-strengthening to the greater personality (Frederick, 1992).

The case presented next is that of the treatment of a severe obsessional phobia reported by Erickson and Kubie (1939/1980). Erickson was aware of the adaptive nature of alters or ego states in severely dissociated patients (Erickson, 1959; Erickson & Kubie, 1939/1980). He (Erickson & Kubie, 1939/1980) worked therapeutically with a 20-year-old college student named Miss Damon.

Case Example: Miss Damon

Miss Damon suffered from severe obsessional fears that doors were being opened. She checked doors compulsively at home and at school. She also had "an intense hatred of cats." She had also volunteered to be a subject in some experiments in hypnotism at a time when her obsessional fears were beginning to expand. She did this "without any conscious or deliberate therapeutic intent" (Erickson & Kubie, 1939/1980, p. 231).

Milton Erickson worked experimentally with Ms. Damon. She was an excellent trance subject, and she easily developed amnesia, hand levitation, and arm catalepsy. Erickson suggested that he would call her Miss Brown when she was in formal trance. On the following day she was observed to neglect her work in favor of autohypnosis, hand levitation, and arm cata-lepsy for which she had no reasonable explanation.

Erickson suggested automatic writing as a way of discovering what was transpiring. After a session of automatic writing, Miss Damon looked at her production and wondered if she had really written it. Without her awareness, she automatically wrote "No." Erickson then discovered that he was communicating with a second personality, Miss Brown. Miss Da-mon was unaware of Miss Brown's existence, and Miss Brown wanted it that way because she had memory material and information she did not want Miss Damon to know because it would be too frightening to her.

Erickson worked with Miss Damon and her ego state, Miss Brown, in ses-sions that totaled 12 hours. He established a therapeutic alliance with Miss Brown. Eventually information that Miss Damon had been lost when she was 3 emerged. Miss Brown guided Erickson into using crystal-gazing to help Miss Damon have a hypnotic age regression. Miss Brown even specified exactly when the problem would be solved.

She also helped Miss Damon recall a traumatic incident that had taken place when she was 3. It involved her being lost and her grandfather's al-lusions to doors and a muskrat that appeared in the pantry when he was a child and, like Miss Damon, also lost. The recollected material explained to Miss Damon's satisfaction her phobias and compulsions. The experi-mental therapeutic process resulted in the permanent cure of Ms. Damon's obsessional phobia.

This case is discussed with the case of Jacques, which is presented next.

Case Example: Jacques

Jacques was a practicing psychiatrist who had thought that his several stints of psychotherapy over many years had given him a fair amount of insight into himself. He had begun to commute to Canada to participate in a research project; when he was in Calgary, he stayed with his mother who lived nearby. This arrangement put Jacques and his mother into much more contact with one another than had existed for many years.

Jacques was quite surprised one day while he was doing a Century Run (a 112-mile bicycle trip in a day). As he peddled furiously up a hill, he heard a voice talking to him; it seemed to be saying something like: "You can do that all you want, but you will never get away from me!!!" It is no surprise that he pulled off the road and, in the shade of a tree, contemplated what was going on as the voice continued. "You have ignored my existence for too long, and it just isn't going to be that way anymore." Jacques, who was tall, wiry, fair complexioned, fair haired, and blue eyed, became aware of the mental image of an 8- or 9-year-old child with dark hair. He was leaning against a wall with a smirk on his face that said he knew something Jacques didn't know. "And he had vampire teeth and a grin to go with them ... perhaps, even a cape."

Jacques' first thought was that he was going crazy. He said to the strange manifestation, "Who are you?" The answer was, "I am Conrad, and you had better pay attention to me. Know this as well. I am a shape shifter. I can take many forms. I am power. My power is anger ... I am so fucking mad, so goddamned mad at the people who abused me that I could kill them!!!"

This internal apparition drove Jacques back into therapy immediately, this time with a therapist he knew would be interested in working with his ego states. Jacques described a childhood with an alcoholic father who was absent all the time he was there and of a mother with a considerable amount of bizarre behavior. She washed, powdered, and diapered Jacques and his sister who were bedwetters, until they were in their midteens. She also allowed Jacques to see her in various attitudes of nudity. Jacques developed a terrible and explosive temper that, when it erupted, frightened him because it had caused him to fight on rare occasions. Jacques described a repertoire of dissociative talents. For example, in wartime battle zones, he had put himself to sleep each night by mentally constructing a small castle, piece by piece.

In his next session Jacques brought dreams and described a feeling that the direction of his affective life was in a teeter-totter position now. One hand wants to smash things, and the other is still involved with "You don't have the right." Jacques appeared to have sufficient ego strength for us to begin ego-state exploration immediately. When Conrad was activated, he appeared in the form of a beautiful black stallion; he was delighted that I had decided to take him seriously. He told me that he had a purpose and that it was to liberate Jacques from his mother. Jacques had to grow up and face who he really was. He, Conrad, knew a lot that was out of Jacques' awareness.

Another part was activated, Snoopy, who was childlike like a plush animal. He was the part that Jacques had been in active mental communication with since childhood. Snoopy's function was to be a container for all the pain in Jacques' life. Several other ego states were also activated. There was Pet, who was like a buddy, and yet another, Anthony, who envisioned Jacques' future in a positive way and wanted to lead him there. Finally, there was an animal ego state, a bull named Red Charger, who was a source of power. All the ego states were terrified of Conrad. Nevertheless, internal diplomacy was utilized, and all the parts agreed to enter the same internal room with the other parts. This degree of movement in the direction of integration by the parts was a wonderful feeling for Jacques. At the end of the session he reported being both amazed and delighted at the "feeling of them being in the same room."

After this session Conrad appeared to Jacques again while he was drying off after a swim. He agreed to give Jacques some of his power because he, Conrad, felt so lonely. As Jacques told me about this incident, the phrase came into his mind: "I was used!!" In trance work Jacques saw his mother, partially nude, telling him that he could, in the whole world, rely only on her. A flurry of other painful scenes followed this, and Jacques felt overwhelmed.

I suggested that Jacques might want to construct a more comprehensive container for the pain and terror; he then visualized a mountain and a spring. After he achieved greater clarity about his inner place, all the parts placed the pain and terror into the mountain, now working together.

Later in the session, Jacques told me that he was overjoyed at the ego states' working together, like a family or a group of good friends. It was clear that this had been ego-strengthening for him at a time when trauma memory material was emerging at a great rate. Conrad and the other parts were now very close.

One day while Jacques was engaged in trance work, he told me, "Conrad wants to give more now." After a series of visualizations the patient began to cry. "I must have realized as a kid that I never had a sense of love or nurturance, and that was why Conrad was created." Convinced and strengthened by Conrad's love for him and by the engagement of the ego states in joint efforts and joint revelations, Jacques is deeply involved in his therapy, is functioning better than ever, and feeling good about himself at a time when emerging trauma material could have been a serious problem for him had he not had a little help from his friends.

Conflict-laden ego states help in Ego State Therapy in the following ways:

- The ego state saw an opportunity for change and directed the greater personality into it.
- The ego state formed a therapeutic alliance with the therapist.
- The ego state held and contained valuable memories that the greater personality could not tolerate without damage to her self-esteem.
- The ego state was protective of the other ego states and paced the revelation of traumatic material to the ability of the greater personality to tolerate it.
- The ego state may have provided a screen memory for a more traumatic situation, utilizing this symbolic and less threatening mode of problem resolution.

(Frederick, 1996d)

There are other ways in which ego states can strengthen the greater personality. Sometimes ego states formed in one trauma may often step in to protect the greater personality from other similar traumata. This kind of dissociative response is one in which the ego state acts much like a circuit breaker that keeps the greater personality and less developed parts from irretrievably blowing the circuits though the development of psychosis or successfully suicidal behavior.

The clinical material of Jacques shows how we can, without any difficulty, discover many ego-strengthening characteristics and behaviors of conflict-laden ego states and utilize these precious resources in our therapeutic work. Apart from any ego-strengthening aspects, many therapeutic situations are greatly facilitated by ego-state approaches. The dividend of closely working with conflict-laden ego states, so as to capitalize on their gifts and talents, is that it incorporates ego-strengthening into the therapeutic model from the beginning. As Erickson recognized in working with Miss Damon, the first step in working with a personality part is to form a therapeutic alliance. When the therapist does this, ever mindful of the adaptive nature of all ego states, a chord is struck within the internal system, signaling the beginning of a reign of cooperation. The therapist, through forming those initial alliances, communicates to all the ego states the kind of interaction she seeks. That interaction is not based on a master–slave, a scientist–specimen, or a "big healing/poor little you" model. Rather, it is the dynamic of cooperation and sharing. The internal resources of the ego states of the therapist cooperate with those of the patient.

The ego states respond to receptiveness of the therapist by pouring forth abundant resources, usually from the time of their first contact. Indeed, sometimes conflict-laden ego states are so laden with resources such as information, memory experiences, affects, problem-solving abilities, and backbone that they can no longer remain quiet; they anticipate therapy and drive patients into therapy, even if, at times, they must frighten them to do so. This is what happened with both Miss Damon and Jacques. In each case the ego state with awareness of the need for solutions prompted an individual into treatment who was not even aware of having a problem.

Ego states like Conrad often utilize an amazingly creative bag of tricks such as threats, overwhelming affect, the assumption of various forms, and threats to activate patients into taking the steps that are needed for healing. It is possible that some therapists might even have viewed Conrad as a malevolent ego state (Beahrs, 1982b; Frederick, 1996a; Watkins & Watkins, 1988) bent, at best, only on protecting the patient. Both malevolent ego states (Beahrs, 1982b; Frederick, 1996a; Watkins & Watkins, 1988, 1997) as well as silent or non-verbal ego states (Frederick, 1994e) contain and can offer many resources for the greater personality. For example, Conrad, although a protector, was clearly also a shover, pushing and shoving Jacques into really examining unresolved material aroused by his recent contacts with his mother. Like Erickson's Miss Brown who directed the greater personality to become a volunteer subject in experiments with hypnotism, he saw an opportunity for change and directed the greater personality into it.

Both Miss Brown and Conrad held valuable memories that the greater personality could not tolerate at first without being overwhelmed or suffering damage to his or her self-esteem, and both personality parts paced and metered the traumatic memory experiences so that other ego states as well as the greater personality could tolerate and metabolize the information without undue damage to their self-esteem. This kind of regulation, frequently attributed to Internal Self Helpers, is also a most valuable capability of conflict-laden ego states.

The therapeutic alliances that ego states form with the therapist are often mirrored in their alliances with other ego states whom they have previously experienced as alien or not belonging to the internal family or for whom they have felt disdain, contempt, or fear. As ego states approach one another, communicate, enter into cooperative ventures, and continue to proceed along the path to integration (Phillips & Frederick, 1995), it is as though their resident internal resources both grow and become accessible in a geometrically increasing fashion. In the case of Miss Damon, automatic writing and crystal gazing were the facilitators for strengthening; in the case of Jacques, assembling the ego states in a common room where their work could be pursued with a sense of community was the catalyst for their rapprochement. Fraser (1991, 1993) has called this the Dissociative Table Technique.

In emphasizing the utilization of conflict-laden ego states as internal resources, the therapist is working with what is closer at hand and what is already available. We consider this an organic form of Ego State Therapy that works with what is presented and at hand. Ego states are always there within the personality, like family members or old friends. As Virginia Woolf's character, Bernard, so aptly said in her novel, *The Waves*: "Some people go to priests; others to poetry; I to my friends" (Woolf, 1931/1959, p. 266). It usually is not difficult for us to get a little help from our friends. As with most things we need in life, we just have to ask for it.

The next chapter enters further into the realm of projective/evocative ego-strengthening as it examines ways in which the use of time and time distortion can activate powerful inner resources and provide invaluable information about the clinical status of the patient and the efficacy of her therapy.

Chapter 5

The Utilization of Time as a Vehicle for Projective/Evocative Ego-Strengthening

Time preoccupies the Western mind in a most pervasive way. We perceive it as inexorable and waiting for no man. Most of us would be helpless without our clocks and watches, and most of our concepts of psychological and developmental process are thought of in terms of time. Although we would like to claim that we are enlightened, we usually think of time in an Aristotelian sense. "Time," Aristotle told us, was "the measure of motion in space." He was referring to objective time—the time of the physics of his day. Subjective time is the material of art, psychotherapy, and post-Newtonian physics. Freud's liberation of mankind from linear time into the timelessness of the unconscious was faithfully rendered by Dali when he used limp watches in his famous painting, *The Persistence of Memory* (1931). H. G. Wells (1895) fictionalized mankind's view of a more plastic time when he wrote about *The Time Machine*, as if in anticipation of Einstein's theory of relativity (1905, 1916), which allowed us to understand that the relativity we are aware of in subjective time is, in a way, mirrored by other kinds of relativity in objective time.

The concept of time consciousness also became the subject of philosophy's attention, and Husserl's (1906) work on the subject, and that of his student and successor Heidegger, seeded a revolution in philosophy known as phenomenology. Artists had always viewed time as a malleable and supremely subjective experience. Jorge Luis Borges (1941/1964) described this intimacy of time and human experience: "Time is the substance from which I am made. Time is a river which carries me along, but I am the river; it is a tiger that devours me, but I am the tiger; it is a fire that consumes me, but I am the fire" (p. 234). Our subjective experience of time, Borges seems to be saying, is an integral part of our identities and an expression of who we are.

Milton Erickson (1901–1980) grew up in this dynamic, changing atmosphere in which concepts of time were becoming radically altered. He was a child of Freud, Jung, and Einstein, and his early life experiences with the pliability of time perception remained with him as he became interested in what kinds of beneficial shaping could be given to the time distortions produced by hypnosis.

DOI:10.4324/9781003442585-5

In 1948 Cooper published a seminal paper on time distortion as a phenomenon that could be produced by hypnosis. Two years later Erickson joined Cooper in a second publication on the topic (Cooper & Erickson, 1950), this one much more extensive. In this paper the authors concluded that: (a) time distortion in hypnosis is a phenomenon that can be reduplicated in the majority of subjects; (b) time sense can be altered to a predetermined degree, and that although activity occurring in time altered states may appear to the subject to be proceeding at a rate perceived as natural, it occurred at rates that were rapid when measured by clock time; (c) the subjects did not falsify their reports retrospectively; (d) the subjective experiences of distorted time included an experience of continuity; and (e) thinking in distorted time occurs more rapidly than in "world time" and may actually be superior in nature to "waking thought."

Erickson wrote the special section in which he discussed the psychological and psychiatric implications of his and Cooper's experimental work. He regarded Cooper's discovery as new, big, and significant. Cooper and Erickson published their book, *Time Distortion in Hypnosis*, in 1959. In it Erickson revealed that he had successfully used time distortion (time condensation) with a patient before Cooper had published his initial report on the topic. Erickson remained fascinated for the rest of his professional career with the many possibilities that time distortion could offer distressed individuals.

In one of the clinical cases Erickson reported in his and Cooper's (1959) book, he described the used of time distortion (time expansion) as a mechanism for helping several patients hypnotically age regress to a number of traumatic incidents within a 20-second interval. In another case report Erickson introduced the concept of using time distortion in such a way that *only* the unconscious mind would know what had transpired.

Ego-Strengthening with Positive Hypnotic Age Regressions

We now join two Ericksonian themes as we move into the topic of projective/evocative age regression. These are the demonstrated ability of hypnosis to distort subjective time and the concept that the unconscious mind is a vast reservoir of available and accessible resources. It is to the accessible unconscious resources that are based in the past that we now turn our attention.

Age Regression

The individual who experiences *age regression* is having some kind of subjective experience of the past. Age regression occurs in a spectrum that ranges from the ordinary, naturalistic events of reminiscence in human life to the dramatic flashbacks of posttraumatic stress disorder (PTSD). Reminiscence is somewhere at the heart of nonhypnotic psychodynamic psychotherapies. Age regression can also be used as a therapeutic technique designed to take the patient back, to a greater or lesser degree, into some experience in his perceived past. It has been used by many therapists and in many kinds of therapies. Age regression offers numerous possibilities for helping the patient discover hitherto unknown resources and internal sources of problem material whose discovery may aid in its resolution. Janet (1897, 1919/1976) used hypnotic age regressions with his patients at the turn of the century. It became a popular technique with clinicians who worked with war neuroses after both world wars (Grinker & Spiegel, 1945; Simmel, 1944; Watkins, 1949; Wingfield, 1920).

There is considerable debate as to whether hypnotic age regression is real. Subjects may produce regressions that are simulated, partial, and complete. Some subjects may experience *revivification* (Kroger, 1977; Watkins, 1987), which is a regression that is experienced as an actual reliving of a recalled event, rather than simply remembering it. Watkins (1987) has reviewed various theories for why hypnotic age regressions occur. The *age-consistency theory* hypothesizes that subjects will recall certain aspects of the past and will also regress to a psychological level of development consistent with the time of the recalled events. Brown and Fromm (1986) espouse this view: "it is a partial reinstatement of earlier modes of functioning and behavior. For instance, age regression to infancy can sometimes yield infant reflexes, such as the plantar, the sucking, or the grasping reflex ..." (p. 32).

Brown and Fromm (1986) have noticed that (a) affect regresses during hypnotic age regression, (b) there is cognitive perceptual regression, and (c) regressed subjects may return to a primary childhood language unused since childhood. However, they remind us that none of this means that age regression is an exact return to earlier modes, because regressed subjects may respond at higher developmental levels on one hand, or may act more childlike, overplaying the situation on the other. They cite Greenleaf's (1969) observation that it is typical of any age regression, even in the most highly hypnotizable subject, for there to be fluctuations between genuine elements of retrieval of the past and role-playing.

There are also *role-enactment* theories that view hypnotic age regression as a form of dramaturgy, as well as interpersonal theories that are based on deeper interactions between the patient and the therapist in therapy. According to Watkins (1987):

> The reality of hypnotic age regression remains controversial, especially among experimentalists. Therapists, however, use it widely and consider it a valuable tool, especially in hypnoanalysis. It is possible that the intensive, regressed hypnotic relationship which inheres in a therapist-patient interaction does not obtain in the more artificial laboratory setting. If so, clinicians and experimentalists may not be observing the same phenomena.
>
> (p. 76)

We have found age regressions to be invaluable for ego-strengthening as well as for uncovering. However, we do not use the pure concept of *memory* or *memories* when working with our patients. Without dishonoring the relevance and importance of material from the past for the patient or failing to help the patient work out the implications of such material for himself, we also acknowledge certain necessary realities. They include the following: we were not present at the time; memories can be distorted in the stages of acquisition, storage, and retrieval; and we cannot decide what really happened for the patient. Consequently, we call all material produced with age regression *memory material* (Phillips & Frederick, 1995) or *memory experiences* produced by patients. The topic of memory is presented in greater detail in chapter 13.

Techniques of Age Regression

Age regression can be accomplished in a naturalistic fashion ("Can you recall what your brother said to you that made you feel so angry with him?") or can be formally structured ("Perhaps you can tell me more about that time when you had been so successful on your first job"). Many therapists within the non-hypnotic psychodynamic tradition, as well as many Ericksonian therapists, frequently employ naturalistic age regressions. Often they are desirable preambles to more formal procedures that may be introduced later in therapy.

There are many ways to do formal hypnotic age regressions. However, it is important to recall that age regression may occur spontaneously, to a greater or lesser degree, once the hypnotic state has been induced. Direct suggestion can also produce age regression in many patients. Other valuable methods include imagery and fantasy, ideomotor approaches, and the affect bridge.

All too often therapy is stereotyped as a situation in which the patient's only contact with his past consists of digging up painful or unpleasant material. Most patients have a plenum of positive memories that can be accessed in therapy and utilized as resources. Too frequently the emphasis in therapy is on the use of age regression for uncovering work and abreaction, and too seldom is its usefulness for strengthening the patient explored. We use both structured and unstructured positive age regressions for ego-strengthening, and we do this in a variety of ways, some of which are described next.

Structured Positive Age Regressions

The structured age regression is one in which the therapist directs the patient to a specific time in his life. This could be a time when problems had occurred or when the patient was engaged in successes, wonderful experiences with relationships, or great productivity or creativity. Regression to particular positive experiences is a predictable way the therapist can guide the patient into an ego-strengthening aspect of the past.

Case Example: Martha

Martha was a 49-year-old woman who came to therapy because she felt depressed, fearful, and stuck. She felt that her life had become routine and uninteresting. However, she was quite fearful of making any changes. She said that she was interested in using hypnosis to help her solve her problems. She entered trance very easily and experienced vivid imagery in her inner world.

Martha's history had featured wonderful experiences of travel in Europe when she was in her 20s. She referred to this time as "The most exciting time of my life!" In a hypnotic session I (SM) gave Martha the specific task of returning mentally to that time when she was in her 20s, traveling abroad, and feeling adventurous and engaged with life.

When Martha emerged from the trance state, she appeared to sparkle with a new vitality and began to talk about how she could recall, so much more vividly, how much more she had enjoyed life then. I had told Martha while she was in trance as well as later that this time of her life was important for her to remember and reexperience. She would be able to bring back that spirit of curiosity and adventure into her current life. She was told that whenever she felt fearful about asserting herself in her present life, she would discover that she had an urge to picture her 20-year-old self in Europe.

In a subsequent session Martha appeared more animated and related several incidents in which she had been able to assert herself and ask for something she wanted without feeling fearful. Over time, Martha began to make major changes in her life. She got a new job, bought a house, and formed a new relationship with a man who loved to travel.

Unstructured Positive Age Regressions

Unstructured age regressions are often quite powerful experiences for patients. They are evocative in the sense that they call on resources in such a way that the decision about what kinds of positive memories will appear is left up to deeper levels of mind. They are also projective in that they are not the result of an agenda imposed by the therapist. They allow both the patient and the therapist to learn more about what is important to the patient. In general, we recommend that any therapist begin such an exploration naturalistically.

Generally Pleasant Experiences.   Most patients have certain positive experiences in their pasts and have positive experiences in their present as well. Too often, we, as therapists, tend to lose track of our patients' positive life experiences as we become immersed in pursuing their pathologies. There is also what appears to be a built-in resistance within many patients to speak of the pleasant and positive unless the therapist pursues it. Some simply do not believe that therapists in general want to hear about their ordinary positive experiences. Others may blatantly inform their therapists that to talk about their pleasant experiences is a waste of money. For some patients positive material is avoided because, if they begin to share it, they feel they might grow closer to the therapist, and this could be threatening. Yet positive experiences from the past, even the recent past, can be ego-strengthening. It is desirable for the therapist to begin to help the patient get in touch with positive memories by using naturalistic approaches. Positive reinforcement through shows of interest on the therapist's part is valuable, as are questions that may lead into positive details.

Case Example: Nell

Nell was referred to me (CF) after her youngest son, the light of her life, had died from a brief and unexpected illness. When she had discovered she was pregnant with Tom, she had thought: "Now I have somebody to love me." Tom did love her very much and in his adult years he remained involved with Nell and her third husband.

After her son's death Nell entered into pathological bereavement; she had lost her primary nurturing figure. In time she developed a Major Depression. When I first saw her, she was unable to have any view of her future whatsoever, and she offered little in the therapy sessions. It was as if she were waiting for me to pull her out of a terrible place she had no particular wish to leave. The therapy sessions were laborious for Nell and me. She wanted to please me but could not get in touch with anything positive. I wanted to be a good therapist but felt ineffective and constantly wondered what I could do that would be an improvement on what I was already doing inasmuch as it felt as if I were doing nothing. Nell feared, I learned later, that I would become frustrated or bored with her and give up on her case.

One day I discovered that Nell had an interest in excellent food and fine wines. I then began what I have come to call "Menutherapy." At every opportunity I encouraged Nell to elaborate the details of meals she wished she had enough energy to prepare, meals she had out, and meals she had prepared and/or eaten in the past. This discussion of food allowed Nell to begin to come in touch with positive experiences in her therapy sessions. The positive memories about food eventually served as a pathway along which she was able to find wonderful memory experiences of Tom. These brought her joy, and they also put her in touch with her feelings of grief. Nell was able to cry in a new way.

The detailed discussions of food with Nell helped pull her out of the paralysis of grief and depression she experienced. It also helped move her toward more participation in the therapeutic alliance; she began to see me as a fellow gourmet with whom she might be able to collaborate successfully in the work of her therapy as well. The utilization of her own resources—the positive memory experiences or positive regressions—showed Nell that she was not as completely empty as she had imagined. Finally, the "Menutherapy" afforded her a safe and acceptable way of obtaining some nurturing in her therapy.

There is no question that naturalistic age regression can help patients tap into many rich and useful positive memories from the past. However, with the introduction of direct hypnosis, the activation of these resources can be deeper, more complete, and often more profound.

Revivification of Positive Memory and Mastery Experiences. Good therapists know the value of helping patients access positive memory material of past successes and mastery experiences as well as prior encounters with meaningful interpersonal events of healing, creativity, and spirituality. Naturalistic invitation to such memories is meaningful and strengthening for many patients. However, there are patients who just draw a blank when they are asked to recall their greatest successes. There are patients who recall these kinds of experiences but do not seem to be in touch with much of the positive affect that was present when these experiences originally occurred.

It is with these patients that hypnosis can be particularly useful. Patients in formal trance can be asked to recall such experiences. For example, a patient could be helped to enter trance and then asked to recall "the most successful event in your life." When the patient begins to access this kind of material, he is experiencing a true hypnotic age regression age. If he becomes deeply immersed in the experience, he will revivify it, and it will have a more profound influence on him. As with all age regressions, it is important to assist the revivification by directing the patient's focus to the particular details involved in the memory material. The therapist might help with such comments as: "Where are you? Who is with you? ... you can look around you and see the large picture, too.... What you are wearing.... How does it feel ... I wonder if you can realize now ... that although lives have many ups and downs ... and not all of life is lived, or can be, at such a peak.... that this experience belongs to you ... and that nothing can ever take it away from you." Scripts for this kind of age regression can be particularly powerful when they evoke affect. It has been noted that affect, in turn, can enhance memory (Bower, 1981). With this kind of structured, positive hypnotic age regression that is so effective in revivifying positive memory, the spotlight can be turned on many ego-strengthening areas in patients' lives.

These structured age regressions are both evocative and projective. Many patients experience degrees of internal emptiness and impoverishment, may be depressed, and may even be somewhat dissociated from their resources. All of our patients are living in the negative past to some extent while dwelling in a dissatisfying present. Those who are able to revivify have become infinitely wealthier.

Indeed, the infusion of positive energy from resources from which they had been alienated may be revitalizing for them, filling them with life instead of emptiness and vacancy. The projective message from patients who are not able to produce positive memory material is that they may be close to emotional bankruptcy; many of these patients need direct, suggestive ego-strengthening techniques (Phillips & Frederick, 1995).

Recalling and Revivifying Nurturing Figures from the Past.   We often observe that some of the most powerful events in therapy occur when the patient is helped to come into direct contact with his unconscious mind. This direct contact with the unconscious, in terms of the resources from the past, can be profoundly meaningful. This is particularly true with patients who are not able to produce a great deal in the positive memory department naturalistically, with those who appear to have little awareness of unconscious processes, and with those who are not psychologically minded and need significant evidence that there is more going on than what is seen on the surface.

Perhaps some of the most profound therapeutic events available to patients with hypnotic techniques of age regression are those that are directed to reexperiencing positive nurturing figures from childhood and adolescence who are outside the parental sphere (McNeal & Frederick, 1993). McNeal (1986) described her observations that regression to positive nurturing figures had been helpful to a number of patients. McNeal and Frederick (1993) reported further clinical success with such positive hypnotic age regressions. We view them as "an often overlooked resource" (McNeal & Frederick, 1993, p. 173). The purpose for excluding parents from this kind of age regression resides in the probability that patients have more conflict about their parents than about other childhood nurturing figures.

Script for Age Regression to Significant Nurturing Figures

Life is very complex. Sometimes we have hard times, and sometimes we have better times. Some of our experiences are wonderful ... and as we go back into the past ... we can remember times when we were very, very much alone ... times when it seemed no one cared for us ... times when we had conflicts with our parents ... and nobody seems available ...

In most human lives, though ... it's really wonderful how it happens ... when we are children ... little kids, there are other people around ... sometimes we have really forgotten them ... grown-ups who are there for us ... who have done special things with us ... maybe just a smile, or a word of encouragement ... maybe a special appreciation ... or a trip ... just a treat ... or a good time ... or even a look of admiration and appreciation. People in the neighborhood ... people in the extended family ... the school teachers ... the janitor ... maybe someone at a church ... in a camp ... maybe someone you met in a store one day. Just take your time, allowing these images, thoughts, and feelings to come into your mind.... When you have a sense that this experience is complete, all you need to do is let your "yes" finger lift.

These people who have given these things to you from the past are with you now in the present, and will always be with you as part of your strength and confidence, as a reflection from the world to you of your uniqueness and your value. And you can remember, and you can notice now, how good it made you feel to be with the people you've recalled. Just let your self experience how good it felt ... and know that you can bring these feelings back with you from the past into the present.

(McNeal & Frederick, 1993, pp. 173–174)

These memory events can be almost universally accessed, and the experiences usually contain powerful images, thoughts, and strong affect. For most patients positive age regressions are identifiably evocative of unconscious resources and are noticeably ego-strengthening.

The experiences that are reported by the patient are often deeply significant in psychodynamic terms. In this sense the technique is also projective in nature, as there is no way of predicting ahead of time what kind of material will come into the patient's awareness during this ego-strengthening exercise.

(McNeal & Frederick, 1993, p. 174)

These experiences are also projective because they give us a window into the patient's childhood perceptions of self and others and allow the therapeutic process to view the nature and degree of some of the patient's available internal nurturing resources.

We have not had any negative experiences with our patients when using this technique. However, we would caution clinicians that it is always possible that techniques designed to tap resources could, in certain severely traumatized patients, evoke negative, traumatic age regression. Consequently, we recommend that formal positive hypnotic age regressions and revivifications be conducted only by therapists who have been trained to handle negative material should it emerge.

Hypnotic Ideomotor Activation of Resources From the Past

The Nature of Ideomotor Signals. It is within the arena of hypnosis that the inseparability of the mind and the body can be clearly seen. One of the most basic and easily accessible evidences of this seamless connection is the ideomotor response. The term *ideomotor* refers to an involuntary motor activity of the body that is the direct result of a thought or idea. Rossi and Cheek (1988) have noted that it had its first "scientific" demonstration by Chevreul (see chap. 10).

The term *ideomotor* has been replaced by many with the more accurate term *ideodynamic* (Rossi & Cheek, 1988). Both indicate the connection of mental process with the active, dynamic functioning of the mind–body. In clinical hypnosis ideomotor signals are frequently used to communicate with deeper levels of consciousness that are outside the patient's awareness. This provides both the patient and the hypnotherapist with a means of communication in trance and a safety net, because the signals can be used to pace treatment as well as make important determinations about what direction it should take. Ideodynamic healing, a therapeutic approach that utilizes ideomotor responses of the body in various ways, is a powerful ego-strengthening tool that promotes resolution and healing at an unconscious level. Since the healing, reorganization, and reintegration is done outside of awareness, ideomotor signals are used to establish communication, signal willingness to enter into a healing process, and indicate unconscious access to problem areas as well as resolution. Ideodynamic healing is discussed in chapter 10.

The precise nature of ideomotor signals is not known. Some simplistic therapists naively assume that ideomotor communications are always concrete and truthful and that there is an exact parallelism between specific true unconscious content and ideomotor signals. Fortunately for all of us, the unconscious mind is more complicated than our 10 fingers. In our experience ideomotor signals are not always accurate any more than free association is seen to be accurate. Ideomotor signals can even lie. However, on the main, they still remain one of the most practical methods for accessing many aspects of what is going on within deeper levels of mind. An additional benefit is that they provide opportunities for the patient to communicate without speaking. When patients are speaking in trance, ideomotor signals can indicate the presence of internal conflict. For example, the patient may be reporting a certain kind of memory experience with great confidence while the finger signals are saying "no." What the "no" could mean might then become the focus of therapy.

There is a variety of ways to establish ideomotor signaling. Usually ideomotor signals are established on the patient's fingers. This is a convenient location that is easy to observe. However, patients may display ideomotor signaling in other parts of the body in the form of involuntary movements or somatosensory responses, such as flushing or tingling. The observant hypnotherapist will detect many of these; it is possible much of the time to have these kinds of signals transferred to the fingers by a willing and cooperative inner mind.

Although many hypnotherapists assign fingers for "yes" and "no" to patients, it is recommended that they be allowed to develop naturally. A certain number of patients will develop ideomotor responses that cause the finger to lift automatically; however, many patients respond *ideosensorily*. This means that their mind–body communication is sensory rather than motor. Instead of being aware of movements in their fingers, they are aware of sensory changes such as numbness, heat, cold, increased sensitivity, tingling, and so on.

Ideomotor signals are used by hypnotherapists at every level of development. Their use allows the therapist to develop communication and rapport with deeper levels of personality. In this way the therapy can become more comprehensive. The lack of voluntariness of the signal is often impressive to patients. It may change their belief systems profoundly when they discover that there are levels of personality they have not been aware of that wish to communicate with them and to help them. Frederick (1995c) has a practical set of instructions for eliciting ideomotor signals that can later be used within a therapeutic context:

There are several approaches to establishing ideomotor signals. Some therapists assign these signals to certain fingers. We prefer a more permissive and projective orientation. This permits deeper levels of mind to be more spontaneously expressive. We believe this to be of assistance in further strengthening the therapeutic alliance.

How to Establish Ideomotor Signals.   The following list explains how to establish ideomotor signals:

1. Establish rapport and help the patient enter light trance. Be sure to have the patient place his/her hands where you can see them.
2. Ask the patient to mentally picture the word "Yes" and to allow him/herself to think and feel "Yes ... Yes ... Yes."
3. Then ask the patient's inner mind (or unconscious mind, inner self, inner guide, etc.) to cause a "yes" response to develop in one of the patients' fingers. Describe what that response could be: "That response is a different kind of a feeling in one of your fingers. It could be a decreased sensitivity ... or an increased sensitivity ... or, that finger might just feel different in some other way ... it could tingle ... or feel lighter ... or heavier ... just take all the time you need for that signal to develop ... and when it does develop, you can let me know which finger it appears in by just lifting that finger a bit."
4. Repeat the procedure to establish a "no" signal as well as a privacy signal that can be used if the patient's inner mind needs an "I don't know" or an "I don't want to tell you" response.
5. Establish the accuracy of the signals by asking questions about the date, the season of the year, etc.
6. Once ideomotor signals have been established, they can be used for ongoing communication with the patient's deeper levels of consciousness for a variety of purposes. For example, they can be used to help activate positive inner resources such as positive memories or positive aspects of personality. They can also help the hypnotherapist enter hypnoanalytic exploration in a safe way. Ideomotor signaling is also a part of a deep unconscious form of healing known as ideodynamic healing.

(Frederick, 1995c, pp. 1–2)

Ideomotor Activation of Positive Progressions

Once the therapist has been able to activate a patient's ideomotor signals and to tell the difference between "yes" and "no," he can then communicate with the inner mind and request an activation of positive resources from the past for which the patient has no conscious awareness. The effects of this kind of projective/evocative intervention can be quite dramatic. Frederick (1995c) has clear instructions for this kind of activation. Although hypnotic age progressions are not discussed until later in this chapter, the use of a hypnotic age progression is included in the exercise.

Instructions for Facilitating Ideomotorically Activated Positive Age Regression.   Frederick (1996h) listed the following instructions:

Ideomotor activation of positive age regressions is a powerful, frequently dramatic, projective/evocative ego-strengthening technique. It evokes or activates inner resources; it produces material whose specifics are unknown to both patient and therapist beforehand; and are consequently projective; and it offers the patient dramatic evidence of the working and power of the unconscious mind. The steps for this procedure are simple:

1.) Ask the subject/patient (subsequently referred to here as "N") to think of an issue or problem he/she would like some help with. If you are doing this in a class practicum it is recommended that you use a generic issue such as "Becoming a better therapist."
2.) Establish ideomotor signals.
3.) Ask N's "inner mind" if it would be willing to produce some positive memory material from an earlier time in N's life that would be helpful in the successful resolution of this issue.
4.) If there is a "yes" signal, ask the inner mind to go ahead and produce the positive memory material and to signal with the "yes" finger when that experience is completed.
5.) If time permits you may wish to repeat (3) and (4), asking this time for an even earlier time in N's life that would be helpful, etc. This can deepen the experience greatly at times.
6.) Although it is not part of an age regression technique, it is often useful to the patient to complete this experience with an unstructured age progression. While the subject/patient is still in trance, ask the inner mind if it would be willing to go forward in time to allow N to see how things will be in the future when the issue has been resolved.
7.) If, after (3), you get a "No" signal, ask if the inner mind is willing to give some information about what has to be done before it could give the positive memory material.
8.) Re-alert the subject patient and ask for feedback.

(p. 1)

Ego-State Activation of Positive Age Regressions

Just as the greater personality can activate positive age regressions either with direct suggestive techniques of hypnotic age regression or by ideomotor activation, so also can individual ego states activate positive memory material that can be strengthening to them and/or to the greater personality. The ideomotor script presented previously can be easily modified. Instead of asking the inner mind to be helpful, the therapist asks, "is there a part of N that would be willing to produce positive memory material?" This is in keeping with the axiom in ego-state work that any technique that can be used with an individual patient can be used with an ego state.

Hypnotic Age Progressions that are Projective and Evocative

Structured Age Progressions: Mental Rehearsal and End Result Imagery

Phillips and Frederick (1992) noted that Hartland (1965, 1971), Gardner (1976), Dimond (1981), and Stanton (1989) used future-oriented suggestions in therapy that were ego-strengthening and often involved mastery. Hammond (1990d) regarded structured hypnotic age progressions to be "goal-directed hypnotherapy techniques" that are "compatible with Alfred Adler's teleological or future-oriented approach to treatment [Ansbacher & Ansbacher, 1985], wherein people are perceived as being basically goal-oriented" (Hammond, 1990d, p. 515). According to Hammond there are various terms for views of the future in his review of the literature:

> *Age progression, time projection, pseudo-orientation in time into the future, mental rehearsal, process imagery, goal imagery, success imagery, end result imagery* are all terms that have been used in a rather fuzzy and sometimes interchangeable manner in hypnosis. All of these terms refer to future-oriented work, but they are not all synonyms for the same thing.
>
> (Hammond, 1990d, p. 515; italics added)

Among techniques for structured, future-oriented work is *mental rehearsal*. Hammond views this hypnotic technique as being parallel to its cognitive-behavioral counterpart. The therapist helps the patient mentally enact the steps required for the accomplishment of a future activity. This kind of structured age progression has been called *process imagery* by Zilbergeld and Lazarus (1987) because it requires that the process through which a goal is realized be visualized and rehearsed step by step. This kind of structured imagery can be particularly useful when issues of performance are at stake; they are commonly used by athletes (Unestahl, 1983), performing artists (McNeal, 1986), and individuals taking examinations (Zilbergeld and Lazarus, 1987). We discuss their uses further in chapter 11.

Hammond (1990d) considers *end result imagery*, *goal imagery*, and *success imagery* as mental processes in which one pictures or imagines oneself in the future, after the goal has been achieved, and he wisely points out that trance is not required for this kind of imagery. Visualizing the end result has become a popular technique in the positive thinking movement and is also utilized in the same kinds of performance situations where mental rehearsal is appropriate. Therapists frequently guide patients into end result imagery when they speak about goals, the future, and the changes therapy will bring.

Unstructured Hypnotic Age Progressions

Pseudo-Orientation in Time: The Erickson Model

Hammond classifies Erickson's (1954) pseudo-orientation in time as being a kind of end result imagery that has been made much more powerful because it takes place in deep trance. Erickson dipped into the tradition of "fortune-tellers, gypsies, and soothsayers" (Phillips & Frederick, 1992, p. 99) when he taught subjects in controlled hypnotic experiments to enter trance by staring at crystal balls that were held above eye level. Later, Erickson had deep trance subjects "project themselves into the future in order to gain an understanding of the behaviors necessary to reach their therapeutic goals" (Havens, 1986, p. 258). His subjects gazed at a series of internally visualized (or, as he termed it, *hallucinated*) crystal balls within each of which they could see another successful step in the accomplishment of their goals. He then produced hypnotic amnesia for what had transpired in hypnosis as he felt that *only the unconscious* mind really knew what the individual's achievable goals might be. The purpose of the amnesia was to keep the conscious mind from contaminating the process.

Erickson believed that most unhypnotized persons could not generate accurate projections of what was needed to achieve goals or necessarily know what goals were truly attainable for them. He believed the conscious mind was capable of generating fantasies that were unrealistic and evaluations that were incomplete or off the mark. Erickson (1954) believed that, for most individuals, the hypnotic state alone could provide the necessary objectivity within which they could perceive accurately their own capabilities. Erickson believed dissociation to be the mechanism for hypnotic age progressions (pseudo-orientation in time).

Erickson gave additional help to the unconscious minds of his subjects in his pseudo-orientation in time experiments; he also gave what was tantamount to a posthypnotic suggestion—that they would indeed perform the desirable activities they had seen in the crystal balls. Subsequently, the subjects rather automatically began to perform the actions and to achieve the results they wished in ways that seemed natural and spontaneous to them.

In their review of the literature, Phillips and Frederick (1992) noted that de Shazer (1978) successfully used a somewhat similar technique with two patients who had sexual dysfunction. He had his subjects picture successful sexual experiences in hypnotically visualized crystal balls. Havens (1986) also used a similar future orientation in "the remarkable transformation" (p. 260) of a depressed, inhibited, and colorless young woman into a calm, assured, assertive, and outgoing person. Havens (1986) reported using his variation of Erickson's technique, which he called *posthypnotic predetermination of therapeutic progress,* in a variety of clinical situations.

Solution-focused therapy, with its emphasis upon a projected future and the *miracle question* (de Shazer, 1985, 1988; O'Hanlon & Wiener-Davis, 1989), is related to Erickson's concept of pseudo-orientation in time.

"Back From the Future": The Dolan and Torem Models

Age progressions can be structured so that the patient is guided into communicating with an imagined future self who may be healthy and is certainly presumed to be wiser. Dolan (1991) uses a technique in which the patient is asked to consider the possibility of suggestions or advice from herself at a later date, when she will be older "and presumably wiser." Dolan described how she might get a patient in touch with this kind of age progression:

> Imagine that you have grown to be a healthy, wise old woman and you are looking back on this period of your life. What do you think that this wonderful, old, wiser you would suggest to you to help you get through this current phase of your life? What would she tell you to remember? What would she suggest that would be most helpful in helping you heal from the past? What would she say to comfort you? And does she have any advice about how therapy could be most useful and helpful?
>
> (p. 36)

Dolan then asks the patient to write a letter to the older, wiser self. In this letter she describes her difficulties. Then the patient is asked to write a reply from the perspective of the older, wiser self to the patient in the present. This letter will contain "comfort, advice, and helpful instructions about getting through this period of life based on what she has learned from old age" (Dolan, 1991, p. 36). Dolan also allows for the possibility of the patient consulting an imagined deceased relative or friend who is presumed to be supportive.

Torem (1992) developed his version of a highly structured hypnotic age progression which he has called the *Back-From-The-Future* technique. The technique has the following steps:

• The therapist must understand the patient's condition and life circumstances before undertaking the technique, and the patient must have learned how to do self-hypnosis.

- A discussion must take place before the hypnotic session into which the age progression is introduced. The therapist learns in this discussion what kind of image or images would represent to the patient "a better, healthier desired, or at least, acceptable setting" in her life.
- Trance is facilitated— "age progression is hypnotically facilitated by 'time travel' into a specific time in the future."
- The therapist deliberately enhances the future experience for the patient by guiding the patient into a focus upon "visual, auditory, touch, smell, and taste senses." This may create a "vivification" of a future event.

(p. 83)

These experiences are amplified by ego-strengthening suggestions of Hartland (1965, 1971) and Torem (1990) that emphasize "positive thinking and positive feelings of joy and pride in reaching a solution to a specific problem. This is also accompanied by suggestions for a sense of health, strength, accomplishment, and a sense of inner resourcefulness and creativity in coping with life's stresses" (Torem, 1990, p. 83). The therapist then directs the patient to store all the positive experiences and feelings and to internalize them.

As the patient is being brought back hypnotically to the present, she is told that she is taking with her, as a special gift, the "positive images, sensations, and feelings" that she is now bringing "back from the future" to help guide her into healing and recovery at every level of mind. Either during the hypnotic experience or after this experience and a discussion of it, the patient is given her homework assignment: to write about her experience. She will then read what she has written at her next therapy session.

Torem (1992) has found that this technique is of special value in replacing "symptoms of futurelessness, helplessness, and hopelessness" (p. 83) with "a sense of new hope, strength, inner resourcefulness, self-mastery, and a belief in one's recovery" (p. 83).

Torem's technique is extremely powerful for many reasons. One is that a view of the future that is enhanced with sensory components of sight, hearing, touch, and so on may become a true vivification. That is, that patient may actually relive the experience in a quite vivid way. This aspect of the experience is projective/evocative in that it ignites combinations of inner resources that manifest themselves in the experience. In addition to this, potent direct suggestion is added at a time when the patient is highly "programmable" because of her deep involvement in a hypnotic experience. The additional direct suggestion that she is bringing back a manifold of gifts with her into the present that can work at deep levels of mind brings resources from the future into the present. The patient's participation in discussion, self-hypnosis, and writing and reading about the experience reinforce it further.

The possibilities for hypnotic variations of this technique are very real. Patients can be asked to imagine the details of a future goal achieved, told that their very awareness of this kind of material from their unconscious minds has liberated it into the present, and prompted to reinforce their imaginative experiences by writing and discussing them. Although such interventions will be helpful with certain patients, it is doubtful that they will ever have the strength of the hypnotic technique.

The Future Self: The Napier Model

Nancy Napier (1990) has conceptualized the self as a complex system of parts including resource parts, of which "… the most versatile and useful is the future self" (p. 110). Napier claims to have been influenced by Ericksonian thinking. In trance she spontaneously encountered her own future self, and she has translated this into an exercise or script that can be used by many. The script is projective/evocative in the sense that there are many opportunities for patients to respond to it with their own material. Our only concern about the use of the script is that it invokes an *inner child*. This is a concept that has become very popular. However, from our standpoint, there is no *inner child*. There are internal child ego states that cannot ever be reduced to just one inner child part. Care must be taken in using this script prematurely with certain dissociative patients because the allusion to the "inner child" could activate child ego states who might be traumatized and incapable of participating in the exercise. We use Napier's (1990) script with certain patients with modifications to accommodate our ego-state orientation. Where the Napier (1990) script uses the term *child*, we substitute the words *some parts* or *parts of yourself*. We are careful not to use the word *child* as, at times, the part can appear as something else, such as an animal, a space creature, or as an adult.

It is important to keep in mind that Napier (1990) has emphasized *the essence and quality* of the impressions that occur during this experience. This is much more important than obsessive emphasis on the completeness and accuracy of the imagery obtained in trance. Here is Napier's (1990) script:

Discovering Your Future Self

From the back of your mind to the front of your mind, allow an impression to emerge, **now**, of a path. It represents your optimal life path, or whatever journey you're undertaking now.

Imagine yourself walking along this path. Notice the surface underfoot, is it hard? Soft? … What color is it? … Become aware of the feel of that surface as you move along …

Is the path a straight path? Can you see ahead in the direction you're going? Does the path curve? Go uphill? Downhill? … Simply become aware of the nature of the path and accept whatever comes to mind.

And, how about the surrounding environment? Notice the colors, shapes and textures around you …

Are there natural sounds and natural smells that come to mind? …

You might notice whether you're in sunlight or shade. Are there patterns of light and shadow that capture your attention? ...

You may find that there is a special feeling in the air itself. There may be a sense of anticipation, or curiosity, or even a kind of magical sparkle in the air. Simply notice how it feels as you walk along ...

This is your optimal path. It represents an important journey in your life, a journey you have decided to take ...

Remember that your conscious mind is a passenger on this journey. Allow it to wonder what you will discover as you go along.

Allow the child to join you now. Remember that this is the child's path as well. If you have mixed feelings about having the child there with you, just accept what comes into your experience. It's all important information about the quality and current state of your internal relationship with the child in you ...

You might take a moment, now, to become aware of the state of mind of the child who has joined you. This might be a child within you've met many times, and whom you know very well. Or, it may be a child who is new to you, a child who is ready to emerge now and become part of your healing process ...

Whatever the child's state of mind, simply accept it. You may be surprised to discover that there will be times when the child is even more eager than you are to go down the path. The child is perfectly safe here, so you can allow that child to run or explore, or to stay close.

If you discover that you or the child are reluctant to go forward on your optimal path, give yourself permission to wonder about what beliefs or fears may be holding you or the child back, now ...

If there is a protective part that is frightened by the prospect of going forward, make a note of it. Later, when you have time, you might want to work with the protective part to resolve any fears or beliefs it may have that it is dangerous to go forward ...

For now, move ahead a bit along the path, simply noticing how it feels to go forward ...

Take a moment, now, and look back and see how far you've come. You might also become aware of the quality of the environment you've left behind.... Of what it used to be like to be there. You might be surprised at how far you've come ...

And, now, look forward again and begin to move ahead on your optimal path. Be sure to keep the child in your awareness, offering encouragement if it's needed.

Remind yourself that every step you take on this path is a step towards something you seek to achieve ... towards healing, empowerment, recovery. Let yourself know that each step along the path represents an affirmation to your unconscious that you want to move forward in your life, that you are moving.

Notice, now, that coming towards you from on up the path, from where you have yet to travel, someone is approaching. That someone is your future self, the part of you that has already made this journey ...

Simply let some impressions come from the back of your mind to the front of your mind as the future self comes nearer. Give yourself permission to just let the impressions come, with the thought that you can analyze them later, if you want.

Take a moment now to notice ... what kind of person is this? ... What is this person wearing? ... What do you notice about this person that is different from your present-day self? What do you think of this person? ... Are you comfortable or uncomfortable with your experience of your future self?

Take a moment, now, to become that person. Notice how it feels to be inside your future self ... What is it like to be that person?

Take a moment, now, to experience where, in your body, you feel the power and the stability of that future self most strongly. Your body is learning something important about how to create this experience as a reality in your present-day life ...

Once your body learns to recognize the feeling of being the future self you can recall that feeling often. Your body will remember.

If you were able to look at the world through the eyes of the future self what would you see? ... How would the world be different from the one you experience as your present-day self

Now, from the perspective of the future self take a moment to look at the present-day you, standing there. What feelings do you experience as you look at your present day-self through the eyes of this wiser, more mature part of you?

Remember the future self has learned much more about love and self acceptance than you know in your present-day consciousness. You may discover a feeling of love for yourself that is richer than what you've experienced before.... Or you may have some other experience that is deeply meaningful for you at this time in other ways ...

For a moment, now, become aware of how the child responds to the future self and how the future self responds to the child ...

Simply allow the response to be whatever it is right now. Use every opportunity to convey acceptance to the child. It's okay for that child to have honest feelings.

Perhaps for a moment, now, you might allow the future self to convey to the back of your mind anything that would be helpful for you to know in the present. Perhaps the future self would be willing to convey to you an impression of the next step you need to take in healing or resolving a situation, or in promoting a particular development. Remember to leave this alone consciously.... Simply let the back of your mind receive whatever the future self wishes to communicate. In your own best time and your own best ways, the unconscious will convey to your conscious mind whatever impressions are most helpful.

The memories of the future self become the blueprint for your journey, the map that you will follow unconsciously to get you from here to there.

Take a minute or so of clock time, now, to let the future self give you whatever impressions may be available. That minute of clock time can be all the time you need to receive whatever will be helpful for this journey.

As your present-day self now, perhaps you could ask your future self to become your guide.... Each day, you face many choices so that each takes you more surely towards your optimal future. And, if you like your future self and feel positive about your experience, you might want to say to the future self often, "I want to be you" ...

For now, it's time to come back, so leave a part of you on that path, moving forward with the future self and the child within. As you come back, remember that there is a part of you always on that path, always moving forward on your journey, no matter what your conscious mind may be doing, no matter what your day-to-day demands require of your attention.

Give yourself the suggestion, now, that by the time you open your eyes, you'll be as alert as you need to be for whatever is next on your agenda. Take a moment to wiggle your fingers and toes and come all the way back, now, and take a few minutes to write down your experience.

(p. 125; reprinted with permission)

Unstructured Hypnotic Age Progressions: The Phillips and Frederick Model

Phillips and Frederick (1992) became aware of the frequency with which hypnotic age progressions occurred spontaneously or in light trance or reverie in psychotherapy sessions. They began to use hypnotic age progressions that contained practically no structure with patients in formal trance as well. Phillips and Frederick (1995) view suggestions for age progressions as existing on a spectrum. At one end of the spectrum are the most structured, such as those found in rehearsal or imagery of goal achievement. The moderately structured suggestions, such as Erickson's (1954) crystal ball technique of pseudo-orientation in time, are in the middle of the spectrum. At the farther end of the continuum are suggestions that are relatively unstructured and sometimes indirect or even spontaneous. They do not view hypnosis as always being necessary for age progressions: "It is our experience that age progressions may be used with equal effectiveness in normal waking states without trance induction or can be further used by the therapist to induce an informal or more naturalistic trance experience" (Phillips & Frederick, 1992, p. 101).

Phillips and Frederick (1992) believe that unstructured hypnotic age progressions possess a hitherto unsuspected array of advantages: Positive age progressions are ego-strengthening; this can be especially true for the patient because the material of the progression comes from within her own plenum of internal resources rather than from a therapist. Unlike Erickson (1954), Phillips and Frederick (1992) do not want their patients to dissociate from the age progression material or have amnesia for it. Instead, it appears that they have striven to promote conscious–unconscious complementarity: "when an individual achieves a positive view of the future in a hypnotic state, she/he is already viewing an ego that has become more positively enhanced through the mirror of the mind" (Phillips & Frederick, 1992, p. 100). Positive age progression material can be evoked by the patient mentally when needed for anchoring, as an emblem of hope that can be reviewed periodically for ego-strengthening, or as symbolic of internal changes that are anticipated in the future. Like Erickson (1954), Phillips and Frederick (1992) believe that age progression experiences can be integrating, that they "also may serve as a valuable way of integrating abreacted material, affect, aspirations, and other therapy experiences" (p. 106).

Phillips and Frederick (1992) have identified the previously unrecognized clinical prognostic value of hypnotic age progressions. The nature of the progression can act as an indicator for the therapy process. This discovery was foreshadowed by the work of Rossi and Cheek (1988) who used hypnotic age progressions routinely with their psychosomatic patients. When patients could not generate views of a future time when symptom resolution had occurred, they were thought to need more preparatory work. "From this perspective, age progressions can serve as a barometer that can let the therapist know something about the direction of therapy" (Phillips & Frederick, 1992, p. 106). For example, patients who cannot generate positive age progressions may be struggling with ego impairment, may be immobilized by depression, or may be in the grips of a negative transference or a negative therapeutic reaction. The inability of a patient to generate a positive age progression should alert the therapist to evaluate the situation carefully.

The presence of a negative hypnotic age progression is an indicator that something more is needed in therapy. The elicitation of hypnotic age progressions in depressed and suicidal patients has previously been a technique that has been thought to be fraught with the danger of creating a self-fulfilling prophecy (Brown & Fromm, 1986). Hammond (1990d) has also cautioned that age progressions should be approached with caution in the depressed patient.

Phillips and Frederick (1992) recommend the use of hypnotic age progressions with most patients. Negative age progressions mean that treatment needs to be reevaluated because some additional element is needed. That element could be increased frequency of sessions, family therapy, support groups, 12-step work, a change in medication, or even partial or total hospitalization. Correct patient–therapist match needs to be included here as well.

It is our experience that hypnotic age progressions are invaluable prognostic tools; we use them frequently with our patients. We also educate our patients about the prognostic function of the age progression experiences in terms of how their therapy is going at the time as opposed to what its ultimate outcome shall be.

The Philips–Frederick model of unstructured hypnotic age progressions is ego-strengthening that is both projective and evocative. It allows the patient's deepest beliefs about himself to surface as resources. Because of the prognostic value of this kind of age progression, even negative progressions are resources. Therapists using this technique should be cautioned that amnesia is undesirable and depotentiates its usefulness. This is reemphasized because apparent misunderstandings about this matter can arise (Kessler & Miller, 1995).

Case Example: Nell (continued)

Nell continued to be incapable of distributing her son Tom's ashes. She agreed to have a complete medical work-up because her energy had been progressively diminishing, and she was having recurrent respiratory infections. A diagnosis of chronic fatigue immune deficiency syndrome (CFIDS) was made. The appearance of this illness was linked by her internist to leaking silicone breast implants that had replaced her breasts when she had had successful cancer surgery years earlier. After Nell had the implants removed, silicon granules were extruded into her scar tissue and appeared in her sweat.

Nell was no longer able to work. In her therapy, she continued to report behavior in which she acted like a door mat for any and all who wished to use her as such, and she continued to have serious symptoms of depression. She remained incapable of producing any kind of age progression. I (CF) continued with Menutherapy. Each time I saw Nell, I mentally reviewed what kinds of changes might be advantageous to her therapy and considered what kinds of interventions I could make that might be helpful to her. I did direct suggestive ego-strengthening, and I utilized the "Inner Strength" technique (McNeal, 1986, 1989; McNeal & Frederick, 1993). I also guided Nell through a hypnotic imagery exercise for grieving.

Although Nell continued to be symptomatic, I had a strong sense that I had become her lifeline, and that I had come to replace Tom as her nurturer. After her sessions I felt quite fatigued, and I had a strong subjective sense that she was borrowing my ego. One day Nell called me to say that she really wanted help. She said that up till then she had just been seeing me because that's what everyone had told her she needed to do, but that now she wanted the therapy for herself.

Nell initially had almost no memory of her childhood. Gradually her story unfolded with the help of uncovering hypnotic techniques including Ego State Therapy. She had been the child of alcoholic parents who had left her as an infant and a small child in the care of an older brother who resented her. She was locked in dark closets and physically and emotionally abused by him. Later, her mother attempted to get Nell into the Hollywood circuit as a child actress. Nell produced memory material of sexual abuse by her acting coach at age 4.

As Nell's therapy progressed, she was able to focus on the difficulties in her relationship with her husband. They began attending marriage counseling together for a while but stopped because he believed that he had no problems, would not make any changes, and saw joint therapy as a waste of money. Ultimately, he left her for an old high school girlfriend with whom he had not been in touch for many years.

Nell enjoyed living alone, free from her husband's nagging, and she bought two puppies as companions. One day Nell said to me: "You know, the house is on the market now ... and I have started looking at other houses ... smaller ones. I'm not sure whether I'll still live here at the Lake, but wherever I live, I want a small house like the one I saw yesterday ... with some kind of a view, and a garden ... and a fence for the dogs." She was smiling and her gaze was somewhat unfocused.

Shortly after the session in which she had produced this spontaneous age progression, Nell had occasion to deal with her husband again. This time she was appropriately assertive. This assertiveness then noticeably extended to other areas of her life. Her depression lifted, and she was finally able to distribute Tom's ashes.

In Nell's case it had been essential for me (CF) to *hang in* with Nell while she was unable to produce any age progression experiences (over 2 years). Their absence was not a reflection of an inadequacy in her treatment, but rather a product of her ego deficits.

Case Example: Patricia

Patricia had been periodically depressed and was quite unhappy about her job. She was also dealing with menopausal symptoms. When I (SM) asked Patricia to produce a view of the future, she reported that she could see nothing but darkness. Patricia and I decided that she should be evaluated for hormone replacement therapy as well as for the advisability of taking antidepressant medication.

Patricia was placed on Prozac (fluoxetine) by a psychiatrist. Her gynecologist started her on hormonal replacement therapy as well. Subsequently she was asked to have another view of the future. This time she saw herself as poised and confident as she lectured to her group of students.

Unstructured Age Progressions in Urgent and Emergent Situations

There is a long-standing tradition for the utilization of hypnotic techniques to manage urgent and emergent medical situations such as "highway accidents, severe burns, cardiac arrest, surgical shock, and in many cases health crises ..." (Frederick & Phillips, 1992, p. 90). One particular kind of hypnotherapeutic intervention that has been found to be particularly valuable in emergency situations is the hypnotic age progression. In addition to reports of their usefulness in medical emergencies (Rossi & Cheek, 1988), they have been documented as quite useful in psychiatric emergencies as well. Kluft (1983) and Torem, Gilbertson, and Kemp (1990) reported the successful use of hypnotic age progressions in the emergency management of Multiple Personality Disorder (MPD; now called Dissociative Identity Disorder, DID) patients. Torem (1987b, 1989) also reported on the utilization of hypnotic age progressions in a number of psychiatric crisis situations, including severe depression and dissociative regressions. Frederick and Phillips (1992) have reported their effectiveness as interventions with acute psychosomatic situations.

Patients facing the overwhelming physical symptoms of psychosomatic disorders as well as patients in suicidal and other serious psychological crises are often in life-threatening situations. Their conscious beliefs, often repeated and invested with highly charged views of frightening and dismal futures, offer nothing to help them weather their crises, and they reinforce negative belief systems already associated with their illnesses. Frederick and Phillips (1992) concluded that patients in such situations, who are usually generating negative age progressions at the conscious level, do not know what their deepest beliefs might truly be. The hypnotic age progressions helped put them in touch with the strong internal resources of their deepest positive inner beliefs. The resultant ego-strengthening and integrative effects helped stabilize patients so that they could do further necessary psychodynamic work concerning their illness.

It is safe to say that few of us living in today's complex and rapidly changing technological society really know the nature of our unconscious beliefs about many matters. There are probably several reasons for this that are recognizable to hypnotherapists. One has to do with a lack of objectivity that frequently appears to exist at the conscious level. Another involves the usual inaccessibility of deep unconscious information to the conscious mind. Thus, Erickson's (1954) belief that the conscious mind was not capable of knowing what an individual's attainable goals might be takes on special meaning in the presence of life-threatening acute situations and emergent crises.

Hypnotic Age Progressions: The Ego-State Perspective

Another reason we might be uncertain about what we believe is that different aspects of our personality might hold totally different beliefs about the same topic.

We commonly call such a situation *ambivalence*. However, this ambivalence can be a reflection of internal personality conflict, or ego-state conflict as described in chapter 4. From the standpoint of Ego State Therapy the ego is in a state of integration when the component ego states are working together harmoniously and sharing their consciousnesses. At such times, there might appear to be more unanimity of belief systems. However, the very complexity of the human personality is intended by the metaphor of ego states. The ego states can be thought of as holding the totality of the personality's affect and impulse (McNeal & Frederick, 1995). It is not surprising that variation and contradiction can be present at times, even in the most integrated individuals. Patients in psychosomatic and other psychiatric emergencies are seldom well integrated.

The calm, objective mind that Erickson (1980b) respected so much as a premier problem-solving resource does not exist in many individuals, even in the hypnotic state, because they have such poor ego strength and, because of developmental difficulties, lack the ability to soothe and calm themselves (McNeal & Frederick, 1994). They may be able to enter trance; however, once they are there, their minds continue to race, and often much time is required for deepening.

The ego-strengthening properties of hypnotic age progressions (Phillips & Frederick, 1992) may lie, partially, in their ability to offer anchors of internal support and safety by putting the patient in touch with deep internal resources on a fairly rapid basis. They may also ego-strengthen because they possess innate self-soothing abilities (McNeal & Frederick, 1994) and may even offer the patient a mechanism for transmuting and containing frightening affect (McNeal & Frederick, 1995), integrating abreacted or conflicted material (Phillips & Frederick, 1992), or bridging "the gap between insight and the actualization of change" (McNeal & Frederick, 1993, p. 177). The following case examples are from Frederick (1995d).

Case Example: Geoffrey

Geoffrey had been sent to me (CF) by his family physician for the treatment of depression. Geoffrey had "maybe accidentally" driven his car off the road, wrecking it. Just before the accident he had been looking at Lake Tahoe and thinking of a friend who had drowned when they were both children.

Geoffrey's clinical picture and history were compatible with a diagnosis of Bipolar Disorder, and a SPEC scan performed by the neurologist to whom I had referred him confirmed this. However, Geoffrey's childhood had been traumatic (he recalled ongoing, brutal physical abuse from his alcoholic father and strange kisses from his paternal grandmother). We agreed that there might be posttraumatic issues as well and that in his therapy we would be sensitive to this possibility.

Geoffrey's wife, Linda, was a source of great concern to him as she had many psychotic features including religious delusions (and possibly hallucinations). As she anticipated leaving Geoffrey for a man whose affections for her existed only in her own mind, she impulsively cashed their IRAs so that she could take half the money and "feel more financially secure." The events of the session I describe here occurred shortly after Geoffrey had learned from his accountant that Linda's cashing of the IRAs had cost him nearly $10,000—money he had put aside to buy a richly deserved new car. Linda had also inherited a great sum of money and announced to Geoffrey that she was leaving him in mid-June and taking their son Jasper with her to another state. She also continued to tell him repeatedly that she had had a message from God that he would be dead by June because he had failed to "mature in Christ." Geoffrey had found himself believing her.

Three nights before his session Geoffrey was awakened from a sound sleep by a loud explosion in his head. He thought that some terrible physical event had occurred within his brain such as a lethal stroke. He stayed in bed late the next morning, experiencing his thinking as fragmented. It is interesting that he did not get in touch with me or with his family physician.

When he was able to tell me about the events of the previous week, Geoffrey also told me that he thought he was losing it, that is, having a mental breakdown that was going to necessitate hospitalization lest he "lose control" of himself. I was able to focus on a therapy theme that had been emerging—a pattern that indicated that he appeared to believe he had to suffer alone and not ask for help when he felt overwhelmed. As we continued to find out more about what was going on with him, I asked him if he had had any angry feelings. At this point he looked as if he would explode. "So that's it! That's what was going on!" Geoffrey connected the explosion in his head that had awakened him with his angry feelings, but now he faced another problem. "What do I do with all this?"

I helped Geoffrey use the hypnotic technique, the silent abreaction to release this negative affect. With this technique the entranced patient is guided to a remotely placed rock pile. There he/she wields an imaginary sledge hammer, breaking and smashing the rock and shouting anything he/she wishes mentally while recalling the incidents and people who angered him. As Geoffrey worked silently on the rock pile, I noticed that his face was red and sweat glistened on his forehead. His facial expressions displayed fury. When, after a very long time, he gave me the signal that he was finished, I led him away from the rock pile and invited him to have an unstructured hypnotic age progression.

When Geoffrey came out of trance, he told me about his experiences at the rock pile and how totally caught up he felt in these feelings. In the age progression he saw himself with his son in the pacific northwest in the autumn. The leaves were turning. I was somewhere in the scene. Geoffrey was amazed at how much better he felt, how much serenity he was experiencing, and how much hope he had.

At the following session he showed that he had maintained his even keel. This time an age progression resulted in the therapist being replaced by a blonde woman who was his partner. His son, still present, was 11 or 12. He saw his wife spinning in a circle in the air, looking terrific with yet another of her face lifts, connected to her narcissism rather than to them.

Case Example: Patsy

An earlier stage of Patsy's case has been reported elsewhere (Phillips & Frederick, 1995). Patsy suffered an industrial injury and was diagnosed with bilateral carpal tunnel syndrome and reflex sympathetic dystrophy (RSD). She had also developed a major depression and displayed many signs of a dissociative disorder.

Patsy's emotional symptoms were directly related to her stress level with which they fluctuated. However, the severe pain she experienced as a result of the RSD appeared to be a result of the worsening of her physical condition. There was a reason for this: although they authorized her psychiatric treatment with me, the new insurance company that handled her worker's compensation case would not authorize appropriate treatment for her physical condition. About a month before the episode described below, Patsy had received a copy of a letter her orthopedist had sent to the insurance company. In it he told them that he was withdrawing from her case because they would not authorize the treatments he had prescribed as necessary and he could not continue to assume responsibility for treating her.

Patsy subsequently made contact with a physician she knew. He took her into his pain clinic without insurance authorization and made it clear to her that he would arrange for her to see a reflex sympathetic dystrophy (RSD) specialist at Stanford if she did not improve. Pain control had always been a significant part of our work, and, in spite of a great deal of resistance to self-care, Patsy had worked on increasing her comfort at home quite successfully with glove anaesthesia. Although she was a dissociator, we had never been successful in getting her to dissociate the pain or to utilize other pain control maneuvers.

Because of the worsening of her physical condition, the pain had outgrown Patsy's ability to control it. She began to entertain suicidal thoughts. Three days before I saw her, she had had to go the hospital emergency room because her hands had become grossly swollen and painful. At home she told her husband that she would end her life soon if she could not get relief.

I believed Patsy to be genuinely suicidal when I saw her. After we had discussed her situation, I invited her to enter trance. This was an interactive trance in which I reminded her that she had told me she believed there was a physician somewhere who could help her with her hands. I then activated her ego states, with whom I had been in contact for some time. They were shy and presented themselves as lights of different colors. In this session the Red Light who carried Patsy's anger was activated. This ego state communicated through Patsy's lips that her rage with her former employer, the insurance company, and the insurance company's attorneys and others was making her condition worse. The Red Light did not want to give up this anger, and was not interested in the silent abreaction (see chap. 14 for a description of this technique).

I (CF) helped Patsy to have an Inner Love experience (a projective/ evocative ego-strengthening technique that is described in chap. 9). This was quite successful. (Please see a description of the application of this technique in Patsy's case in chap. 9). I decided to increase Patsy's relaxation and ask her to have an unstructured hypnotic age progression: "Just let your mind drift forward effortlessly into time to a time when all of these medical problems have been resolved." Patsy's response was dramatic.

"I don't know how I know this but I do know that there's a research project on RSD at Stanford and that they will help me. I'm on a beautiful cloud now, Cloud Nine. I don't think I've ever felt so relaxed, ever. There is a golden light on me and it's warming me. I've never felt this before. My right hand is hurting me really bad, but I don't care at all.... This is the best I've ever felt ... my left hand is hurting like a son of a bitch, but it doesn't matter."

I checked ideomotorically whether this was a view of the future. The answer was "Yes." I asked if any particular part had sent this future experience. The answer was "Yes." I asked which part had done this. The answer floated into Patsy's mind. "It's the Red Light ... it's decided to help, to change the anger into this. I can keep positive thoughts now." Other parts indicated that they were now less frightened of the Red Light and would be more able to work together to produce dissociation of pain as well as hopefulness.

After Patsy was out of trance, she reported having had a profound and dramatic experience, of having perceived a positive future and having been given something to hold onto until it was realized.

There is probably no time when beliefs are more crucial in the outcome of a series of events than in medical and psychiatric emergencies. The power of belief to control a person's well-being was noted by Walter Cannon (1957), the physiologist who is known for his work with the autonomic nervous system. Cannon reported how native tribesmen could sicken and die as a result of their beliefs that the curses of witch doctors leveled at them were lethal. Cannon (1957) attributed this *voodoo death* to the overwhelming action of the parasympathetic nervous system on the physiology of the afflicted tribesmen.

During emergencies the integrity and existence of the psychological and/or physical organism is threatened, and fight-or-flight mechanisms are activated (Cannon, 1957). Although it would be desirable for ego states concerned with mobilizing the individual in the direction of survival to preponderate, the unfortunate truth may be that the most childlike and frightened ego states may prevail at such times. Their messages may be conveyed with great sonority so that their voices of fear and panic may drown those of the more mature ego states who constitute a reservoir of inner resources for the patient in an emergency. At such times the patient may not be able to recognize positive, resourceful ego states that may be present because these ego states are communicating in a variety of nonverbal ways (Frederick, 1994e; Frederick & Phillips, 1996). It is also possible that destructive ego states whose need is to purvey negative messages of doom and destruction may be activated (Frederick, 1995d).

The hypnotic age progression often gives the patient an opportunity to bypass both immature and negative ego states and reach the deepest reservoir of mature ego states associated with strength and survival. When they cannot be accessed, this is a prognostic sign that something additional is needed in the treatment situation. It was Frederick's (1995d) most recent experience that it can be profitable to discover which ego state or states has produced the negative progression so that this can be used as a springboard for further work.

The hypnotic age progression also ego-strengthens because it affords greater objectivity to the internal family and to the patient as a whole. Ego-state involvement in the treatment of reflex sympathetic dystrophy (RSD) has been reported by Gainer (1992). In the case of Patsy it would seem that the age progression at this crisis point in her life became a fitting stage upon which a heretofore malevolent ego state had an opportunity to turn insight into change—a function of many ego-strengthening procedures (McNeal & Frederick, 1993).

Geoffrey's and Patsy's cases illustrate the self-soothing attributes of age progressions as well as the greater objectivity afforded by the hypnotic state. Like Patsy, Geoffrey entertained negative beliefs about the future on a conscious level. He felt hexed by his wife's prophecies that he would die and had begun to live them out symbolically through his symptoms. In the emergency age progression he saw himself alive long after the time of his prophesied death, supported by therapy as evidenced by the presence of the therapist and having a good experience with his son. In the progression the following week he saw himself continuing to live and having moved into a normal life with a new life partner.

Hypnotic age progressions are vital, dynamic tools for dealing with psychiatric and psychosomatic emergencies. Positive age progressions soothe, produce greater objectivity, and allow frightened and negative ego states to be reassured by more stronger and more mature ones, and promote integration. They may also be, at times, the vehicle for the resolution of ego-state conflict. Negative hypnotic age progressions also give messages that are relevant to healing (Phillips & Frederick, 1992). In this case the message—a prognostic one about the therapeutic situation—should always be explained to the patient. In urgent and emergency situations they can be of inestimable value if the hypnotherapist is willing to summon the healing messenger of time.

The next chapter looks at another powerful projective/evocative ego-strengthening technique: Inner Strength. It examines the nature of the ego that is being strengthened by ego-strengthening procedures from several theoretical viewpoints.

Chapter 6

The Ego

Its Composition

When we discuss ego-strengthening, one might wonder what it is we are talking about. What is the ego-strengthening process? What is the structure and function of the ego, and to what ego are we referring? There is a myriad of different concepts and definitions of the ego, and different theories look at ego development through different lenses. Here we review some of the major theoretical orientations about ego development in general and how developmental arrests can produce pathologies that impel individuals to seek psychotherapeutic treatment. Ego-strengthening is then considered in the context of psychotherapy that seeks to repair developmental arrests through strengthening the ego.

Cognitive Development

Cognitive development refers to the mental functions involved in understanding and dealing with the world around us: perception, language, concept formation, abstraction, problem solving, intelligence, and thinking. When a child is born she comes into the world with a central nervous system that has synthesizing functions (i.e., mental equipment) ready to organize perceptions and responses to the environment. This innate organizational process offers the substratum for the structure of the ego (Horner, 1995). One of the major contributors to our understanding of organizational processes was Jean Piaget who systematically studied cognitive development in young children.

Among Piaget's contributions were his descriptions of the complementary processes of *assimilation and accommodation, differentiation and integration. Assimilation* involves taking in new experiences and modifying them to fit with existing mental structure, whereas *accommodation* changes or adjusts preexisting structure to correspond to perceptions of reality. Experience is organized into patterns that Piaget called schema. Through the process of generalization, the schema comes to represent a class of experiences that, as the capacity to discriminate reality increases, may be divided into several new schema (i.e., the schema of a person may be divided into male and female). These schema form the basis for concepts of self and object, good and bad

DOI:10.4324/9781003442585-6

self, good and bad object, and other object relations concepts (Horner, 1995; Piaget, 1936/1952).

Piaget is credited for tracing cognitive development systematically and comprehensively through developmental stages as the child grows and continuously interacts with her environment. Piaget studied children through extensive naturalistic and experimental observations. Mussen (1963) summarizes Piaget's stages as beginning with *sensori-motor operations* involving coordination of reflexes and responses and moving into the stage of *concrete operations*, where imagery, symbolic functions such as language, and intuitive thought begin to develop. Dealing with verbal expressions of logical relationships requires *formal operations* that a child normally develops around the age of 11 or 12. This ability to apply logical rules and reasoning to abstract problems is "the essence of intellectual growth" according to Piaget (1936/1952), and is fully developed by the age of 15. Perceiving, reacting, responding, assimilating, accommodating, generalizing, differentiating, integrating, and verbalizing are all cognitive organizing functions of the ego.

Psychosexual and Psychosocial

Freud (1923/1964) referred to the ego as "a coherent organization of mental processes" to which "consciousness is attached." He went on to say that

> … the ego controls the approaches to motility: that is, to the discharge of excitations into the external world; it is the mental agency which supervises all its own constituent processes, and which goes to sleep at night, though even then it exercises the censorship in dreams.
>
> (p. 7)

Freud believed that some of the ego was unconscious and not sharply separated from the id. He viewed the ego as the part of the id that has been modified by the influence of the external world, and brings the influence of the external world to bear upon the id, substituting the *reality principle* for the *pleasure principle* of the id. Perception is to the ego as instinct is to the id. The ego represents reason, whereas the id contains the passions.

The third part of Freud's structural model is the superego. According to Freud's model, the superego emerges from the process of the resolution of the Oedipus complex. The superego is the internal representative of our relations to our parents—that is, what we admire and fear, and take into ourselves.

Freud (1923/1964) described the ego as having strengths and weaknesses:

> The ego develops from perceiving instincts to controlling them, from obeying instincts to inhibiting them … however, we see this same ego as a poor creature owing service to three masters and consequently menaced by three

dangers: from the external world, from the libido of the id, and from the severity of the superego.

(p. 46)

The ego is also the seat of anxiety and fears of being overwhelmed or annihilated. The ego employs the defense mechanisms to ward off threatening affect. The task of psychoanalysis then is to increase the efficiency of the ego in its internal mediation tasks and to enhance its effectiveness in the world.

Hartmann's Conflict-Free Sphere of the Ego

Freud's emphasis on the importance of the ego became the impetus for ego psychology which expanded the concept of the ego even further. Anna Freud (1936/1946) enumerated a number of defense mechanisms that the ego employed to deal with anxiety created by the pressure of id impulses and unconscious wishes. Because these defenses were seen as resistances in analytic treatment, even more attention became focused on the development and functioning of the ego.

Heinz Hartmann (1961) was an ego psychologist who emphasized the autonomy of the ego. He believed that some of the functions of the ego, such as memory, perception, and motility, do not develop from the frustration of drives but are developed autonomously from birth. In contrast with Freud's view, that the ego emerged out of the id, Hartmann saw the ego as developing separately. Summers (1994) described ego development in Hartmann's theory as having two sources: inborn "apparatuses of *primary ego autonomy*" and the frustration of the drives, resulting in *secondary autonomy* (Hartmann, 1961). Hartmann theorized that the ego is a group of functions that include defenses and adaptive, healthy mechanisms that he referred to as the *synthetic function* of the ego. Since these ego functions exist apart from frustration and conflict, he called them the *conflict-free ego sphere.*

Hartmann is considered to be a transitional theorist because he was the first to make a strong case for the importance of reality and the development that comes from the infant's interactions with the environment and the adults in her environment (Greenberg & Mitchell, 1983). He was interested in delineating the mechanisms that enabled human survival. He set the stage for later modifications of drive theory by elaborating and adding to it without completely abandoning classical drive theory.

Object Relations and Self Psychology

The elaboration and expansion of classic psychoanalytic drive theory into different models such as ego psychology, object relations, and self psychology has produced new terms and redefinition of older terms. To understand the similarities and differences among these various theoretical approaches, it may be helpful to distinguish among some of the terms that are sometimes used inter-changeably. Hamilton (1988) defines an *object* as "a person, place, thing, idea, fantasy, or memory invested with emotional energy" (p. 7). An *internal object* is a mental representation, an image, idea, fantasy, feeling, or memory pertaining to a person, place, or thing, whereas an *external object* is an actual person, place, or thing. Freud introduced the term, and Klein (1948) developed one of the earliest theories of *object relations* or the relationships between internal fantasies of the self and internal fantasies of objects.

Object Relations

Freud first introduced the term *object* to mean the object toward which the impulse is directed (Fairbairn, 1954). Melanie Klein's conceptions of *internalized objects* led to theories of *object relations*, involving relationships of the ego to its internalized objects. Whereas Klein (1948) focused on unconscious fantasies of internalized objects, it was really Fairbairn (1952, 1954) who extended the theories to include the relationships of the ego with objects that were internalized from the child's actual relationships with its caregivers in the real world.

According to Greenberg and Mitchell (1983), Klein departed from Freud. For Freud libido and aggression, not love and hate, are the origins of experience; for Klein love and hate are the basic motivational forces within the system. In Freud's model, the ego is neutral in relation to the drives, and the task of the ego is to mediate among the id, the superego, and the outside world. For Klein, the ego is involved in internal dynamic struggles involving love and the life instinct. Klein's ego is derived from the life instinct; as the ego becomes more identified with love, the id becomes identified with hate. The ego is identified with good objects and fears the destruction of itself and all good objects by the id.

In contrast to Freud's psychosexual stages, Klein used the term *positions*. This term referred to patterns of anxieties and defenses. The Kleinian positions reflect different patterns of loving and hateful relations with others. The *paranoid-schizoid position* organizes loving relations and hateful relations as separate from each other. The mechanism of splitting involves fantasies of an object as good or bad. In the *depressive position*, loving and hating are unified, and the object is recognized as a whole person who can be both good and bad. According to Klein, it is the working through of the depressive position that strengthens the ego, by growth and by assimilation of good objects.

Fairbairn replaces Freud's libido and aggression as motivational principles with libido and reaction to libidinal frustration. Fairbairn's libidinal ego is the part of the ego that has not given up unsatisfied longings of infantile dependence. It is hopeful, and, in its attachment to an exciting object, clings to unfulfilled longings for contact with the mother. "The anti-libidinal ego is the part of the ego that becomes the repository for all the hatred and destructiveness which accumulate as a consequence of the frustration of libidinal longing" (Greenberg &

Mitchell, 1983, p. 166). The anti-libidinal ego becomes identified with maternal rejection and withholding. This part of the ego is an internal saboteur and can produce self-destructive behavior. In Fairbairn's model, the protagonists in internal struggle are relational units, consisting of a portion of the ego and a portion of the child's relations to the parents, experienced as internal objects. Through internalization of good objects it would be possible, eventually, for the ego to release its attachment to internalized bad objects. Fairbairn appears to espouse a parts theory of the ego (see chap. 4).

The theories of Winnicott (1953, 1956/1958, 1962/1965, 1975) are important in terms of how psychotherapy can modify object relations. These are considered further in chapter 7.

Definition of the Self

Developmentally, the ability to discriminate differences in objects precedes the ability to be aware of oneself as a separate entity distinct from her mother. The concept of *self* is also an internal mental representation pertaining to one's own person. It is biological in that it is in the body and has visual, kinesthetic, and emotional components. Self-representations are private but can be described and may be conscious or unconscious. The self is the sense of *me* in object relations theory (Hamilton, 1988).

Hamilton (1988) defines *object relations* as "the interactions of the self and internal or external objects" (p. 13). Object relations units consist of a self-representation and an internal object-representation connected by a drive or affect. Developmentally, the earliest is the *selfobject*—the blurring of self and other, which is characteristic of symbiosis. Self psychology is a particular branch of object relations theory of which Kohut (1971) is the best known proponent.

Self Psychology

Self psychology theorists categorize psychological structure as *self-object experiences* (Wolf, 1988, p. 28). Here *selfobject* is defined as the "subjective aspect of a self-sustaining function performed by a relationship of self to objects who by their presence or activity evoke and maintain the self and the experience of selfhood" (Wolf, 1988, p. 184). Selfobject experiences (St. Clair, 1986; Wolf, 1988) are those that give cohesion to the self. In simpler language this means that the individual internalizes her interpersonal experiences with others. Pathology results when the environment fails to be appropriately responsive. This creates a structural deficit. The goal of treatment then is "to strengthen the self so that the person is willing and able to actively plunge into the rough-and-tumble of everyday life, not without fear but nevertheless undeterred" (Wolf, 1988, p. 102).

Repair of the structural deficit through the therapeutic relationship strengthens the structure of the self so that the person can tolerate "less than optimal selfobject experiences without a significant loss of self-esteem" (Wolf, 1988, p. 102). A strengthened self will be able to integrate previously dissociated affects and develop whole object relationships (i.e., object constancy). A strengthened ego integrates good and bad aspects of self-representations and good and bad object representations. The world is no longer black and white, and split object relations are replaced by whole object relations. The self-psychology framework emphasizes the empathy and understanding provided by the therapist as essential in repairing structural deficits and strengthening the self.

Definition of the Ego

According to Hamilton (1988) the ego cannot be experienced subjectively because it is "the observer within the observed." The ego *functions* (i.e., it perceives, thinks, acts, etc.). It is the organizer of experience, not the organization, nor the self. In *The Ego and the Id* Freud (1923) discussed the concept of the ego as having an organizing function and as equivalent to the self. Freud did not distinguish between ego as organizer and ego as system or self as described by Hamilton (1988).

Hartmann (1961, 1965), considered the founder of ego psychology theory, elaborated on the concept of the ego and considered it to be both system and organizer without distinguishing between organizer and organization. He viewed the ego as "the agent of centralized functional control" (Hamilton, 1988), and "emphasized the functions of differentiation, synthesis, integration, and balancing in the realms of perception, cognition, impulse control, and motor function" (Hamilton, 1988, p. 22).

Other object relations theorists have had somewhat different concepts of the ego. Summers (1994) analyzed Klein's use of *ego* as analogous to the concept of self. Federn (1952) retained Freud's description of the ego and added the concept of *ego boundary* to which Summers has referred as *selfobject boundary*. In his self-psychology theory Kohut (1971) essentially discarded the concept of ego, and Kernberg (1982) also is ambiguous concerning the ego as self and as system.

Archetypal or Transpersonal

In abstracting Carl Jung's writings about the phenomenology of the self, Campbell (1971) shows Jung to view the ego as "the complex factor to which all conscious contents are related. It forms, as it were, the centre of the field of consciousness; and in so far as this comprises the empirical personality, the ego is the subject of all personal acts of consciousness" (p. 139). The ego arises from the "collision between the somatic factor and the environment, and once established as a subject, goes on developing from further collisions with the outer world and the inner" (Campbell, 1971, p. 141). The ego is responsible for all successful attempts at adaptation. "It is the ego that serves to light up the entire system, allowing it to become conscious and thus to be realized" (Jung, 1964, p. 162). The total personality that includes unconscious processes is called the self and includes the ego as a part of the whole. Jung believed that the self can only be completely grasped through the investigation of one's own dreams. Consciously coming to terms with the self comprises the process of *individuation*.

The unconscious, according to Jung, is divided into the *personal unconscious*, where the contents are collected over the lifetime of the individual, and the *collective unconscious*, whose contents are archetypes present from the beginning. Those archetypes capable of exerting the most disturbing influence on the ego are the *shadow*, the *animus*, and the *anima*. The *shadow* can be known from exploring the personal unconscious, because it contains the *dark* aspects of personality. The *anima* represents the feminine element in a man's personality. The *animus* is the masculine element in a woman's personality. They are usually projected on others and appear in dreams. The ego, which contains the *complexes*, must come to terms with the unconscious and allow the *transcendent function*, which is the coming together of conscious and unconscious mental contents (Jung, 1964). The ego and the unconscious mind engage in dialogue and wrestle with each other, much as two people with equal rights might do (Campbell, 1971).

There appears to be some similarity in the manner in which Jung conceptualizes the archetypes and Federn's (1952) concept of ego states. Jung saw the archetypes as patterns of instinctual behavior from the collective unconscious. They could be thought of as corresponding to ego states that develop as part of the normal process of growth and maturation.

Jung was also interested in the transpersonal in the sense of spirituality and man's connection to a higher power in the universe (see chap. 15). He has written on "the spiritual problem of modern man" and the differences between Eastern and Western thinking (Campbell, 1971). He observed that the goal of some Eastern religions is to dispense with the ego, but he believed that would be impossible because there has to be someone there who is observing and meditating. He felt that emphasis on an egoless mental condition was a reflection of Eastern religions' need to deemphasize the importance of the ego. From this standpoint, the person need not be identified with the mind or even consider consciousness to be all that important. Primarily, Jung emphasized that individuals in the Western world tend to become overly concerned with acquisitions in the external material world, rather than with one's inner or transpersonal world.

Ego-Strengthening

In this book, the *ego* is defined as the agent or organizer, while the *self* applies to the organization or system that is experienced or perceived by the ego. The ego can be thought of as the "I" and the self as "me."

Ego-strengthening from a classical Freudian viewpoint extends the sphere and control of the ego over the id and superego as it is freed from early life conflicts (Freud, 1932/1964, 1940/1964a). Hartmann (1961, 1965) emphasized the healthy adaptive ego functions including the conflict-free sphere of the ego. From his perspective, ego-strengthening could occur as a natural developmental process. With the emergence of ego psychology, the ego was then considered to have a central role in personality organization; the degree of health or pathology depended on the ability of the ego and its strength to handle conflicting demands of the id, superego, and reality (Summers, 1994).

Federn's (1952) concepts of ego states and Watkins and Watkins' (1997) development of ego state theory (see chap. 4) would explain ego-strengthening as increasing the interplay between positive, healthy ego states and extending their influence over more childlike and less constructive ego states, such that the more positive ego states are executive more of the time (Frederick, 1992). The maturation of ego states also strengthens the ego.

From the Jungian point of view, ego-strengthening would involve facilitating the ego to be stronger than the pressure of the unconscious so as not to be overwhelmed and taken over by unconscious processes. The analyst can be a mediator in this process. The goal of Jungian analysis is to strip away the *persona*, the mask created from the collective psyche—so the person can arrive at individuation or self-realization (Jung, 1964).

Ego-strengthening has to do with the process of extending the scope and influence of the ego and increasing the effectiveness of ego functions. When ego-strengthening has occurred, the organization of ego functions has become stronger and more capable, and the self is experienced as stronger, more adequate, and more effective in coping with both the internal and external worlds. When a person speaks in terms such as, "I have found myself," "I've come back to myself," and "I now have faith and trust in myself," she is expressing her awareness of a stronger sense of self, and we can assume that ego-strengthening has taken place.

How ego-strengthening occurs has to do, developmentally, with the creation of psychological structure. Object relations theorists believe that humans are innately oriented toward object contact (Fairbairn, 1952, 1954, 1958). The development of self-structure in this view is a product of the internalization of attachments in the form of object relationships (Fairbairn, 1958; Summers, 1994), so that the way the child perceives and responds to the environment is critical to the formation of psychic structure. According to Summers, *pathology* is a product of distorted object relations that interfere with the structure and functioning of the self. The goal of treatment then is to "change the structure of the patient's object relations in such a manner that the self can function more effectively" (Summers, 1994, p. 361). Interpretation of and provision for a new relationship are the tasks of the object relations therapist. The therapist can connect with the patient in a new way, getting in touch with the unengaged parts of the self, confronting the resulting anxiety, and forming a new kind of attachment that results in higher functioning object relations structures (Greenberg & Mitchell, 1983).

We can say that the ego of the patient participates in such a way that successful treatment results in a stronger ego and more healthy sense of self.

Integration of disparate personality parts is also considered to be a goal of treatment. When working with patients with dissociative disorders and when utilizing an ego-state model of treatment, integration and formation of a new identity is the final stage of treatment (see chap. 4). We can say that the regressed parts of the ego and the split-off parts of the ego have become transformed and matured to the point of integration. As the ego becomes stronger, integration becomes more possible and the result of integration is an even stronger ego.

Regression in the Service of the Ego

Guntrip (1969) was an object relations theorist who believed that his concept of the regressed ego marked the final shift in psychoanalytic theory from drive psychology to object relations theory. Guntrip took Fairbairn's concept of the libidinal ego and divided it into an active, oral, and sadomasochistic ego and a re-gressed ego. This division represents the difference between the former—an ego invested in bad object relations—and the latter, "an ego seeking to return to the prenatal safety of no object relations" (Summers, 1994, p. 61). Guntrip believed that all psychopathology had at its core the desire to regress to an egoless state. For analysis to be successful, the therapist needed to reach these repressed long-ings so that the buried personality could emerge into the therapeutic relationship. Since he felt this could only occur when the patient felt safe, Guntrip emphasized the importance of the quality of the therapeutic relationship. According to Gun-trip, the regressed ego was "a product of trauma in the child's longing for love and its offering of love. It is the original unsatisfactory relationship that leads to the splitting-off of the infantile longings into the buried part of the self" (Summers, 1994, p. 63). If this traumatized part is to emerge again, a new relationship must be experienced in which the patient feels safe enough not to fear being injured again. Guntrip's emphasis on the therapeutic relationship was influenced by Win-nicott. However, according to Guntrip, with the patient's emerging individuality comes renewed threat because the regressed ego experiences the object contact from which it withdrew. So the ego again craves regression and fears the very relationship it needs (Guntrip, 1969). The analyst needs to be patient while the patient's ego gradually becomes strengthened and able to tolerate the new rela-tionship. Guntrip's concepts anticipated Kohut's concept of allowing the patient's defenses to form the transference relationship until they can be gradually relin-quished in the context of the new relationship (Summers, 1994).

In writing about clinical hypnosis and hypnotherapy, Brown and Fromm (1986) have characterized hypnosis as *regression in the service of the ego*, a concept defined by Kris (1951, 1972) and applied as an explanation of hypnosis by Gill and Brenman (1959). Kris' concept appears to be similar to Hartmann's (1961) *adaptive regression*, which meant withdrawal into the inner world of imagery, fantasy, memory, and thinking and a return to the external world with improved mastery. According to Gill and Brenman, the patient in a hypnotic trance can let reality fade into the background of awareness, enter into the inner world of imagery, gain insight, and then return to reality, often able to act with improved mastery. Because hypnosis is an altered state, it allows the patient to function more with the unconscious ego and explore one's inner world. It can help the patient to become aware of previously unrecognized resources within herself (Brown & Fromm, 1986).

Because of the regression in service of the ego and increased access to the unconscious, therapeutic results can be obtained faster than in the waking state. However, the patient is also less vigilant and defended, requiring the nature of the hypnotherapeutic relationship to be extremely important—even more so than in traditional psychotherapy. Thus, it needs to be emphasized that the therapist utilizing hypnosis needs to be well trained in both psychotherapy and hypnotherapy.

The Innate Drive for Survival as Reflected in Selfobjects

Classical drive theory viewed the drive for survival as innate and instinctive. Freud believed in only two major classes of instincts: the life instincts or *eros*, and the death instincts, or *thanatos* (Freud, 1923). Eros included the sexual instincts and the instincts for self-preservation. "The emergence of life would thus be the cause of the continuance of life" (Freud, 1923/1964, p. 31).

Object relations and self psychology theory hold that the earliest phase of infancy is a stage of physiological needs and tensions without awareness (Kohut, 1977). The mother responds to the baby and begins the process of formation of the self creating the first selfobject in the infant's experience. The object fulfills a necessary life-sustaining function that the self is unable to provide for itself (Summers, 1994). Then according to Wolf (1988), "The very emergence and maintenance of the self as a psychological structure depends on the continuing presence of an evoking-sustaining-responding matrix of selfobject experiences" (p. 28). Although Kohut (1971) sometimes referred to a selfobject as an external person filling important needs for the subject's self, such as approval and validation, selfobject, as used here, refers to an aspect of the self-image blurred with aspects of an internal object-image as described by Hamilton (1988).

Hamilton (1988) refers to the earliest object relations unit as a symbiotic selfobject in which there is little or no distinction between self and object. Symbiosis is the most undifferentiated selfobject and is traditionally associated with pleasant feelings such as love and the feeling of oneness, fusion, or merging. It is out of this symbiotic state that the self emerges. If the earliest selfobject experiences are empathic and appropriate, a healthy sense of self will develop. If the responses of the external selfobjects are not empathic, developmental arrests and pathology results (Kohut, 1977). Selfobject experiences need to be optimally frustrating—that is, not excessively frustrating or stimulating. If frustration or stimulation is excessive, the self will become threatened, erect defenses, and experience *disintegration anxiety*—the fear of loss of self, which Kohut believed underlines all pathology (Summers, 1994). Kohut felt that selfobject needs continued throughout life and that a goal of analysis is to replace archaic selfobject needs with mature selfobject needs, enabling patients to evoke needed responses from mature selfobjects (Summers, 1994).

Clinical hypnosis can be used to provide selfobject experiences that can be healing by creatively structuring the hypnosis to access positive experiences that may have been forgotten, to reframe experiences in a new way that can facilitate recovery, and to provide experiences that assist with the maturation of selfobjects. Some of these hypnotic techniques were reviewed in previous chapters, and others are described in this and future chapters.

Synthesizing aspects of Kohut's and Jung's theories, Gregory (1997) used the term *archetypal selfobject* to refer to selfobjects from the collective unconscious that can be activated by various hypnotic techniques. This suggests that it is not only the infant's experience with the maternal figure that forms early selfobject experiences, but that certain selfobjects are innate and due to the evolution of the species.

Inner Strength

The concept of *inner strength* is part of the vernacular of the common man. It is not uncommon to hear individuals, whether they would be considered psychologically minded or not, use the term inner strength to describe their sense of internal resources available to them upon contemplation of a particular action. We think of inner strength as psychic structure created through ordinary maturation and development. Psychotherapeutic interventions that are ego-strengthening enhance the patient's ability to feel and access resources within oneself (see chap. 2). Presenting these interventions when the patient is in a hypnotic trance is a way to enhance their effectiveness. The hypnotic state allows for the increased access to imagery, fantasy, emotion, and memories during a period of decreased defensiveness and increased receptiveness.

Preparing the Patient for the Hypnotic Experience

As discussed in chapter 2 considerable preparation is needed before introducing the use of hypnosis. The therapeutic alliance needs to be well established and the therapist needs to have taken a thorough history. The patient needs the opportunity to disclose possible reservations, fears, and concerns about the hypnotic experience. After a comprehensive discussion, the patient must sign an informed consent for hypnosis (see appendix). In most instances the therapist would first introduce the patient to hypnosis by doing an induction for relaxation and then comprehensively discuss and assess the patient's experience. We evaluate hypnotizability to discover the patient's hypnotic talents in a series of various hypnotic experiences. It is helpful to have ideomotor signals established.

Whether to use the Inner Strength technique depends on clinical judgment about the nature of the patient's personality organization, the history, diagnosis, therapeutic relationship, and stage of treatment. It can be most useful when the relationship is well established. The Inner Strength experience can be an appropriate therapeutic intervention for helping to establish safety in the therapeutic hour and facilitate the development of ego strength required for the ongoing work of psychotherapy.

The Inner Strength Script

The following script is similar to other ego-strengthening scripts that have been developed and published and are available in many sources (see Hammond, 1990d; Hunter, 1994). Most ego-strengthening scripts are highly structured and quite directive. The hypnotic script that follows—that of getting in touch with Inner Strength—is less structured and more projective than most others. It is presented after appropriate induction and deepening has occurred.

Meeting Inner Strength

"I would like to invite you to take a journey within yourself to a place that feels like the very center of your being, that place where it's very quiet ... and peaceful ... still.... And when you're in that place ... it's possible for you to have a sense of finding a part of yourself ... a part that I will refer to as your Inner Strength.

"This is a part of yourself that has always been there since the moment of birth ... even though at times it may have been difficult for you to feel ... and it is with you now.... It's that part of yourself that has allowed you to survive ... and to overcome many, many obstacles in the past.... Just as it helps you now to overcome obstacles wherever you face them.... Maybe you'd like to take a few moments of time to get in touch with that part of yourself.... And you can notice what images ... or feelings ... what thoughts ... what bodily sensations are associated with being in touch with your Inner Strength.... And when those images, or thoughts, or feelings or bodily sensations, or however it is coming to you, are clear to you in your inner mind, and when you have a sense that the experience is completed for you ... then your 'yes' finger can raise.

"In the future, when you wish to get in touch with Inner Strength ... you will find that you can do so by calling forth these images, thoughts, feelings, bodily sensations, and that by so doing you will be in touch with Inner Strength again.

"And when you're in touch with this part of yourself, you will be able to feel more confident … confident with the knowledge that you have, within yourself, all the resources you really need to take steps in the direction that you wish to go … to be able to set goals and to be able to achieve them … and to have the experience that dreams can come true. When you're in touch with this part of yourself, it's possible to feel more calm, more optimistic, to look forward to the future." [At this point particular goals, which the patient has shared with the therapist, may be *stated*.]

"And in the next days and weeks to come, you may find yourself becoming calmer and more optimistic about your life … and you will find that any time during the day it will be possible for you to get in touch with your own Inner Strength by simply closing your eyes for a moment, bringing your hand to your forehead, evoking the image of your Inner Strength, and reminding yourself that you have within you … all the resources that you really need. The more you can use these methods to be in touch with your inner strength, the more you will be able to trust your inner self, your intuition, your feelings, and will be able to use them as your guide."

(McNeal & Frederick, 1993, pp. 172–173)

Inner Strength Experiences

Patients are encouraged to share their experiences after coming out of trance. They are asked to describe whatever images, feelings, thoughts, bodily sensations, memories, and so forth that were perceived to be manifestations of Inner Strength. A variety of experiences has been described and reported. A visual image of an idealized and strong self of the same sex is commonly reported. The image may be action-oriented, as in seeing oneself dancing, running, or performing an athletic feat. Sometimes the patients may be reliving successful experiences or remembering times of feeling calm and safe, perhaps with certain people, at times older family members, often no longer living. Some patients see religious imagery such as the Virgin Mary, Virgin of Guadeloupe, or works of art depicting saints and meaningful religious figures. Sometimes places such as a beautiful underground cavern, a mountain meadow, or a mountain top appear. For some people, the Inner Strength experience is sensory, such as a calm feeling within, or a surge of energy, or, in one case, an erect penis. Others have kinaesthetic experiences such as a heightened sense of muscle strength.

Some see only abstract shapes or swirling colors and lights. The experience is almost always reported as being quite profound and meaningful. Some have even described it as a spiritual experience where they felt they had been in touch with their higher power. Many patients report complex, multimodal experiences of Inner Strength that combine imagery, affect, and somatic experiences. Once in a while a person has a negative experience. This also has important projective meaning and provides significant information to the therapist, as the following case illustrates:

Case Example: Clara

Clara, a 23-year-old college student, requested that I (SM) help her use hypnosis to aid her in habit control. When she came out of trance, she reported that her response to the Inner Strength technique was that she experienced herself in a warm bath. The water in the tub was red from the blood flowing from the cuts on her wrists. She reported feeling warm, relaxed, and content.

Following this experience, she began to reveal the extent of her suicidal ideation, which she had not previously disclosed and had felt too ashamed to tell me. Focus on the transference and renegotiation of the therapeutic alliance ensued. She agreed to a psychiatric evaluation and was prescribed antidepressants. When she was stabilized, we repeated the Inner Strength technique, and she had a completely different experience. She went to a beautiful place she had been before in the high desert of California and experienced herself as calm and strong.

Among other negative experiences is the failure of patients to have Inner Strength experiences. When this occurs, we reassure the patient and give her an audiotape of the hypnotic session. She is asked to use it at home, where she will be under considerably less pressure to perform perfectly. In most instances the patient reports a good experience at home and is then able to have subsequent Inner Strength experiences in the office.

Inner Strength as a Path to Self-Care

Patients are encouraged to use the Inner Strength technique on their own between sessions. We recommend that the therapist audiotape the trance induction and the Inner Strength script. The patient then has a transitional object to take with her. Self-hypnosis can also be taught so that the patient put herself into trance, evoke the image of Inner Strength, and remind herself that she has within her own inner strength that is there for her when she needs it. The patient can also be instructed in several methods of self-hypnosis including one that is very brief and can be used in most any situation with eyes opened (see chap. 7).

When a patient has been taught to use self-hypnosis or has a hypnosis audiotape to play, she is much less likely to call between sessions and less likely to feel helpless, dependent, or powerless. Therapy may be briefer because the patient is developing methods of accessing her own inner resources and feeling empowered, rather than only depending on the strength of the therapist.

Inner Strength With Ego States

The Inner Strength technique is one that can be freely adapted to ego states. It is particularly useful in strengthening ego states enough for them to take another step in the direction of mastery. This could include such things as developing a new skill, moving further into uncovering work, or braving obstacles that keep them separated from other ego states. Somehow the strengthening this technique brings helps certain ego states develop "a more mature perspective" (McNeal & Frederick, 1993, p. 254).

These ego states are able in turn to inspire other ego states to behave in more adult ways. Frederick and McNeal (1993) have suggested that both the message of Inner Strength and the energy of Inner Strength appear to be incorporated by certain ego states when the technique is used. They compared this with the strengthening that Shakespeare's Henry V gave to his English forces before battle against overwhelming odds. Somehow the English yeomen were inspired, as it were, breathed into, with the strength and determination of the young king who asked them to fight both for him and for an archetypal English figure: "for Harry and St. George!"

In addition to an internalization of the archetypal strength of Inner Strength, another model that may be at work comes from family therapy. When a family member becomes stronger and more differentiated, the family system may respond positively to this change (Bowen, 1978; Kerr & Bowen, 1988; Satir, 1983). It would appear that a certain modeling has taken place within the family system. One thing that tends to increase is communication—both within the system, as well as with the rest of the world. The healthier internal family seems to respond to positive change within its members in the same way.

Frederick and McNeal (1993) reported on cases in which the use of the Inner Strength technique with individual ego states resulted in the removal of specific symptoms. They had selected ego states that (a) were capable of entering into therapeutic alliances, (b) could have hypnotic experiences, (c) were motivated to give up the symptoms, and (d) agreed to participate in the Inner Strength experience offered them at the time.

The question of whether symptom removal is advisable needs to be examined on a case-by-case basis. At times it is necessary because of external factors. One of Frederick and McNeal's (1993) patients had an ego state that was threatening to discontinue therapy if it received no relief. Another of their patients, whose case is also reported in some detail (McNeal & Frederick, 1993), was under the pressure of her insurance money running out, and the ticking of her biological clock in terms of her ability to have a child—something an addiction to Nicorette (polacrilex) prevented.

Case Example: Irene

Irene was a 25-year-old woman who was referred to me (SM) by a colleague for treatment of her seemingly intractable depression. She had been placed on Prozac (fluoxetine), which had produced little change in her symptoms. She was interested in hypnosis. When the therapeutic alliance was in place, the Inner Strength script was utilized while she was in trance. The experience was calming for her, and she reported a sense of finding a peaceful space within, accompanied by a visual image of a beautiful green, leafy glade.

As therapy progressed, I also introduced Ego State Therapy, and she was able to identify specific ego states responsible for her depression: a young, frightened, and very needy child state who was frequently angrily berated by a part called Gertrude, an introject of Irene's mother. Future projections and the ego-state work produced a vague and indistinct ego state she called "Newi" (new Irene) for a new emerging part that was beginning to feel stronger and healthier.

Although her depression lifted, she continued to feel shaky about whether she could trust and rely upon her inner resources consistently enough to feel more optimistic about the future. She was struggling with ideas about what kind of work she wanted to pursue and wondered whether she could make long-term decisions that would be appropriate for her.

When she was in trance and had accessed the Newi ego state, I asked the part whether it would like to experience the Inner Strength technique, and the part indicated consent with a "yes" finger signal. I introduced the Inner Strength script to this part. When Irene came out of trance, she exclaimed that the Newi part became more clear and distinct and seemed larger and more real to her. She also had another image that she wanted to capture in a painting. The following session she brought in a painting of a girl in a boat held by a giant hand—a painting which to her expressed her feeling of being guided by the new part of herself that could make decisions that would be right for her.

Currently, the depression Irene had experienced continues to be in remission. She is excited about starting graduate school this fall and embarking on a course of study that will prepare her to work with children.

Frederick and McNeal believed that their results called for an exploration of the further uses of the Inner Strength technique with ego states. This technique has found its way into the established literature (Phillips & Frederick, 1995) for the treatment of posttraumatic and dissociative conditions.

Chapter 7

Internal Self-Soothing and the Development of the Self

Many individuals who seek psychotherapy are deficient in their ability to calm and soothe themselves. Some experience overwhelming anxiety and feel unable to cope, fearing that they may be going crazy or having a nervous breakdown. Trauma survivors in particular may have difficulty calming themselves. Some prospective patients may be so well defended that they are not in touch with their feelings, but are behaving in ways that are maladaptive; others may feel blocked from achieving satisfaction and success in their lives. There are a number of ways pathological self-soothing can occur.

Addictions

Those who use or abuse alcohol or drugs are sometimes said to be medicating themselves. We know that specific amounts of alcohol or certain drugs reduce anxiety and promote relaxation. For self-conscious, shy, and inhibited individuals who are apprehensive in social situations, alcohol consumption is widely accepted. Other drugs such as marijuana are used by people who want to mellow out. Prescription drugs such as mild tranquilizers and sleeping pills can be overused by those who have difficulty relaxing and experience insomnia. Small amounts of most of these substances are rarely harmful, especially when used as prescribed, but when these prescribed substances are used in excess, habituation and addiction may result. Addiction is most likely to occur when the individual does not know other methods of producing the desired state of relaxation.

Compulsive overeating can also function as an addiction. Patients who have eating disorders characterized by excessive intake of food will often describe how they use food to anesthetize themselves and enter an altered state of consciousness, where they can tune out, relax, and go to sleep. Eating can also be a distraction from unpleasant feelings.

Smoking cigarettes has been shown to produce relaxation even though physiological arousal also results. In a stressful situation, a smoker will want to smoke more, although to the casual observer the chain smoker usually appears to be restless, nervous, and agitated. Other forms of addiction that do not involve

DOI:10.4324/9781003442585-7

substance abuse or chemical dependency include watching television, surfing the Internet, running and other sports, gambling, as well as compulsive sexuality. Depending on how *addiction* is defined, many activities could be viewed as addictions if they interfere with normal everyday functioning and prevent the individual from appropriate self-care, productive work, playfulness, creativity, and appropriate relationships with others.

Transference Manifestations of Pathological Self-Soothing

In the course of psychotherapy, certain patients may become excessively dependent on the therapist for calming and soothing. If patients request extra sessions and call frequently between sessions, they are usually unable to calm themselves; they turn to the therapist for comfort and reassurance. Some patients may attempt to provoke boundary violations, wanting to be held, hugged, or caressed, believing that the therapist's physical touch will succeed in calming them down. These patients are reacting as if they were infants and the therapist were their parent who could fulfill their fantasies of a loving, nurturing caregiver who would always be there to comfort and support them.

When overwhelming positive transference is present, the patient may become obsessed with the therapist, who becomes the center of his world, and the patient behaves as if he were starving to death for love, approval, and specialness (Frederick, 1997). This kind of transference can disrupt treatment: The patient seeks real-life gratification of the transference wishes and resists participating in the therapeutic alliance (Greenson, 1967). The therapist's countertransference feelings are activated and he is tempted to gratify or reject the patient. Both the therapist's interventions and failure to intervene are likely to be interpreted as rejection by the patient (Frederick, 1997).

Patients who are victims of trauma can be expected to repeat certain aspects of the trauma in the transference. Herman (1992) discusses the demands made on the therapist by the trauma survivor as expressing the need for an omnipotent rescuer, given the terror and helplessness the victim has experienced. In addition, trauma survivors may have cognitive and emotional deficits (Fine, 1990; Fish-Murray, Koby, & van der Kolk, 1987; Herman, 1992; McFarlane and van der Kolk, 1996; Terr, 1991), which produce transferences that reflect developmental failures as well as symbolic repetition of the trauma (Frederick, 1997).

Reenactment of Trauma

Enactment, according to Hegeman (1995), is a form of communication of unconscious material in treatment. *Reenactment* is "the replaying of dissociative relations in the here and now, usually at first without the recognition of their developmental significance" (Hegeman, 1995, p. 195). For reenactments to be recognized as communication, the therapist needs to be aware of countertransference feelings and understand how trauma keeps the patient "frozen in time" (Reis, 1993). Hegeman (1995) distinguishes repetition compulsion from reenactment in that the latter has an automatic, dreamlike quality and the awareness of choice is absent.

When reenactments in the transference occur, the desire for comfort from the therapist can quickly turn to fear and anger when the therapist does not comply with needs for gratification; he may then become perceived as the abuser. The therapist can easily become seen as "the rapist" (Rose, 1986). Part of the difficulty that many patients have in being able to calm and soothe themselves is that they may be transferentially reenacting a portion of the trauma in which they have been helpless and immobilized. It is extremely important in working with trauma survivors to handle the dynamics of transference and countertransference cautiously and skillfully.

Causes of Inadequate or Maladaptive Self-Soothing

The Overburdened Self

Wolf (1988) has described a pathological state of self called the *overburdened self*. This self:

> did not have the opportunity to merge with the calmness of an omnipotent selfobject. Therefore, such individuals lack the self-soothing structures that protect the normal individual from being traumatized by the spreading of his or her emotions. Even gentle stimuli cause painful excitement, and the world is experienced as hostile and dangerous.
>
> (p. 72)

Patients who have experienced abuse or neglect in childhood are often unable to feel good and function without depression because they lack internal mechanisms for balanced psychological functioning. They characteristically experience themselves consciously or unconsciously in terms of the responsiveness of others to them (Wolf, 1988). Such patients are prone to strong dependency on the therapist to supply soothing and calming for them. These patients may experience intense subjective discomfort and varying degrees of loss of energy and vitality if their internal structures lose cohesion as a result of regression. Under stress they can become disorganized; with too much stress, disintegration of the personality can produce psychotic states. Patients who lack cohesive internal structures may complain of feeling empty and of having low self-esteem, anxiety, or depression, and a sense of worthlessness.

The Role of Trauma

There are many different theories about the role of trauma: what it is, how it occurs, and what are its effects. Psychiatric diagnostic classification systems are constantly being revised to include new research results about the nature of trauma and how individuals are affected. Patients who seek treatment are sometimes dealing with acute trauma involving death, destruction, or loss, whether through personal loss (death of a loved one, major surgery, serious illness), acts of violence (domestic violence, victims of robberies, assaults, rape), or the consequences of natural disasters (tornadoes, floods, earthquakes). More often, however, our patients are dealing with the after effects of childhood abuse and neglect—physical and sexual abuse, that can lead to serious developmental delays and mental illness and more subtle emotional abuse and neglect leading to less extreme but equally serious neurotic and characterological disorders. There are several major theoretical beliefs about the role of trauma in inadequate self-soothing.

Freud (1920/1961) theorized the presence within the individual of a protective barrier against external stimuli that he called the *stimulus barrier* (Reitschutz). He believed that protection from being overwhelmed by external stimuli was necessary for the healthy functioning of any organism. In his view trauma represented a breach of the stimulus barrier.

> *Protection against* stimuli is an almost more important function for the living organism than *reception of* stimuli. The protective shield is supplied with its own store of energy and must above all endeavour to preserve the special modes of transformation of energy operating in it against the effects threatened by enormous energies at work in the external world—effects which tend towards a levelling out of them and hence towards destruction.
>
> (Freud, 1920/1961, p. 27)

Freud (1920/1961) believed that internal stimuli are treated by the stimulus barrier as if they were external stimuli, and the stimulus barrier only permits fragments of the intensity of the original stimulus to be transmitted to the organism. In Freud's later thinking, the stimulus barrier was perceived as a precursor of the ego (Freud, 1940/1964a). Hartmann (1961) also believed that automatized activities serve as a stimulus barrier in the mental apparatus. In contrast with the biological or instinctual emphasis, later developments in Freud's thinking, further evolutions in concepts of the ego psychologists, and later the object relationships theorists placed greater importance on the role of the mother or primary caregiver in providing the stimulus barrier for the developing human infant.

Khan (1963) elaborated on the function of the mother's role as a protective shield. He argued that "cumulative trauma is the result of the breaches in the mother's role as a protective shield over the whole course of the child's development, from infancy to adolescence" (p. 290). When the mother fails in this protective shield role with significant frequency, the child experiences impingements, which he has no means of eliminating, and "they set up a nucleus of pathogenic reaction" (Khan, 1963, p. 298). According to Khan, some of the effects can include premature and selective ego development, interference with development of a differentiated separate coherent ego and self, false identification with the mother, disruption of the synthetic function of the ego, and interference with development of the bodyego and sense of self.

Horner (1995) has extended Khan's ideas into an object relations framework and has addressed inadequate mothering in early years of life as depriving the child of a sufficient protective shield. This leaves the child in the position of being subjected to repeated traumatic states that interfere with the development of ego organization and the synthesis of a cohesive self-representation.

Kluft (1984a) recognized that inadequacies of the stimulus barrier can be a perpetuating factor in the creation of Dissociative Identity Disorder (DID). He believed that the status of the stimulus barrier and the presence or absence of restorative experiences through parental protection, nurturing, and soothing influence whether pathological dissociation will occur later on in a traumatized child's life.

These theorists emphasize the role of trauma as disrupting normal development in the child such that systems and structure for coping with stimuli from the environment are undeveloped or only partially developed. This failure to develop produces psychic structure that is fragile and can lead to personality disorganization under stressful conditions later in life. Thus, understanding the role of the parent or caregiver early in life is of the utmost importance. Then we can be prepared to discover what strategies and interventions of the therapist will be most helpful in the healing process.

Deficiencies in Internalized Objects

Freud's (1926, 1964) later development of his theories of anxiety and trauma and the beginning of ego psychology placed increasing emphasis on the role of the environment (i.e., the mother and the need for help in situations of helplessness where trauma is involved). Freud described two types of anxiety: anxiety as an automatic response to the occurrence of a traumatic situation, and anxiety as a signal of impending trauma (Khan, 1963).

Horner (1995) has also distinguished traumatic anxiety from signal anxiety. "*Traumatic anxiety* overwhelms the ego, while *signal anxiety* sends a message that something bad is about to happen, and if adequate defenses can be mobilized, the something bad can be averted" (Horner, 1995, p. 337; italics added). If the defenses fail, anxiety escalates to panic and a traumatic state ensues. Anxiety as a signal comes from the gradual internalization of the comforting functions of the primary mothering person so that the experience of distress is consistently followed by the experience of comfort before a traumatic state can develop. Ideally, the *good-enough-mother* (Winnicott, 1962/1965) can intervene frequently and appropriately enough to provide internalization of an adequate protective shield and so build an adequate stimulus barrier for the child.

Problems with both the child and the mother can interfere with development of the stimulus barrier. The mother may feel powerless to alleviate pain and illness in the child or may lack empathy for the child's suffering (Horner, 1995). Khan (1963) differentiates between "gross intrusions of the mother's acute pathology" (p. 291) and what he terms as *maladaption* to the infant's "anaclitic needs" (Khan, 1963, p. 291). In the latter situation, breaches in the mother's role as a protective shield are not traumatic singly but accumulate over time as to "bias" ego development, and "become embedded in the specific traits of a given character structure" (Khan, 1963, p. 291). So the results of this type of cumulative trauma can only be known in retrospect at a later time.

According to Winnicott (1958) the mother is motivated by her "primary maternal preoccupation." Khan (1963) sees the protective shield role as "the result of conflict-free autonomous ego functions in the mother" (p. 295). If the mother has personal conflicts that intrude, the result can be a shift away from the protective shield role to that of symbiosis or rejective withdrawal. The reactions of the infant depend on the nature, intensity, duration, and repetitiveness of the trauma (Khan, 1963). Many theorists have discussed the effects of inadequate or destructive parenting. Rather than summarizing that vast literature here, we discuss therapeutic interventions that can be reparative of damaged ego development and underdeveloped psychic structure.

Hypnotic Interventions for Internal Self-Soothing

All the considerations about introducing hypnosis to the patient discussed in chapter 2 and chapter 6 apply here as well. The therapeutic alliance needs to be well established and the patient should be encouraged to express whatever fears or reservations he might have. Experiences of hypnotic phenomena can be provided with the goals of relaxation and enjoyment of the trance-induction process. Ideomotor signals and other methods of communication within trance can be implemented.

Establishing Body-Based Points of Reference for Relaxation

For the patient who feels overwhelmed, anxious, and unable to calm himself, the experience of progressive muscle relaxation can be enormously helpful. Guiding the person to pay attention to tensing and relaxing muscles throughout his body can facilitate shifting attention from his thoughts to his bodily sensations, naturally bringing about a decrease in obsessing and worrying. The person begins to focus more on the present and his immediate subjective experiencing and less on his fears or negative thoughts.

Helping the patient focus simply on breathing—to breathe slowly and deeply, to take some deep breaths and let the air out slowly, to breathe naturally and notice the air coming in and going out, to notice each inhalation, each exhalation, and the quiet spaces in between—comprises one of the most versatile techniques, something the patient can do at any time or place. Other kinds of suggestions can be paired with suggestions about breathing as the following script illustrates.

The Internal Self-Soothing Script

The Inner Strength technique described in chapter 6 has intrinsic self-soothing properties and has been modified to emphasize calming and soothing as follows:

I would like to invite you to take a journey within yourself to a place that feels like the very center of your being ... as you pay attention to your breathing you can notice that in between each inhalation and each exhalation there is a moment of quiet space ... and you can know that you have within you this same quiet space ... that place where it's very quiet and peaceful and still. And when you're in that place ... it's possible for you to have a sense of finding your shoulders ... your neck ... your arms ... your chest and ... abdomen ... your thighs ... and legs, how even the tiny muscles of your face and head have relaxed ... the muscles around your mouth ... your jaws ... your eyelids ... forehead ... all the muscles of your scalp. How wonderful it is just to take a slow deep breath ... and let it out ... and you know, that just the way you can enjoy that comfort in your body, you can let yourself feel, now, a deep peacefulness of your spirit, your feelings ... and it's even possible that you may notice that certain images float into your mind that are beautiful or that are specially comforting to you ... in this peaceful, calm, special place inside of you ... or perhaps you will find that this place itself is a place within that you can so calmly explore ... for sights ... sounds ... for its sense of safety. In this place you can just take a few moments and enjoy how good your body feels.

Now I would like to invite you to meet a part of yourself ... a part that I will refer to as your Inner Strength. This is a part of yourself that has always been there since the moment of birth ... even though at times it may have been difficult for you to feel ... and it is with you now. It's that part of yourself that has allowed you to survive and to overcome many, many obstacles in the past ... just as it helps you now to overcome obstacles wherever you face them ... Maybe you'd like to take a few moments of time to get in touch with that part of yourself.... And you can notice what images ... or feelings ... what thoughts ... what bodily sensations, or however it is coming to you, are clear to you in your inner mind, and when you have a sense that the experience is completed for you ... then your "yes" finger can raise.

When you're in touch with this part of yourself it's possible to feel more calm, knowing you have the capacity to comfort and soothe yourself whenever you need this calming and soothing.... And when you're in touch with this part of yourself, you will be able to feel more confident ... confident with the knowledge that you have, within yourself, all the resources you really need to take steps in the direction that you wish to go ... to be able to set goals and to be able to achieve them ... and to have the experience that dreams can come true.

When you're in touch with this part of yourself it's possible to feel more optimistic, to look forward to the future. (At this point particular goals, which the patient has shared with the therapist, may be stated.)

And you will find that any time during the day it will be possible for you to get in touch with your own Inner Strength by simply closing your eyes for a moment, bringing your hand to your forehead, evoking the image of your Inner Strength, and reminding yourself that you have within you ... all the resources that you really need. The more that you can use these methods to be in touch with your Inner Strength, the more you will be able to trust your inner self, your intuition, your feelings, and will be able to use them as your guide.

(McNeal & Frederick, 1994, p. 11)

The following case example is from McNeal and Frederick (1994):

Case Example: Jennifer

Jennifer, a 28-year-old woman, was referred to me (SM) by her therapist who felt that she and Jennifer had reached an impasse in therapy. Considerable therapeutic time had been expended in exploring and processing Jennifer's relationship with her parents. She had recently visited them for the first time after a long interval of her having had no contact with them, and she felt quite disillusioned about the visit, especially about the quality of her interaction with her parents. The experience felt superficial to her. It lacked the warmth and intimacy she had hoped for. She became more depressed after the visit and blamed herself, feeling that she was a failure. She admitted to a preponderance of "negative self-talk," which drove her deeper into the depression.

Jennifer had also been attending a 12-step group and was having trouble dealing with her spirituality and the concept of a higher self. She said she felt God was out there somewhere but not inside of her. She felt even more stuck, discouraged, and depressed.

Jennifer was interested in hypnosis and was a good subject. The Inner Strength script was used with her. When she came out of trance, she reported being impressed at the vivid imagery she had experienced. She had been able to find a center of calmness, and she had also been able to establish a safe place.

In her next session she reported observing how much negative self-talk she used when she felt distressed. Each time she noticed she was doing this, she accessed her sense of Inner Strength and calmed herself. Jennifer felt that the Inner Strength technique, which was powerful for her, also fulfilled her spiritual need. For the first time in her life, she could feel that she did have within herself something that was positive and good.

The Ego-Strengthening Effects of Transitional Objects and Experiences

The use of transitional objects (Watkins & Watkins, 1997) and other transitional phenomena (Baker, 1983b, 1994; McNeal & Frederick, 1994; Morton & Frederick, 1997a; Phillips & Smith, 1996; Smith, 1995) in therapy has the potential to help the individual advance developmentally into a more independent person with a stronger, more adult ego.

The developmental sequence in which transitional phenomena emerge is well known. Initially, the infant lives in a state of psychological fusion or symbiosis with his mother. From his point of view, he and the mother are the same being (Winnicott, 1953, 1960/1965, 1971). There are no distinctions between *me* and *not me*. This can be thought of as an illusion (Cwick, 1989) of omnipotence that bears no reference to the true state of affairs.

Time brings to the infant further development of his central nervous system and sense organs, better coordination, and increased motility. Little by little, the infant begins to move in the direction of separation from his mother. The mother abets these moves because she must, of necessity, eventually frustrate the infant. A phase of disillusionment ensues.

To negotiate the alien waters of independence, the infant produces a second, creative illusion whose purpose is to serve as a kind of a life raft between the earlier symbiosis and independent functioning. This is the transitional space, the first *not me* object. The illusory nature of this space lies in the fact that the child perceives it as part of himself, whereas it is, actually, a part of the environment.

Winnicott (1953, 1960/1965, 1971) tells us that it is within the transitional space that the transitional object and transitional activities occur. The transitional object is endowed by the imagination of the child with nurturing and soothing properties originally connected with the mother. Typically, the child clings to such transitional objects as teddy bears, blankets, and pacifiers. He may also engage in transitional activities such as musical melodies and play activities. McNeal and Frederick (1997) have noted that there is a wide range of transitional phenomena available to the child such as "… certain places, times of the day, particular aromas and kinesthetic experiences, and so forth" (McNeal & Frederick, 1997, p. 6). Within the transitional space the child begins play activities (Cwick, 1989; Giovacchini, 1996).

As soothing functions are eventually internalized, transitional objects gradually lose their functions (Horner, 1995). With the passage of time the original transitional objects lose their significance to the child. Transitional activities enter the mainstream of the individual's entire cultural field as part of continued growth and development. However, identifiable transitional processes continue to occur in play and creativity as well as interpersonal interactions between the self and the other (Rose, 1978; Winnicott, 1971).

Transitional phenomena are of great importance in the therapy of patients who engage in symbiotic and dependent transferences. They can be noticed when the attachment to the therapist/mother is given up (Baker, 1983b; Greenbaum, 1978). Often patients have transitional experiences that are pathological and limited in both range and variety. These include the use of the body in autoeroticism and other compulsive sexual activities, addictions to drugs and food as well as to fantasy, and addictions to certain settings, rituals, and objects— sometimes even objects that have been preserved by the patient from childhood (Sugarman & Jaffe, 1987).

Because the normal range of transitional experiences is therapeutically desirable, it is necessary for the therapist to be able to identify them when they occur, to activate them, and to utilize them. We believe that it is frequently essential to teach patients how to take on these functions. For many developmentally compromised patients they are *corrective emotional experiences* for glaring deficits. Often these must be dealt with in therapy before any uncovering or integrative work can take place.

Emotional deficits are not limited to the greater personality. Some ego states may be fixated in or have regressed to the symbiotic/omnipotent stage. Some ego states may produce their own transitional phenomena, but they may not be frequent enough, sufficient, or adequately shared. Others may act as internalized transitional objects that resist integration, while still others may need, initially, to have their transitional experiences supplied by the therapist (McNeal & Frederick, 1997).

Hypnotherapeutic Approaches With Transitional States

Hypnosis has unique qualities that make it well suited for providing transitional adventures. Among them are time distortion and a sense of timelessness, relaxation, and greater access to imagery and memory material. Many hypnotic experiences, like transitional experiences, are occasions for play, fantasy, and creativity (Giovacchini, 1996; Winnicott, 1971). The resources of primary processes (Brown & Fromm, 1986) and conscious–unconscious complementarity (Gilligan, 1987; Morton & Frederick, 1997b) are more accessible to the patient.

Cwick (1991) believes that hypnosis seems to "recapitulate Winnicott's phase of illusion" (p. 32). Indeed, we have suggested (McNeal & Frederick, 1997) that the hypnotic state is often experienced as a transitional state and that transitional states are always, in some sense, hypnotic experiences.

When hypnosis is introduced into the therapeutic situation, it usually enhances the patient's associations to the presence of soothing and nurturing transitional experiences within the therapy setting. Deepening in trance can enhance its transitional qualities, and this trance within a trance can become another kind of direct transitional experience, particularly for ego states. Because the therapeutic process is interlaced with direct and indirect hypnotic experiences and mutual trance, it can provide transitional safety for the management of the patient's overwhelming and chaotic affect. The unique ability of hypnosis to produce transitional imagery has been reported by Brown and Fromm (1986), who have found this rich internal resource to be of particular value with suicidal patients. They have noted that transitional images can lead to transitional relationships.

The patient often comes to perceive the therapist's office as a significant place within which the calming transitional phenomenon of trance itself occurs. "Eventually, the patient's simply entering the therapist's office may trigger a transitional sense of well-being. The office, the trance state, the pacific and comforting 'hypnotic voice' of the therapist, all may become a triggers and a symbols for subsequent transitional experiences" (McNeal & Frederick, 1997, p. 7).

Case Vignettes

A patient, Joyce, after experiencing several sessions of hypnotherapy, settled into her chair, and said to me (SM), "I already feel I'm becoming relaxed, just from sitting down in this chair."

Another patient, Marcella, who regularly used trance in her therapy, entered my (CF) office with her dog, Scarlet, settled into the patient chair, sighed with relief, and began to enter trance as she described her dog's pleasure at her turning her car into the office parking lot. "She couldn't wait to get here."

Ego states may have reactions similar to those of the greater personality.

Case Vignettes

Carol, a physician, told me (SM) that an ego state, Baby, felt safe in my office, and knew that when she was there she could be secure enough to reveal her fears.

An anxious ego state that had been activated hypnotically asked me (CF) for a deeper trance because he was not sure the other ego states liked him

and he desired the comfort of the trance experience to balance their per-
ceived disapproval. In "deeper trance," he interacted playfully and crea-
tively with a new safe place; there he was eventually able to think of an
original way of approaching the ego states who "might not like him." This
ego state was encouraged to enter a deeper state of soothing relaxation
as a way of accessing his creative problem-solving abilities in the future.

The Interpersonal Interaction With the Therapist

The effectiveness of hypnosis in working with severe emotional deficits can be more easily understood in the light of Smith's (1984) description of the development of a special transference relationship when hypnosis is used repeatedly. This *special transference* is quite archaic in that the patient's infantile object relations patterns are replayed. Smith (1995) believes that because of the *special transference* the hypnotherapeutic relationship is a prime locus for the development of an interpersonal transitional space. In the therapeutic situation the therapist can be viewed as a transitional object per se (Baker, 1983b, 1994), or the interpersonal hypnotic relationship between the therapist and the patient can take on transitional significance (Baker, 1994; McNeal & Frederick, 1994; Phillips & Smith, 1996; Smith, 1995). Morton and Frederick (1997a) have formally defined this interpersonal transitional relationship between the therapist and the patient as *interpersonal transitional space*. Baker (1983b) had noted earlier that the therapist can facilitate intrapsychic transitional phenomena such as hypnotic dreams within the patient.

A manifestation of a purely *intrapsychic transitional process* is the perceived imaginal space that exists within the inner world of the patient. It has been described in terms of safe place imagery that is transitional for the patient and that can evolve and become elaborated upon by the unconscious of the patient in the course of therapy (Morton & Frederick, 1997a).

Intrapsychic Transitional Space

Morton and Frederick (1996, 1997a) noted that most processes in psychotherapy are described in terms of the temporal. The element of the spatial is frequently ignored in discussions of psychotherapy, yet every human being has a life of memory and the imagination that is somehow conceptualized as being within. Many individuals, especially those who have survived trauma (see chap. 13) or cumulative trauma (Khan, 1963), may have a difficult time finding soothing and comforting within their inner worlds. Many trauma victims display, to a greater or lesser extent, dissociation and amnesia (van der Kolk, 1984). The memories and imagery that they are able to find there areoften frightening and disruptive; at times it is also intrusive. Moreover, many do not appear to be able to use fantasy in a constructive way. As is seen in chapter 13, cognitive difficulties are rampant in this population because trauma has been a disorganizing influence (van der Kolk, 1986) on neurological, psychological, biochemical, and cognitive processes (Morton & Frederick, 1996, 1997a). Further, their emotional development has been stunted and their perceptions of themselves are distorted. Morton and Frederick (1996, 1997a) have described this group of patients as having disorders of self-integration. They do not possess the *internal holding environment* necessary for the containment and management of affect. They cannot self-soothe, and they have little access to healthy transitional experiences.

Morton and Frederick (1996, 1997a) have theorized that the inner world of imagery, fantasy, memory, and thinking acts as a central regulating factor (Hartmann, 1961, 1965) within the psyche. They believe that hypnosis can extend the patient's ability to learn to access his inner world and there to develop the valuable tools of imaginative thinking, learning, and mastery. Brown and Fromm (1986) thought that "The inner world makes possible a two-step adaptation process: temporary withdrawal from the external world followed by a return to the external world with improved mastery" (p. 221). Hartmann (1961) used the term *adaptive regression* for this process. "In the context of a therapeutic alliance with the hypnotherapist, such adaptive regression via hypnotic trance can facilitate ego-strengthening in the patient by potentiating inner resources needed for coping, transformation and integrative processes" (Morton & Frederick, 1996, p. 5).

The development of trust, structure, and constancy in the interpersonal relationship with the therapist can be an essential precursor to the patient's being able to develop areas of safety within. Morton and Frederick (1996, 1997b) have observed that patients who are severely compromised emotionally can create, embellish, and expand their safe places in such a way that the safe place becomes a transitional space for them.

A review of the hypnosis literature seems to indicate that intrapsychic space has indeed been a neglected child when it comes to discussions about transitional phenomena ... the intrapsychic is turned to by the patient for self-soothing and stabilization in a way that promotes a more autonomous sense of self. That is to say, it serves the same functions as the transitional phenomena that have been previously identified by Fink (1993), Phillips & Frederick, (1995), Smith (1995), Sugarman and Jaffe (1987), and Winnicott (1971). The hypnotic accessing and ongoing modification of the intrapsychic space promotes the healing of the patient's imaginative capacity, her receptivity to inner experiences and her confidence in creating. The patient can experience a continuity of being that is ego-strengthening through her interactions in and with this metaphorical environment. As the patient develops confidence in her ability to access this place, especially through self-hypnosis, her sense of self-as-agent is enhanced. This space reflects to the patient that there is within her something safe and positive and good; a place in which and through which the patient can explore and risk and initiate interactions with her various ego states. In a valuing context, the patient learns a new way of learning and experiences pleasure in creative problem-solving. For as long as it is needed as a transitional state, the intrapsychic space is cathected and meaningful.

(Morton & Frederick, 1997b, p. 12)

Morton and Frederick (1996, 1997b) recommend the use of art productions in therapy as extremely helpful for patients in terms of defining, particularizing, and appreciating the *intrapsychic transitional space*. The development of the intrapsychic transitional space is an example par excellence of utilization in psychotherapy. Morton and Frederick believe that development of this rich internal resource offers the patient a way out of his frightening and dismaying versions of the inner world into his own plenum of resources that grow within the therapeutic setting. Patients who learn to find growth-promoting transitional spaces deep within themselves experience what Ricoeur (1955/1965) has referred to as "a redemption through imagination" (p. 126).

Both *intersubjective* and *intrapsychic transitional phenomena* can be amplified and developed in psychotherapy, more so when hypnosis is introduced. It is our observation that the development of transitional relatedness between therapist and patient strengthens and improves the therapeutic alliance. We believe that the alliance is also made stronger and more effective when the transitional experiences occur as a result of interactions that take place within *mutual trance* (see chap. 3). An example of how mutual trance can enhance the therapist's sensitivity to the patient's need for transitional experiences follows.

Case Example: Marcella

Marcella, an attorney, was immersed in an intense, lengthy, and stressful preparation for an important legal case. In the past such concentrated work always produced flurries of severe migraine headaches, sleeplessness, and other anxiety symptoms. I agreed with Marcella that we would do only ego-strengthening work and no uncovering while she was involved in this preparation of her legal case.

In trance four young ego states (ages 3–5) could be activated. They displayed behavior that suggested they were very frightened. Each ego state lived alone in a separate cave in the face of a cliff. From each cave could be suspended a ladder. Each ladder could also be rolled up and withdrawn into the cave. One day I (CF) told the patient that we would do something very different. I helped her enter deep trance with profound muscle relaxation and instructed her to proceed mentally to a beautiful meadow. At the far end of the meadow, I asked her to see a pond in the center of which was a giant daisy. It was at least two stories tall. As she approached the daisy pond she could see the large green stem of the daisy, the dark green leaves, and the brilliant yellow petals. The center of the daisy was described as a large, soft chocolate brown comfortable place. The waters of the pond were crystal clear and semibuoyant. I invited the patient to climb up the daisy and slide down a petal into the crystalline waters of the pond. Almost parenthetically, I invited the four little ego states to join in the fun.

After this trance experience Marcella reported that the little ego states had been there and had had a terrific time. I taped this session for Marcella, and I gave her the posthypnotic suggestion that she would return to the daisy pond on a regular basis. During this experience I wondered why I had selected the Daisy Pond, and simultaneously knew that it was exactly what the patient and her ego states needed.

This was the first time Marcella had been able to prepare such a case without any migraines or anxiety symptoms. She slept well each night. In subsequent sessions the child ego states were much more accessible for communication and finally agreed that they trusted me enough to undertake some exploration.

The resonating therapist can guide both ego states and the greater personality into transitional spaces, both interpersonal and intrapsychic. Marcella's transitional experience is an example of this. This transitional experience was the result of the therapist and the patient engaging in interpersonal mutual trance. The therapist was able to experience unconscious activation of her own internal family to introduce a playful and creative intrapsychic transitional space for the patient. This space was so preposterous that it bypassed the resistances of the child ego states and gave them "an invitation they could not refuse." It is possible that the right experience for the patient's child ego states would not have been supplied had the therapist not been open to her own unconscious information.

We have discovered that certain technical maneuvers assist us in creating transitional spaces (intrapsychic and interpersonal) that we sense our patients need. These include *tone of voice, introduction of specific imagery* for patients who are incapable of producing sufficiently nurturing images, direct suggestion to participate actively with the trance imagery, *metaphor*, suggestions that *patients may discover other* wonderful places within, as well as suggestions that patients enjoy their own creative safe places. We also use *direct and indirect suggestion* before formal trance and at times without formal trance. These are *seeding* maneuvers. We utilize posthypnotic suggestions that the patient access his transitional space with ease in and out of the therapy hour. With certain patients the post-hypnotic suggestions include the use of audiotapes.

There are patients who are so frightened and impoverished that they do not have flexible and nurturing safe place imagery. Because we always attempt to utilize as many of the patient's own resources as we can activate or identify, we favor the use of *positive hypnotic age regressions* and of *hypnotic age progressions* that have transitional qualities with such patients. Both age regressions and age progressions can be introduced outside of formal trance; they can also be activated in formal trance as well as ideomotorically. They can help these kinds of patients begin to have transitional experiences in therapy in a natural and nonthreatening way.

Much of the value of transitional experiences that come about through positive age regression lies in the significant connections that have been shown to exist between memory and affect (Bower, 1981; Watkins, Matthews, Williamson, & Fuller, 1982). Affects can produce memories, and, conversely, memories can produce affect. Transitional experiences are primarily thought of as affective experiences because affect is their essential element. However, transitional phenomena are often multimodal in nature, possessing sensory, cognitive, imagery, and kinaesthetic components.

Nash (1992) has reported that he and his colleagues (Nash, Drake, Wiley, Khalsa, & Lynn, 1986; Nash, Johnson, & Tipton, 1979; Nash, Lynn, Stanley, Frauman, & Rhue, 1985) found that hypnotically age regressed subjects had "freer access to more intense emotions" (Nash, 1992, p. 163). The purpose of their studies was to assess the manner in which subjects who were hypnotically age regressed related to recalled transitional objects. This was in contrast with a control group that had been instructed only to simulate hypnosis. It was discovered that the hypnotized patients had significantly less accuracy in the recall of their childhood transitional objects. However, they were "significantly more spontaneous, specific, and emotionally intense in relation to their transitional objects than the simulating controls" (Nash, 1992, p. 163). No doubt this has to do with the phenomenon of state-dependent learning (Overton, 1978; Rossi & Cheek, 1988). It suggests that the affective components of transitional phenomena in childhood are what are learned, recalled most accurately, and are most significant.

Transitional Phenomena Specific to Ego States

Some transitional phenomena can be addressed to ego states through the greater personality just as therapists sometimes talk through to ego states. Watkins and Watkins (1997) have recommended the use of transitional objects such as teddy bears, which can be given to the greater personality. Such a transitional object is really being given to one or more child ego states. By the same token, the talisman described by Dolan (1991) can also serve transitional functions. It can also be given to one or more immature ego states through the greater personality.

Many ego states are able to produce healthy internal transitional experiences. Often these are more mature and nurturing ego states, and often they can be enlisted as cotherapists during the course of therapy. The greater personality may be frankly enlisted into providing transitional experiences and at times transitional objects for less mature states. When integration has been successful, the greater personality should be able to access areas of comfort, relaxation, play, and creativity with ease. However, it is not infrequent that new functions need to be found within the energy economy of the internal family for caregiver ego states, whose major role has been to soothe and calm. Too much rigidity in such a role can be problematic for ego states and for the greater personality as well.

Winnicott (1971) believed that disruption of the phase of transitional processes in human development could cause them to go underground: "the sequence may nevertheless be maintained in a hidden way" (p. 5). Some ego states may have special relationships to and with transitional phenomena, and this may cause problems in the integration process. According to Marmer (1980) certain traumatic situations may not allow the traumatized individual to use transitional objects in the external environment. Consequently, some ego states, particularly in Dissociative Identity Disorder (DID) patients, may represent internalized transitional objects (Marmer, 1980). Other defensive uses of transitional objects in non-Dissociative Identity Disorder (DID) patients have been reported as well (Stevenson, 1954).

Fink (1993) has cited several cases of DID patients in which alters have performed transitional functions for other alters. It is Fink's belief that alters (ego states) are formed "based on representations of the self or the other, although their connection to their point of origin may become quite disguised" (Fink, 1993, p. 233). According to Fink, alters that are based on the other present the individual with a real and strong sense of the presence of a calming and soothing other. When the alter is based on self-representation, it is experienced as providing access to more soothing, coherent, and capable aspects of self. Fink suggests that certain ego states may remain out of the integration process because in some way they contribute to the general homeostasis of the internal family. On occasion, such internalized transitional objects may actually lose their transitional or temporary function completely, and become, rather, fetishes (Greenacre, 1971), emotional patches that fill a void. Fetishes also differ from transitional objects in that they are frequently associated with sadomasochistic fantasies (Greenacre, 1969).

Ego states engaged in the transitional phenomena described by Fink (1993) are frequently engaged in pathological transitional behaviors, such as compulsive autoeroticism and other forms of sexual behavior, eating disorders (especially bulimia), addictions to drugs and alcohol, and addictions to fantasies, objects, and people. They need to be helped to take a rest. They also need to learn to enjoy a variety of healthy transitional experiences and share these kinds of activities with other ego states. They can also be helped over time to turn over much of the energy of these functions to the intrapsychic transitional space. Further, transitional transferences to the therapist as well as transitional gratifications by the therapist, such as hypnotic dreaming and other interpersonal transitional activities, are of great assistance in such situations. The gradual introduction of self-hypnosis, which ultimately invests the patient with power to produce his or her own transitional experiences, is essential in such circumstances.

It is not uncommon in Ego State Therapy to encounter ego states that have identifiably unfulfilled transitional desires. Often these ego states are born of trauma, and it is essential to their integration into the internal family that their yearnings be identified and dealt with therapeutically.

Case Example: Cynthia

When Cynthia went to her inner world, she was enchanted with it. Every flower, every piece of furniture, and every vista through the windows produced within her deep feelings of security and relaxation. It was here that she met with her ego states. A headless imago of Cynthia's incestuous father regularly appeared among the other ego states. He was known as "Father Head." His body lay within a murky tunnel and could not be released from that tunnel unless the accompanying trauma material was liberated with it. Father Head told me (CF) that he wanted Cynthia to drastically reduce her social activities. "I want her at home, in bed with me." Further investigation revealed that, like Cynthia's father, Father Head had great difficulty calming and soothing himself. Time alone with Cynthia as well as shared sexual experiences with her seemed to be the only things that calmed and soothed him. The patient herself had a long history of poor access to transitional phenomena when not in sessions, and she often used her sexuality as a transitional experience. I challenged Father Head to join me in discovering other ways of calming himself so that he could learn to become a good father to Cynthia.

One day Cynthia brought her daughter and her 4-month-old grandson to visit her inner world in her imagination. Father Head moved over to be by them, and his facial expression softened. He saw the interaction of the mother and the child as wonderful, and he told me (CF) that it was a model for him. In the next session Father Head had moved into proximity with other adult, cooperating ego states. "I'm changing," he told me (CF), "I'm learning how to be a good father."

Within a few sessions Father Head had completely aligned himself with the mature ego states and helped to bring some frightened child alters out of the tunnel. He identified their need for calming and soothing and assisted other ego states in giving this to them. Then Cynthia was able to enter the tunnel herself.

The discovery or creation of transitional phenomena within the therapy session may be critical. However, the patient's willingness to help himself have such healing experiences outside the therapeutic hour may be equally critical. It is a widening of his fluidity in the world. Self-hypnosis is uniquely suitable for helping patients acquire mastery over emptiness, allowing them to relax and self-soothe in the face of tension and anxiety.

This is one of the reasons we advocate the use of audiotapes with such patients. The audiotapes simulate heterohypnosis. However, it is only a simulation, because the therapist is not present to draw out associations, affects, or interpretations. The audiotape produces a true self-hypnotic experience. It is unique in that it supplies the patient with a transitional object (the tape; McNeal & Frederick, 1994) and transitional experiences whose origin is external to the patient (the therapist's voice, the script). It permits the patient to develop both interpersonal and intrapsychic transitional experiences. For these reasons we believe that audiotapes are superior to self-directed self-hypnosis in early stages of therapy.

Within the therapeutic self-hypnotic atmosphere, in which the therapist is available as a transitional object, a facilitator of interpersonal transitional space, and one who helps the patient create and/or recognize his intrapsychic transitional spaces, we believe that all these transitional phenomena merge with one another into what can be called *a matrix of transitional phenomena.* Thus, self-hypnosis recapitulates and reinforces what is done in therapy sessions. The interpersonal becomes incorporated into the intrapsychic and vice versa. They become symbolically concretized on the audiotape. Another desirable form of concretization of these powerful factors can be found in patient art productions and journal entries, which are the products of another form of self-hypnosis. The efficacy of tapes versus self-directed self-hypnosis is discussed further in the next section of this chapter, which is on self-hypnosis.

Therapies that are based primarily on conscious, secondary process modalities often fail to provide patients and ego states with the transitional experiences they require. Indeed, patients can be trained to feel guilty about having the playful, creative experiences that will help them grow. Cognitive-behavioral therapies may not be useful in helping patients make the transition from dependency to autonomy unless the unconscious interactions are transitional in nature. Wouldn't it be a surprise to rational therapists of many kinds to discover that it was their unconscious transactions that were more valuable to the patient than their planned strategies?

Fusional Alliances

There are patients who are so developmentally compromised that they are unable to use transitional phenomena in psychotherapy. The transference that such patients' dissociation forms with their therapists is fusional. It recapitulates the early mother–child symbiosis that precedes the child's ability to develop and utilize transitional phenomena.

Diamond (1984, 1986) believes that fusional components are present in all therapeutic relationships, to a much greater degree with such patients, and to a lesser degree with patients who have better internal structures. According to Diamond (1983, 1984, 1986) the therapist may have to attempt to work with what is going on with the patient at several levels. There is always a real relationship between the patient and the therapist. It is realistic and grounded in the present. Then there is the therapeutic alliance. A patient may have real problems with the therapist (such as finding a time in his own schedule to match a time when the therapist can see him) and still have a good therapeutic alliance. The alliance will spark the patient's creative energies in the direction of finding a way to meet with his therapist. Finally, there are always transferences. Diamond's fusional alliance is much like the relationship formed by Whittaker and Malone's (1953) therapist and Watkins' (1987) resonating therapist.

Self-Hypnosis

Often the patient may be somewhat passive when the therapist induces a hypnotic trance and/or makes suggestions. However, suggestions are frequently more effective when the patient can be taught to use self-hypnosis. In self-hypnosis the patient is able to reinforce the ego-strengthening suggestions and images. This can be done at whatever times are most advantageous for the patient. Self-hypnosis allows the patient to feel a greater sense of mastery and control; he knows that he has methods he can use on his own when he needs them. He is less likely to feel helpless and dependent on the therapist as he becomes more adept in his use of self-hypnosis techniques.

Hypnosis can occur as *heterohypnosis*, which requires two people: the hypnotist and the subject. It can also be done as *self-hypnosis*, which is self-induced. Both these forms of hypnosis are distinguished from *autohypnosis*, which occurs spontaneously and is thought to be adaptive for survival. Sanders (1991) speaks of the ability to enter trance as instinctual or survival-directed and uses the term *archetypal self-hypnosis* to refer to the "template for other trance states that are taught, induced, or triggered by drugs" (Sanders, 1991, p. 5). Trance states such as occur in Posttraumatic Stress Disorder (PTSD) or Dissociative Identity Disorder (DID) are also forms of archetypal self-hypnosis, but are not adaptive. Although initially formed to protect the patient, archetypal trance states become part of a pathological adaptation that can be changed through treatment. Sanders (1991) believes these spontaneous trances form the model on which other trance states, particularly self-hypnosis, can be developed.

Historically, the antecedents of self-hypnosis go back centuries to the practices of ancient soothsayers, healers, and witches who used rituals and incantations to put themselves into altered states of consciousness. They believed that when they were in such states, they could contact sources of wisdom and power, or spirits of the dead, or could even cast spells on others. In many cultures music and dance, often part of important life passages or initiation rites, have been instrumental in creating trance states in the participants. We know the power of religious ritual to inspire and influence believers. Some religions and spiritual orientations emphasize the practice of meditation, often accompanied by chanting or repetitious mantras that induce altered states of consciousness.

In the scientific tradition, Mesmer introduced the practice of self-magnetism to his patients. Gravitz (1994) has described how D'Eslon, an early supporter of Mesmer, wrote in 1780 about learning self-magnetism from Mesmer. D'Eslon also recounted how Mesmer used self-magnetism to cure himself of a bowel obstruction (Gravitz, 1994). In the 1800s self-magnetism was used by practitioners in France and Germany, and later by Braid (Gravitz, 1994). In this century, Coué (1922) wrote about the principles of *conscious autosuggestion* which he believed could develop self-mastery. He is best remembered for his admonition that his patients say several times a day: "Day by day in every way, I am getting better and better."

The experimental study of self-hypnosis was not pursued earnestly until the 20th century. Early studies focused on teaching self-hypnosis for dealing with pain and physical problems. Many single-case studies were reported in the literature, the most famous of which was perhaps that of Milton Erickson (Erickson & Rossi, 1977). He spontaneously began to use self-hypnosis at a young age to deal with congenital physical problems. When he was stricken with polio as a teenager, he used recall of memories in trance of what it was like to walk and run. He was able to temporarily teach himself how to walk again. He learned how to give himself posthypnotic suggestions in self-hypnosis to help him accomplish many other tasks that might have been impossible without the use of self-hypnosis.

Early studies compared self-hypnosis with heterohypnosis (Hilgard, 1977; Johnson & Weight, 1976; Johnson et al., 1983; Ruch, 1975). In general, it was found that untrained subjects did as well in self-hypnosis as in heterohypnosis— that the subjective experience is similar and behavioral scores are comparable. Ruch (1975) concluded that self-hypnosis is the primary phenomenon. Hilgard (1977) also believed that all hypnosis is really self-hypnosis.

An extensive body of research has focused, not on the quantitative aspects, but more on the qualitative or experiential aspects of self-hypnosis, particularly those of highly hypnotizable subjects. This research by Erika Fromm and her associates, termed the *Chicago Paradigm*, has produced an extensive series of studies (Fromm & Kahn, 1990; Kahn & Fromm, 1992).

The Chicago Paradigm

Beginning in the 1970s a series of studies conducted at the University of Chicago examined the nature of self-hypnosis, compared it with heterohypnosis, and later looked at the personality characteristics of individuals who are talented in self-hypnosis. Fromm and her colleagues at the University of Chicago used two kinds of experiential approaches: the subjects' retrospective assessment and an analysis that enlisted subjects as scientific collaborators in understanding their self-hypnotic experiences. In this way, the subjects self-initiated their trances in the absence of a hypnotist and in an unstructured manner.

The research consisted of three phases (Kahn & Fromm, 1992): (a) conceptualization and pilot studies, (b) questionnaires administered and analyzed where subjects were asked to judge what kinds and how much of various hypnotic phenomena they experienced during self-hypnosis, and (c) analysis of self-hypnotic experiences from daily diary content written immediately after each self-hypnosis session.

During Phase 1 differences were found between heterohypnosis (HH) and self-hypnosis (SH). In SH the ego seemed to be subdivided more than in HH (i.e., in HH the ego appeared to be divided into an experiencing part and an observer part). In SH a third part appeared: the "director." Secondly, in SH imagery, both reality-oriented imagery and primary-process imagery seemed to be more important than in HH. In the third place, ego *receptivity* was more prominent in SH. *Ego receptivity* is "a mode of consciousness in which unconscious and preconscious material is allowed to emerge into awareness as the ego temporarily relinquishes deliberate control of internal experience, critical judgment, and goal-directed activity" (Kahn & Fromm, 1992, p. 396). Fourth, only highly hypnotizable subjects were able to distinguish between the two hypnotic states (HH and SH). Finally, findings suggested that the subject's personality influences SH. This was studied further in the next phases.

Results from Phase 2 showed that aspects of trance such as absorption and fading of the generalized reality orientation occurred in both HH and SH. SH also involved free-floating attention, fluctuations in trance depth, and ego receptivity to stimuli coming from within. *Ego activity* directed the process. When subjects in SH shifted back and forth from ego receptivity to ego activity, the experience was heightened. Attention was focused, concentrated, and expansive as well. In terms of content, imagery production was important in both conditions. Age regression was more successful in the HH group, and time distortion occurred in both SH and HH. Personality results suggested that openness, spontaneity, and a seeking attitude were involved in successful SH.

The diary entries were analyzed in Phase 3. In the SH group, ego activity occurred more frequently than ego receptivity. Ego receptivity was found to be more important, however, because it provided the context for aspects of the self to "bubble up" from the unconscious (Kahn & Fromm, 1992). Subjects who were independent, at ease with themselves, spontaneous, and open to new experiences and their own emotions were able to allow more ego receptivity in SH. Imagery production was the most powerful variable and influenced trance depth more than ego receptivity. Subjects who were more attuned to their impulses, outgoing, and more self-actualized experienced the most vivid and profound imagery in SH. HH susceptibility had the strongest correlation with SH, and the authors stated that "the capacity to engage in an altered state is what underlies the ability to engage in either SH or heterohypnosis" (Kahn & Fromm, 1992, p. 401).

Modes of the Ego in Self-Hypnosis

It is important that therapists be aware that there are three possible modes of ego functioning in self-hypnosis. These are *ego passivity, ego activity,* and *ego-receptivity.* These concepts were developed by Fromm and her colleagues (Fromm & Kahn, 1990; Kahn & Fromm, 1992). *Ego passivity* is defined as helplessness in the face of internal demands or environmental constraints. It can be a temporary inability to make decisions or a pathological regression, as in psychosis: In self-hypnosis, ego passivity is present when the patient feels overwhelmed by the imagery he is experiencing and is unable to cope with the conflicted thoughts arising from within himself.

Ego activity, according to Fromm and Kahn, consists of decision making, goal-directed activity, sequential logical reasoning, autonomous functioning, and the erection and maintenance of defenses. In self-hypnosis ego activity is directed mental activity such as decisions, thoughts, or suggestions the patient makes to himself (Fromm & Kahn, 1990). This mode involves choice, free will, defensive mechanisms, and mastery.

Ego receptivity is the mode in which "deliberate control of internal experience, critical judgment, and goal-directed thinking is temporarily relinquished, and an individual allows unconscious and preconscious material to emerge freely" (Fromm & Kahn, 1990, p. 123). It is similar to what is called suggestibility in heterohypnosis and it lends itself to the spontaneous appearance of both transitional and previously concealed material.

When highly hypnotizable subjects were studied in the Chicago Paradigm research, ego activity was the most frequently occurring mode in self-hypnosis, with ego-receptivity occurring frequently as well. Hypnotic susceptibility, trance depth, absorption, and reality oriented imagery were all related to ego receptivity. This indicated that the ego becomes expansively receptive to stimuli coming from within in self-hypnosis. Ego activity directs the experience and may at times overshadow ego receptivity and constrict the experience. A strong relationship exists between ego receptivity and primary-process imagery. "When the ego is receptive, defenses are relaxed, allowing into consciousness the emergence of more fluid associations and of images of a fantastic nature" (Fromm & Kahn, 1990, p. 133). Vivid imagery can be experienced almost effortlessly, and creativity is enhanced.

In terms of personality styles, individuals who like order, certainty, and exact structure in their lives and need reassurance and direction from others may be ego active in self-hypnosis. They may give themselves so many suggestions that they do not allow imagery to arise spontaneously and do not become absorbed in the process or allow themselves to go into deeper levels of trance.

Individuals who were independent, willing to take risks, required little external support, and did not need a high degree of order in their lives tended to be highly ego-receptive and open to their internal experience (Fromm & Kahn, 1990).

This is useful information when using self-hypnosis with our patients because we can be creative and adjust how we structure both heterohypnosis and self-hypnosis in an adaptive manner. We can help the ego-passive patient to use the ego-active aspects of self-hypnosis to create and utilize self-suggestions, enhancing the sense of mastery and control. For patients who are defensive and controlling in their lives, the experiencing of ego receptivity can open them up, allowing for freer and more relaxed responding, which is ultimately ego-strengthening as well.

Clinical Self-Hypnosis

Clinical self-hypnosis differs from self-hypnosis in general in that it is an adjunct to other treatment approaches—individual psychotherapy, group therapy, or family therapy (Sanders, 1991). The therapist teaches the patient self-hypnosis, often through heterohypnosis, directs the patient to use it on his own, and monitors the home practice. This allows the patient to actively participate in his own treatment, collaborate with the therapist, and develop self-mastery and self-care skills. He is encouraged to use it between sessions; with continued practice and mastery of the process, he can eventually use self-hypnosis in many areas of his life.

The therapist helps the patient acquire the practice of self-hypnosis by reviewing the words and images and their meanings that the patient uses in home practice (Sanders, 1991). The home practice is self-induced and self-directed according to guidelines developed by the therapist and patient together; it is adjusted to the patient's style and ego functioning. The procedures may be directive or nondirective, authoritarian or permissive, and structured or unstructured depending on the needs of the specific patient. The practice can serve as a useful reinforcement of hypnotherapy (Sanders, 1991).

Eisen and Fromm (1983) have reported a method of interweaving heterohypnosis and self-hypnosis in creative ways to foster independence in the patient. In the heterohypnosis sessions, the therapist functioned as a dependable parent figure who was supportive and available when that was desirable, but who also encouraged and fostered the patient's efforts to develop his inner resources and ability to function autonomously (Eisen & Fromm, 1983, p. 243).

In their method patients were guided into heterohypnotic trances with inductions and deepening. Ideomotor suggestions and imagery were used. The idea of self-hypnosis was introduced, and patients were asked to practice the hypnotic techniques they had experienced—especially the creative production of imagery, at home. They were encouraged to keep diaries of their experiences, which could then be utilized in further heterohypnosis sessions with suggestions from the therapist for expansion, clarification, and interpretation. The therapist also used the affect bridge technique through free association to "depotentiate, dissociate, and realign emotional responses" (Eisen & Fromm, 1983, p. 245) connected to the patient's images. Patients chose their favorite methods for entering and deepening trance and, after a few sessions, most induced their own trance state in session with little intervention by the therapist. On their own, the patients practiced self-hypnosis four times a day for 20 minutes at a time. Eisen and Fromm (1983) presented case material to demonstrate the following phenomena:

- Splitting of Roles and Self-Nurturing Images. Patients can experience themselves as both child and adult. Often the child image arises spontaneously and the adult image can be brought in to provide nurturing.
- Guided Insight Utilizing Self-Hypnotic Imagery. Therapists can give permission for patients to accept new experiences in imagery resulting in altered perceptions and enhanced creativity.
- Suggesting Images with Strong Positive Valence. The therapist can suggest and reinforce in heterohypnosis images from the patient's self-hypnosis which the patient had felt guilty about enjoying.
- Counteracting Images with Strong Negative Valence. The therapist can counteract images of the "bad self" or "bad parent" with idealized self and object images which the patient can integrate into a more realistic representation.

In heterohypnosis the therapist suggested that themes from self-hypnosis would emerge. Thoughts as they were recorded in the diaries might also come to the surface during moments of relaxation. The patient was encouraged to record these thoughts, along with self-hypnosis material and dreams. These themes and their meanings were then available for revivification and interpretation in the heterohypnotic trance as well as in discussion in the session. In heterohypnosis the therapist suggested that images from self-hypnosis could be reevoked to allow the symbolic meaning to become more clear. At times the therapist suggested images or metaphors from cues perceived in the patient's self-hypnotic material, with which the therapist and patient creatively worked together. Many of the patients on follow-up reported using self-hypnosis successfully at other times in their lives.

The authors emphasized the importance of the patient and therapist working together as active partners in the therapeutic alliance. The therapist could function as a "benign guide" (Eisen & Fromm, 1983, p. 252) to help the patient identify themes and metaphors and discover the relevance of symbols occurring in their self-hypnotic imagery. Eisen and Fromm (1983) stated that the therapist served as a transitional selfobject, a mirroring, empathic parent figure (Kohut, 1971), and a good-enough mother (Winnicott, 1971). The interplay between therapist and patient helped patients develop self-confidence and provided the safety and structure for their independence to grow.

Uses of Clinical Self-Hypnosis

Almost as many uses of clinical self-hypnosis have been reported as for heterohypnosis. A few of the uses include: (a) relaxation, (b) ego-strengthening, (c) skills development and improvement, (d) goal-setting and achievement, (e) pain control, (f) habit control, (g) creativity, (h) management of performance anxiety (public speaking, performing, test-taking), (i) performance enhancement (sports, attention focusing), (j) social anxiety, phobias, (k) self-development and growth.

Specific goals for the self-hypnotic experience are important. Sanders (1991) suggests the following goals: "… to release tension, to gain insight, to find a new solution, to restructure an idea, to heighten positive feelings, to reduce negative feelings, to enhance a sense of self-control, to develop healthy habits, to transform a sensation from unpleasant to pleasant, to remove a symptom, or to substitute a less disabling symptom for a more disabling one" (p. 9).

Soskis (1986) believes that self-hypnosis is most helpful when applied to problems that: (a) are perceived, accepted, and presented to the therapist as problems by the patient; (b) are relatively recent. They may be longstanding if the patient is ready and able to have them diminished; (c) have a central element that can be seen as a subjective experience of the patient; and (d) can be influenced by helpful thoughts or images (Soskis, 1986, p. 24).

Methods for Producing Self-Hypnosis

There are many methods for entering self-hypnosis. Here we focus on several that can be particularly useful as adjuncts to psychotherapy into which clinical hypnosis is integrated.

Self-Hypnosis as an Adjunct to Heterohypnosis. Suggestions made in heterohypnosis (e.g., "And in the days to come it is possible for you to …") are commonly used in self-hypnosis. Posthypnotic suggestions made in heterohypnotic trances can establish anchors or conditioned stimuli for triggering the need to do self-hypnosis. They can also suggest specific situations, conditions, and goals established through collaboration by therapist and patient that link the stimuli and desired behavioral response. For example, "When you find yourself reaching for the refrigerator door, you can take a deep breath, tune into your internal sensations, and ask your body whether you are truly hungry." Posthypnotic suggestions are especially useful when establishing the guidelines for how the patient is going to use self-hypnosis. It is useful to go over those guidelines both in and out of trance.

Scripts and Audiotapes. A multitude of scripts can be used in self-hypnosis. These include both directly suggestive scripts, any number of scripts that combine imagery and/or mastery, and projective/evocative scripts. Many of the scripts provided in this book can be useful. It is valuable to integrate posthypnotic suggestions for self-hypnosis with heterohypnosis. Scripts can be even more useful when they are audiotaped so that the patient has something specific to listen to and can allow ego receptivity to predominate over ego activity.

Hammond, Haskins-Bartsch, Grant, and McGhee (1988) compared self-directed and tape-assisted self-hypnosis. Subjects in the tape-assisted self-hypnosis "produced significantly greater concentration and absorption, less distraction with extraneous thoughts, greater depth, more of a perception of involuntariness, and more changes in body perception (e.g., distortion, loss of awareness of body, feelings of heaviness or floating)" (Hammond et al., 1988, p. 133). Subjects were more convinced they were in an altered state of consciousness different from waking or sleep. They claimed to experience better imagery and find the experience more enjoyable. Subjects using the tape were also less likely to fall asleep than the subjects in the self-directed group. The subjects in both groups rated heterohypnosis as superior to either self-hypnosis condition on experiential ratings. No differences were found between the three groups in response to behavioral suggestions. The authors concluded that patients will experience self-hypnosis as less powerful than their experience of heterohypnosis in the office. The use of a tape reduces the qualitative discrepancy. Another study mentioned by Hammond et al. (1988) was conducted with a group of patients with premenstrual syndrome. On 6-month follow-up it was discovered that these patients were using self-directed self-hypnosis more than the tapes. This suggested that boredom with the tapes had set in. Thus, it appears that newly trained patients will initially rely on the tape, but in time and with further experience will become more independent and self-directed in continued application of self-hypnosis.

In our experience, tapes are useful and probably serve as transitional objects for the patient as they contain our voices and can impart feelings of comfort. Listening to a tape over and over facilitates the internalization process as well. We have heard patients say that they never hear the tape all the way through and wonder what is said at the end. Yet one can often hear in their words evidence that they have indeed taken in the suggestions and now believe them to be their own.

Self-Hypnosis and Ego States

Although self-hypnosis is commonly thought about as a phenomenon that involves the total personality, ego-state implications for producing and experiencing self-hypnosis cannot be overlooked (McNeal & Frederick, 1998). With certain patients who appear to be resistant to self-hypnosis it may be discovered that the resistance does not belong to the greater personality. Rather, it is the obstruction of one or more frightened ego states. Work with these ego states can lead to a disappearance of the resistance to self-hypnosis. By the same token, the therapist also has an opportunity to work with ego states as they are involved in the modes of ego experience in the self-hypnotic state (Fromm & Kahn, 1990). For example, a patient who approaches self-hypnosis from an ego-active orientation to the exclusion of ego-receptivity may do so because of ego-state imbalances. Therapeutic work with ego states has a potential for helping many patients who cannot experience self-hypnosis or who have inadequate self-hypnosis experiences. This therapeutic approach can often enable resistant patients to become productively involved in self-hypnosis (McNeal & Frederick, 1998).

Teaching Self-Hypnosis

Self-hypnosis training is invaluable in promoting self-care. It is especially valuable in helping patients know that there are things they can do to relax, calm, and soothe themselves, and to deal with negative emotions. They can also use it to deal with performance anxiety, to assist themselves in overcoming addictions, and for many other purposes. The sense of mastery and control that comes from successful use of self-hypnosis is definitely ego-strengthening for our patients.

There are a number of excellent books on self-hypnosis. Soskis (1986) thoroughly discusses important consideration and gives step-by-step instructions for therapists teaching self-hypnosis to their patients. Sanders (1991) reviews theory and research as well and provides a comprehensive discussion of clinical self-hypnosis. Alman and Lambrou (1992) provide a manual that can be used specifically by patients who want to learn self-hypnosis.

Before the therapist begins to teach self-hypnosis, it is always necessary for him to carefully evaluate and diagnose the patient, especially if the patient has come to work with hypnosis. The therapeutic alliance needs to be well in place before establishing a therapeutic contract about the use of self-hypnosis as part of the treatment plan. It is important to thoroughly educate the patient about the nature of self-hypnosis. From the beginning, the therapist can seed the idea that self-hypnosis is desirable and that the patient can learn it.

We recommend that the patient be introduced to an experience of self-hypnosis by experiencing heterohypnosis first. In heterohypnosis the therapist can suggest to the patient that he can easily learn to self-induce a hypnotic trance. The patient can then be taught an induction ritual that he can practice in the office. One method that is useful for teaching self-hypnosis is to describe a hypnotic technique to the person in trance. This is accompanied by suggestions for using this technique most effectively. We then re-alert the patient and discuss the technique with him. This is followed by his being able to practice the technique for self-hypnosis in the session. Next, deepening can be explained, demonstrated, and taught to the patient in heterohypnosis. Again, the patient is able to practice this aspect of self-induced trance within the session. When we first teach self-hypnosis to our patients, we ask them to practice the simple and useful goal of going to and exploring a place of relaxation. The transformation of such an internal area can be an important step in the development of the safe place by the patient.

We like to teach several self-hypnosis techniques: self-hypnosis experiences can be of varying lengths and depths. It may be valuable for some patients to be able to produce prolonged and deep trance experiences. One method is to encourage the patient to recline, close his eyes, and do an induction ritual. This is followed by deepening. The patient is then able to become more involved with imagery and suggestions. Patients who use this method may spend 20 to 30 minutes or more in trance.

Another type of self-hypnosis trance work takes place with a brief induction, such as the Spiegel eye-roll induction (Spiegel & Spiegel, 1978), which involves closed eyes. The patient then moves into suggestions and imagery. This can be done in a brief time period:

> You can think of the count of three, where at the count of one, you do one thing, at the count of two, you do two things, and at the count of three you do three things. At the count of one, roll your eyes upward as if looking up at the top of your head, or up at your eyebrows. At the count of two close your eyes, and inhale. At the count of three, let your eyes relax, exhale, and imagine yourself floating. Then you can invoke the image of____ and remind yourself that____.

Patients can be encouraged to do self-hypnosis every day, perhaps several times a day for 10 to 15 minutes at a time. Suggestions can be given by the hypnotherapist both in and out of trance to the effect that, "The more often you put yourself in trance, the easier it is to do, the more quickly you will go into trance, and the deeper you can go." The patient can also be taught to use words, images, and phrases that will facilitate immediately going into trance, such as "Whenever you say, *Relax now*, or *At the count of three, you will experience going even deeper ... one ... two ... three.*"

Certain patients will also need to learn an awake-alert trance. See chapter 10 for a discussion and description of this type of eyes-open trance. It can be helpful to include anchors or conditioned stimuli that, when paired with ego-strengthening suggestions, can later evoke the memory of that trance experience as the following example demonstrates.

Case Example: Ruth

Ruth had been referred to me (SM) by her therapist for hypnosis to deal with the anxiety she experienced while preparing for an exam that was very important for her to pass. We had worked with various relaxation techniques and she had become adept at using self-hypnosis. I suggested that she could have an awake-alert trance experience in which she could bring her hand to her forehead. This would remind her of the relaxation she had experienced during trance and would help her to feel more relaxed. Her therapist later reported to me that Ruth told her, "Hypnosis really works! All I have to do now when I feel anxious is to bring my hand to my forehead and I immediately begin to relax."

We emphasize processing the patient's self-hypnosis experiences with him. It is important to inquire about what kinds of images and feelings emerge. Together the patient and the therapist may take note of themes that appear as well. The therapist may wish to become quite directive and gradually introduce specific tasks into the patient's self-hypnosis repertoire. This is particularly valuable with patients who are ego-passive and may only wish to use self-hypnosis to zone out. With such patients structure is important and the therapist needs to give the patient specific instructions and possibly even make contracts for when, where, and how to practice daily. Other issues may need to be addressed, such as how long the self-hypnosis experience should last, what time of day works best, and what kind of environment is desirable. After the patient has had some time to practice, the therapist can review his experiences and help him overcome obstacles. Resistance to practice can be confronted and handled like any other source of resistance in psychotherapy.

Other patients are more ego-active and seem to take to self-hypnosis like ducks to water. With these patients the therapist is less directive. His job is to help the patient discover what methods work best for him and how they can be used for self-care and therapeutic exploration.

Contraindications for Clinical Self-Hypnosis

Self-hypnosis should not be used with posttraumatic or dissociative disorder patients who have not learned how to produce positive or conflict-free trance states or who cannot adequately control the problematic switching of alters. Self-hypnosis is also contraindicated with paranoid patients who have persecutory delusions, or with psychotic or borderline patients for whom contact with primary-process imagery could be undesirable. It would also not be advised for patients with strong erotic or negative transferences (Soskis, 1986).

It seems obvious that a therapist should not insist on self-hypnosis with patients who have low hypnotic capacity, who are unmotivated, or who use self-hypnosis as a drug to escape reality or to actively resist therapy. Some patients may be tempted to use self-hypnosis as a way of satisfying trauma addiction through repeated access to abreactions, using self-hypnosis as thrill-seeking stimulation.

Some patients will request to learn self-hypnosis as a way to obtain "factually accurate" memories. The same criteria apply for memory work in self-hypnosis as with heterohypnosis. However, with the majority of patients, we believe that the functions of self-hypnosis should be limited to various aspects of ego-strengthening and self-care. We discourage, on the main, the use of self-hypnosis for the retrieval of negative memory material (see chap. 13).

Finally, there will always be those patients who see the use of self-hypnosis as a magical solution to help them quit smoking, lose weight, or easily and effortlessly change other habits. Self-hypnosis is least effective with habit disorders because it is harder to change behaviors than to modify subjective experience. The same kind of lack of self-discipline and ambivalence about changing habits can affect the discipline necessary to utilize self-hypnosis in a productive manner. However, aspects of any habit disorder that can be helped with self-hypnosis include: (a) learning relaxation, (b) increasing awareness, (c) emphasizing choice and self-respect, and (d) ego-strengthening that occurs with successful use of self-hypnosis. Ultimately, clinical judgment is required. Therapists should not use self-hypnosis to do anything that could not be done with other kinds of psychotherapeutic interventions.

Chapter 8

Inner Love

Projective/Evocative Ego-Strengthening With Inner Resources of Love

Although in Western civilization emphasis is placed on such things as mastery, achievement, power, and survival against overwhelming odds as the bases for self-esteem, there is ample evidence that individuals need to be in touch with internal aspects of unconditional love (Mahler, 1968; Spitz, 1965; Winnicott, 1953, 1960/1965, 1962/1965). Spitz (1965) demonstrated that infants who are deprived of elementary loving experiences, as embodied in adequate mothering, fail to develop intellectually, cognitively, and emotionally and, in certain instances (anaclitic depression, marasmus), face a shockingly high mortality. According to Spitz several things can go awry: (a) the child can simply not receive the necessary mothering, (b) the mothering can be abruptly withdrawn, (c) the child may receive mothering that is bad inasmuch as it is commingled with undesirable affective components such as rejection, hatred, and anxiety. It is not only the human animal that requires love. Harlow (1960) demonstrated experimentally that the failure to receive love results in permanent damage to primates in many areas, including their adult sexuality.

Freud (1914/1964) was well aware that love was an ongoing essential element of human life. "A strong egoism is a protection against disease, but in the last resort we must begin to love in order that we may not fall ill, and must fall ill if, in consequence of frustration, we cannot love" (p. 85). However, Freud was not naive about the role of love in therapy. For him, therapy was a strongly intellectual pursuit, and manifestations of the patient's love that might appear in therapy were viewed as transference issues. Nevertheless, Freud's colleague, Ferenczi, advocated more active participation on the part of the analyst and emphasized the role of a loving attitude in the treatment of patients who had suffered early life deprivations (Lorand, 1966). It is interesting that Ferenczi evaluated these approaches in terms of their successes as his life drew to a close. He wrote to Freud that he had come to the conclusion that they had not yielded the results he had anticipated (Ferenczi, 1949).

Over the years, many sad and futile attempts have been made to "love patients back into health." These have been more visible in the treatment of the seriously disturbed patient. Schwing (1940) described her methods in *The Way*

DOI:10.4324/9781003442585-8

to the Soul of the Mentally Ill. She advocated permissiveness and attendance to the bodily needs of her patients, encouraged the development of dependence on the therapist, and attempted to gratify the demands of her patients in direct and nonsymbolic ways, such as feeding and cleaning the patient.

The French analyst Madame Sechehaye (1947) described her work with a very seriously regressed young female schizophrenic patient, Renee. Although this young woman's early treatment with Sechehaye had involved reassurance and bodily contact (Boyer & Giovacchini, 1967), Sechehaye moved into a therapeutic stance of supplying, symbolically, to the patient those things of which she concluded the patient had been deprived. For example, "Taking an apple and cutting it in two, I offer Renee a piece, saying 'It is time to drink the good milk from Mummy's apples'" (p. 51). Boyer and Giovacchini have quoted Sechehaye's (1947) reasoning. We find it valuable to do this as well:

> The "loving mother" had to find something other than the verbal method of psychoanalysis, because the initial conflict had occurred before the development of spoken language and because the patient had regressed to a stage of magical presymbol participation. The only [mode] that could be used was that which is suitable to a baby: expression by the symbolic signs of gestures and movements.
>
> (Sechehaye, 1947, pp. 143–144)

Boyer and Giovacchini (1967) have described the utilization in the ensuing years, by many therapists, of various combinations of the techniques of Schwing (1940) and Sechehaye (1947). For example, Azima and Wittkower (1956) "provided milk, baby bottles, brown clay, and mud to provide a miniature infantile situation in which 'appropriate' feelings can be expressed" (Boyer & Giovacchini, 1967, p. 116). Rosen (1962) also attempted to be openly loving to his patients in his "direct analysis." Although therapists were not infrequently encouraged to engage with their patients in more openly "loving ways" in the 1960s and 1970s, a flurry of lawsuits over boundary violations and other therapeutically inappropriate activities brought an end to this period of permissiveness. These activities are now considered as fads of their times rather than models for meaningful, ethical, and respectful therapy.

Unfortunate trends in the direction of loving the patient into health have continued to appear in the treatment of dissociative patients. Each of the authors has had the experience of Dissociative Identity Disorder (DID) patients refusing to enter or to remain in therapy because we would not play with their alters in the therapy session. Within the hypnosis field Shapiro (1991) has advocated the technique of hypnoplay therapy with alters of Multiple Personality Disorder (MPD; now known as Dissociative Identity Disorder) patients. Although Shapiro (1991) appears, indeed, to be able to conduct her therapy with benefit to her patients, many of her imitators seem to wander into the dark forests where therapists nurture alters directly. In these forests both therapists and patients often become lost.

The belief that regressive techniques are helpful and that the patient can be loved into health has been quite justifiably decried by Fine (1993), Kluft (1993), Phillips and Frederick (1995), and others. Although the problem of too little love in early development is quite real, it is an internal problem that requires internal solutions. It cannot be solved through external solutions. It has long been known that gratifying the patient's wishes through therapist acting out does not produce healing. This does not work and may actually worsen the patient through the promotion of continued regression and boundary violations.

This chapter examines several hypnotic techniques that can help the patient repair deficits caused by lack of love by becoming his own internal parent and/ or by activating inner resources of unconditional love. These techniques rely on the existing internal resources of the patient and can be utilized in self-hypnosis. They do not cause lasting regression or increase dependency in the transference. To the contrary, they are appreciated by patients as valuable techniques that strengthen them into greater self-care and increased self-esteem and self-reliance. These techniques are different from those that emphasize logic and reason; their focus is on affect. We believe that their use may fill a need that is often unattended.

Hypnotic Promotion of Positive Affective States

Many traditional ego-strengthening techniques (Hammond, 1990b) produce profound positive affective responses. Some of these hypnotic techniques emphasize the importance of feeling states in ego-strengthening. Helen Watkins (1990) has spoken of the *life energy* or *the nurturing part*. In earlier papers we (McNeal & Frederick, 1993, 1994) described how conflict-free aspects of personality—Inner Strength and the safe place, could be activated hypnotically and shared with the rest of the personality to strengthen ego states, help produce internal self-soothing, assist with appropriate boundary formation and affect containment, and further the maturation of ego states.

Hypnotic Renurturing and Creative Self-Mothering Techniques

There is a body of hypnotic literature that deals with the development of positive feelings for the self through creatively imagined renurturing experiences (Murray-Jobsis, 1990a, 1990b; Scagnelli, 1976; Scagnelli-Jobsis, 1982). These renurturing techniques attempt to repair or replace something that is damaged or missing through the utilization of the patient's existing inner resources. These techniques can be traced to Erickson's February Man who gave hypnotic suggestions that supplied what had not been present in her early life to an age regressed patient (see chap. 3). According to Scagnelli-Jobsis (1982), who created these techniques in her work with psychotic and borderline patients, there are only four concerns about applying them to seriously damaged individuals:

- Is the patient sufficiently capable of hypnosis?
- Will hypnosis lead to decompensation?
- Will the patient in hypnosis display a preference for fantasy over reality by refusing to terminate trance?
- Will hypnotic work cause excessive dependency to develop?

Scagnelli-Jobsis found that with appropriate patient selection and proper approaches these issues can be discounted. In earlier work with schizophrenic patients Scagnelli (1976) had noted three fears: (a) fear of loss of control, (b) fear of closeness, and (c) fear of the emergence of negative self-concepts. Scagnelli's (1976; Scagnelli-Jobsis, 1982) concerns were not about the introduction of hypnosis, but rather that the clinician who introduces it be well trained in psychotherapy with the seriously disturbed patient.

Scagnelli-Jobsis, later publishing as Murray-Jobsis (1984, 1985, 1990a, 1990b, 1990c), has used hypnotic age regression as the setting into which new suggestions are inserted to provide the patient "… with nurturing life experiences that may have been missed" (Murray-Jobsis, 1990a, p. 326). The following scripts come from Murray-Jobsis (1990a):

Renurturing: Forming a Positive Sense of Identity and Bonding

And then perhaps traveling back to some of those earliest memories of existence, those early weeks and months of existence, and beginning to create within our imagery and within ourselves a positive sense of living and loving, a positive sense of self that should have been, could have been, and would have been if we could have been there together. If I could have been there with you, the infant you, it would have been and should have been all of the good feelings. And we can create these feelings now, at least in part, in imagery.

(Murray-Jobsis, 1990a, p. 326)

The Experience of Being Held

And we can begin to imagine the feelings of being held, feeling the arms, the warm strong arms. The feeling of being held snug and secure, tightly held against the warm soft breast. Feeling the rise and fall of the breast with the rhythm of the breathing, much like the rhythm of the ocean, constant, steady, always there. And the sound of the heartbeat, again like the rhythm of breathing, constant, steady. And the rhythm of the rocking, steady, soothing. And perhaps an awareness of the smell of the warmth of that nurturing body, and the taste of the warm sweet milk. And the feelings of fullness, and satisfaction, and well-being. And the feelings of loving and being loved, and warmth and security, and ease and well-being.

And from these early experiences and memories comes a sense of self that is secure, and loved, and loving. And in this beginning are the very beginnings of the sense of self, of well-being, comfort, ease, security, loving and being loved, and everything being well. And then everything does become easier.

(p. 336)

Murray-Jobsis has also written a script called *Suggestions for Creative Self-Mothering*. This script is one that we often audiotape for patients so that they may repeat the exercise in self-hypnosis. In this method the patient is asked to picture or imagine himself as an infant or a baby and to imagine that he is the parent who will "mother" the child. In our experience, male patients are able to take this task on quite well. A variation on it would be to have the patient imagine that his own mother is doing the remothering, this time the right way. Murray-Jobsis believes that the script for creative self-mothering helps the patient to begin to perceive himself as lovable, and that this can facilitate the process of self-parenting and foster self-love and self-acceptance. The following script is from Murray-Jobsis (1990b) and comes from work done with an actual case. Where the name *Lisa* (the patient's pseudonym) is used in the script, the therapist would insert his own patient's name. Appropriate pronoun changes to accommodate male patients are also to be made.

Suggestions for Creative Self-Mothering

If you could have been the mother of that little girl, you would have loved her as she should have been loved, could have been loved. When you look at that little girl Lisa, you know very well that she really was lovable and that she deserved all the love that every little girl has always deserved. If you had been there to be her mother, you would have done all of the things that a mother should do. You would have held her and cradled her and rocked her and sung songs to her and maybe talked to her of all of the love of poetry, of words, and music. You would have shared with her all of the happiness of running and playing, swinging and moving, all of the fun of living and learning and growing, and all of the fun of growing up strong and healthy and well loved. And little Lisa can still get some of those feelings of love from you, all of the feelings that you can give her, the mothering and the loving that she always deserved. The little girl Lisa was truly lovable, just as the grownup Lisa is now lovable.

(Murray-Jobsis, 1990b, p. 328)

McMahon (1986) has reported using a similar script (with an educational experience with Scagnelli as her source) with patients who were neither psychotic nor borderline, but rather "who did suffer from chronic lowered mood and low self-esteem" (p. 151). McMahon's patients were often stringently self-critical, and quite a few of them had been molested as children. For patients who had been sexually molested, creative self-mothering was an ideal way to become reacquainted with the body. McMahon emphasized the desirability of focusing on many sensory aspects of the hypnotic fantasy to increase involvement. McMahon always discussed with patients the nature of their childhood experiences. Before using the hypnotic exercise, she would inquire of her patients what they would like to change about their childhoods. She felt that the outstanding feature of this renurturing technique was that it gave so much control to the patient. According to McMahon, "Ego-strengthening suggestions which might be disputed if given directly to the patient may be accepted as being descriptive of 'the child' being mothered (and, of course, in this way be integrated into the patient's self-image)" (p. 154).

Phillips and Frederick (1995) have also reported using hypnotic renurturing techniques successfully with posttraumatic and dissociative patients. We currently use hypnotic renurturing with a wide variety of patients, ranging from the most disturbed borderline or severe dissociative patients to neurotic patients who are much like those described by McMahon (1986). We have found them to be extremely valuable, and they appear to be useful with certain ego states as well as with the greater personality.

Case Example: Noah

When Noah first came to see me (CF), he had been hospitalized for a manic episode. He was on an antidepressant medication and carbenazepine. He was able to work as a laboratory technician and phlebotomist, but his poor judgment about completing paper work, notifying the appropriate people about clinical laboratory findings and problems, and his distancing of himself from his colleagues frequently led to his "getting written up." He told me that his work wasn't very good, but that he needed his job to finance what he really loved: his athletic life. He had been an outstanding surfer in Hawaii and was a remarkable mountain bike racer and extreme conditions alpine skier.

Noah lived an isolated life in a separate apartment in his parents' vacation home. Although bike racing and skiing were joyous experiences for him, he lived an otherwise isolated life. Nonathletic entertainment consisted of watching videos, having a few beers, and munching on Fritos. During the first year and a half that we met, Noah was constantly preoccupied with suicidal fantasies and urges. He was afraid to reach out to people, to join groups at work, or to make phone calls that could have resulted in social plans.

It was clear that Noah could well have dissociative difficulties. His mother had been schizophrenic during most of his childhood and had been hospitalized a number of times, sometimes after terrible scenes to which the police were called. She lived alone in a distant geographic region. She sent him "crazy" gifts and garbled letters that were impossible to understand. His father was an analytic chemist who was not in touch with his feelings.

Noah had a sense of being divided and of having parts of him that tripped him up. Hypnotic exploration revealed that Noah had some ego states, but they were nonverbal (Frederick, 1994c) and extremely shy. Noah liked trance work very much. A full assortment of ego-strengthening techniques was used with hi, and he very slowly began to improve. One day he came in and said that he really "wanted to get down to business" in his therapy.

In view of Noah's early life experiences, we planned together to use creative remothering. I taped the session and gave Noah the tape so that he could do further work. The results were dramatic. He began to make friends and to date. Then he began to express himself about his great interest, the English literature of a certain period. He found the courage to take a course at a nearby university. Today, 2 years later, he is in the graduate English department of that university as a candidate for a master's degree, has a teaching fellowship, and has begun to do significant research in his field.

In spite of the fact that Noah has moved to another city, he travels weekly for his appointment. We continue to work with the childlike ego states who are now much more communicative and focused on their fear that Noah's great success could anger his father and that this in turn would result in Noah's father harming Noah. For Noah and for me, it is clear that the creative self-mothering was the turning point in his life.

Murray-Jobsis (1990c) has also written hypnotic script material for discovering the physical body, discovering boundaries, separation-individuation, accepting the imperfect world, and beginning to enjoy separateness. They have been included in the discussion of internal boundary formation in chapter 9.

Other trends in hypnotherapeutic intervention that are aimed at repairing damage and/or correcting developmental arrests or deficits from object relations and self psychology viewpoints (Baker, 1983a, 1983b, 1985, 1994; Baker & McColley, 1982; Brown & Fromm, 1986; Diamond, 1983, 1984) are discussed throughout this book, especially in chapters 7 and 9.

Projective/Evocative Ego-Strengthening and the Hypnotic Activation of Archetypal Selfobjects

A way of regarding conflict-free aspects of personality like the safe place or Inner Strength, that are evoked or activated hypnotically from the reservoir of internal resources, is to consider them as archetypal selfobjects (Gregory, 1997). The archetypal selfobject is a concept of Gregory's that synthesizes some of the theoretical conceptualizations of Kohut and Jung. According to Kohut (1977) the developing infant eventually internalizes the interactions with others that are necessary to her growth and development. Kohut's term for these internalizations is *selfobjects*. Certain *selfobjects* can be thought of as residing within the body of internal resources, and they are constantly evoked by the individual for self-soothing and strengthening during the course of ordinary life.

Jung believed the unconscious mind to be a repository within which can be found the archetypes. These are regarded as transpersonal and part of the collective unconscious (see chap. 6). When certain archetypes are accessed, the individual is able to participate in the transpersonal self and have integrating and at times transcendent experiences. Transcendent experiences are compelling, as Beahrs (1982b) has noted, and "often sought by many individuals" (p. 176). He has noted that expansive mystical experiences could be occasions of healthy, creative dissociation: he has wondered about possible connections among the expansiveness of the mystical experience, dissociation, and phenomena such as the Internal Self Helper (Allison, 1974). When terminologies are set aside, there are broad parallels among Jungian archetypes, ego states and Internal Self Helpers, and Kohut's selfobject representations.

According to Gregory (1997), hypnosis offers a unique opportunity to activate archetypes that provide selfobject experiences that enhance positive feelings and regard for the self. Some projective/evocative ego-strengthening techniques appear to be archetypal in nature. We believe that Inner Strength (McNeal & Frederick, 1993), which is "something like an ego state," is an archetypal selfobject that brings to consciousness all of the power associated with archetypes and all of the self-defining qualities of selfobjects. Encounters with such strong and satisfying internal structures are ego-enhancing and can help advance the treatment of many patients.

Inner Love

As noted in chapter 6, Hartmann (1961, 1965) identified the presence of conflict-free spheres of the ego that appeared to be functioning adaptively in many aspects of human life. Free from conflict and struggle, they permitted the individual to function, grow, learn, and develop despite developmental arrests at other levels (see chap. 10). Most of these techniques emphasize what is both conflict free and somehow tuned into the individual's repository of knowledge and guidance. In their imagery work Bresler (1990) and Rossman (1987) use a conflict-free cognitive aspect of self called the Inner Advisor. Allison (1974) and Comstock (1991) have described the Internal or Inner Self Helper (ISH), a conflict-free alter in Dissociative Identity Disorder (DID) patients that could be of great assistance in the therapy process. The Internal Self Helper has insight, knowledge, and guidance that are unencumbered by conflict.

There are several hypnotic techniques that attempt to activate some aspects of the conflict-free sphere so that they can then be utilized by the individual in a positive way. Watkins (1990) explicitly attributed lovingness to the natural self or higher self of which she helped patients develop awareness in her Exercise for Raising Self-Esteem.

Internal Self Helpers frequently report that they have always been with patient. Gainer and Torem (1993; Torem & Gainer, 1995) located the Internal Self Helper in what they call a *center core* that exists within each personality (see chap. 10). They utilized Inner Advisor visualization techniques with Dissociative Identity Disorder (DID) patients and other dissociative patients to explore the *center core*, and they have characterized it as a conflict-free aspect of the self. They have regarded the center core both as an ego state that is aware of the "experience of unity and wholeness" and promotes it within the personality (Gainer & Torem, 1993, p. 127) and "as a representation of the patient's own inner strengths and resources" (Gainer & Torem, 1993, p. 128). They believe that when the therapeutic alliance is working, the therapist can rely on the center core for information and assistance. For them, the center core can also be represented by the safe place. Like Bresler (1990) and Rossman (1987), they emphasize what is logical and rational in experience.

Frederick (1994g, 1995a) introduced a projective/evocative ego-strengthening technique, Inner Love, as one that put the patient into experiential contact with inner resources of unconditional love. We have been using this hypnotic ego-strengthening technique as another way of helping patients get in touch with available but underutilized internal resources of unconditional love. We believe that the experience of Inner Love is broader than the concept of Inner Strength because it goes beyond a person's concern with elemental survival into the realm of one's relationship, self-worth, meaning, and significance in the world.

Humans need to be able to hold strength, mastery, and a host of other ego functions in a balanced way, but they are not substitutes for love itself. The need to experience love within is particularly crucial for patients whose early life experiences have been inadequate in the areas of nurturing, of internalizing the good-enough mother, and of making the transition to self-care.

Beahrs (1982b) has regarded Freud's (1912/1961) comparison of love with hypnosis as quite significant. Freud referred to a state in which one let go of internal boundaries to experience the other. Beahrs reminds us that there are parallels between what happens when one falls in love and William James' (1902/1961) description of the mystical experience. According to Beahrs (1982b), hypnotic suggestion "can carry the same noetic quality described by James and also felt by one in love" (p. 177).

The following case material illustrates how Inner Love, a hypnotically activated, conflict-free internal energy/structure that is something like an ego state, can profoundly affect patients in a positive way, providing the particular kind of self-esteem enhancement that comes with knowing one is loved. Unlike Inner

Strength, which appears to spring from an innate biological urge to survive, Inner Love requires some prior experience with meaningful and loving interpersonal interactions.

Patient Selection and Preliminary Hypnotic Maneuvers

The selection of patients with whom to use the Inner Love technique deserves consideration as does the timing of this technique within therapy. We do not use the Inner Love technique with patients who have not had significant experiences of love in their early lives. Instead, we would use one of Murray-Jobsis' (1990a, 1990b) techniques.

We use the Inner Love technique with patients who give a clear history of positive and loving interactions but who have difficulty recalling or accessing these resources, especially when they are overwhelmed or depressed. This means that the technique should never be used before careful and thorough history-taking. We like to select patients for this technique who have a clear history of meaningful loving experiences in their lives, who have demonstrated the ability to have positive hypnotic age regressions, who have been able to find a safe place, and who are comfortable with a number of projective/evocative ego-strengthening techniques.

The Inner Love Script

(After the patient has entered trance and been appropriately deepened, the therapist can use this script to help the patient access Inner Love.)

And now, (call the patient by name), I'm going to ask you to take a trip to a place that you have visited before, that place that feels as though it's the very center of your being, that place where it is calm and still ... perhaps you have had other wonderful experiences there ... (If the patient has located a safe place here or met Inner Strength or met an Internal Self Helper here in previous trance experiences, he/she should be reminded of these experiences) ... and in this place it is possible for you to have another experience that will ... be special for you, within ... an opportunity to meet all the love that resides ... within ... within you ... and asks for nothing in return ... all the love that will never impose any conditions upon you ... within ... this is your Inner Love ... it is all the unconditional love that you have ever received ... just because you are you. Now, I'll just count to three to help you focus, and at the count of three you will experience ... your ... own ... Inner Love. (Pause here).

Remember that you may encounter Inner Love as visual images ... or thoughts ... or emotions ... feelings ... or even bodily sensations ... And when you wish to get in touch with your Inner Love again, all you have to do is to quieten yourself like this, and begin to think of some of the thoughts

... or mental pictures ... or emotions ... or bodily sensations that you have today ... and you will find that you are in touch with Inner Love again.

(McNeal & Frederick, 1996, p. 9)

Case Example: Patsy (Continued)

Patsy's experiences with hypnotic age progression have been described in chapter 5, and aspects of her case have been discussed elsewhere (Phillips & Frederick, 1995). She suffered from Reflex Sympathetic Dystrophy (RSD), Major Depression, and Dissociative Identity Disorder. The background for the introduction of the Inner Love technique is given in Patsy's case example in chapter 5. Patsy's most serious crises were private. They came out of her struggle to live in the midst of chaos and pain.

Safety considerations dominated Patsy's therapy. She required medication for depressions and for the management of her posttraumatic symptoms. I (CF) had taught Patsy self-hypnosis for internal self-soothing and pain control, and she was able to have positive age regressions. She used self-hypnosis at home frequently. She also had good Inner Strength (McNeal & Frederick, 1993) experiences.

At the time of the crisis described in chapter 5, I decided that it would be helpful for Patsy to get in touch with internal resources of love and comfort. Later, in trance work, Patsy was able to have other positive hypnotic age regressions to adult figures in her childhood who had been ego-strengthening to her. Patsy had loved her father deeply. (She believed he had not been aware of her childhood abuse. It never happened when he was home.) She also had deep feelings of love for a paternal grandmother with whom she had often spent summers. She recalled her kindness and the fun they had had together in such activities as going fishing together.

After we decided that Patsy might benefit from trance work, I helped her to deepen her trance so that she could get beyond the pain and go to her safe place of relaxation (something that was ordinarily very easy for her). In her place of relaxation I asked Patsy to put her aching hands and arms in a cool creek. This helped somewhat with the discomfort. Then I wondered what central organizing experience she might need to help her integrate enough to function again. I decided to use an Inner Love technique whose purpose was to put her in touch with inner resources of unqualified love at this time in her life when she was feeling particularly deprived and rejected. I took her to that place that felt like the very center of her being and used the Inner Love script.

Patsy was very quiet. Then smiles began to wreathe her face. I paced the experience with her by saying "Uh-huh" from time to time. When the trance experience was complete, Patsy was able to tell me that she had had vivid internal experiences (visualizations, affect, and bodily sensations). She had relived the birth of her son, an only child who had been born to her when she was over 40, she had become closely involved in reliving happy family experiences with her husband and her son. She also relived the experience of her father meeting his grandchild. Although her problems still existed, Patsy no longer felt overwhelmed.

Subsequently, Patsy was able to generate a powerful hypnotic age progression (see the clinical example of Patsy in chap. 5) that was accompanied, for the first time, by the development of an ability to dissociate the pain in her hands from her experience (see chap. 5).

Case Example: Caroline

Caroline, a 40-year-old woman with a diagnosis of Major Depression, had complained about her feelings of emptiness, suicidal thoughts, uncontrollable anger, and periods of despair in which she would cry for many hours without relief. She had been in therapy on and off for many years and was referred by her previous therapist who felt that ego-strengthening with hypnosis might be helpful.

In her therapy with me (SM) Caroline was feeling stuck and as deeply depressed as ever. In therapy she had talked about her relationship with her parents, especially her mother who had been chronically angry and verbally abusive. However, her insights about the causes of depression had not been helpful in easing her distress. She expressed interest in doing some hypnotic work, and after rapport was established and the therapeutic alliance was in place, hypnosis was used for relaxation and for the creation of a safe place. Caroline was readily able to go into trance and was adept at visualizing. She had practiced meditation for many years and felt comfortable allowing herself to experience an altered state of consciousness. She was also artistic and often able to create paintings and sculptures of the visual images that came to her in trance.

Caroline's safe place was an internal cavern with stalactites and stalagmites— a quiet, protected, and safe place. Quite early in our hypnotic work I used the Inner Strength script with her, and she was able to experience herself in the safe place, floating in bright blue water. In a subsequent session she laughed as she displayed a painting of the safe place. Some of the stalagmites were breast-like structures. However, Caroline had not noticed the "back to the womb" characteristics of her visualizations. She spoke of beginning to develop a sense that she had something important within herself—something that felt spiritual, perhaps her higher self.

During a recent session she described a dream of a teacher she remembered who had encouraged her and had been very important to her. She became increasingly aware that there were a few people throughout her life who had been kind to her and who had sustained her through periods when she felt suicidal. The Inner Love script was presented while Caroline was in trance in the following session. Upon coming out of trance, she reported that she had a beautiful experience. She experienced bodily sensations of feeling "warm, soft, and fuzzy" like an "infant in sleepers." The visual image was one of lying on a soft yellow pallet floating in the bright blue water. This was the first time she had experienced having some support while floating in the water. (One wonders if this might have been symbolic of a placenta, a life-preserver, etc.)

The Inner Love experience produced an important shift in Caroline's perceptions of the support available to her in her present life. She began to notice and emphasize the presence of friends, colleagues, and relatives who were loving people in her life. Her depression is now in remission, and she has made some leaps forward in her work, winning acknowledgment from her coworkers. At the same time she is more and more able to see herself as a worthwhile person with much to offer.

Patients experiencing Inner Strength (McNeal & Frederick, 1993) often report oceanic and mystical experiences as well as internal self-soothing. We speculated that just as certain patients might be quite dissociated from their own inner strengths, so also might some patients be dissociated from their own inner resources of feeling loved and cared for. Although we know that some children are so deprived of love in their early life experiences that they may even die from the consequences of its lack or loss (anaclitic depression, marasmus; Spitz, 1965), most patients who come to our offices have had a certain amount of nurturing in their lives. Additionally, we have assumed that they also carry within themselves archetypes of unconditional love.

The major issues with the employment of archetypal selfobjects (conflict-free ego states) are the when and the how of helping the patient connect with them as well as the selection of patients for whom they might provide substantive help. As we have noted, there are contraindications to the use of the Inner Strength technique (McNeal & Frederick, 1993). Manic or other grandiose ideation, certain other overt psychotic syndromes, paranoid trends, and severe obsessive-compulsive symptoms that could cause the patient to become entangled in doubts about whether he had "done it right" should give the clinician serious pause before introducing Inner Strength (although we have found that Inner Strength can be most valuable with certain patients with obsessive compulsive disorder; Frederick, 1996c).

We (McNeal & Frederick, 1996) have found the Inner Love technique to add a powerful element to the treatment of patients who are unable to get in touch with their feelings of being loved or having been loved and for whom a significant experience of love at a transpersonal level could serve as a force, heretofore missing, for healing and integration. In our experience, the Inner Love technique adds a dimension to ego-strengthening that is not supplied by other projective/evocative ego-strengthening techniques.

The Inner Love technique should never be used with patients as an initial ego-strengthening maneuver. There is no way of knowing what the patient's capacity for such an experience might be until careful evaluation has taken place. This evaluation includes a good history, observation of the patient's behavior in therapy, and critical examination of the patient's response to a series of hypnotic tasks that are inherently ego-strengthening. Most patients respond so well to these tasks that they will not need the Inner Love technique. None of the projective/evocative techniques needs to be limited to the greater personality (Frederick & McNeal, 1993).

We recommend that patients with evidences of inadequate nurturing be helped to engage in a whole repertoire of projective/evocative ego-strengthening techniques. For example, we use unstructured hypnotic age progressions and hypnotic age regressions to positive events and figures from the past. We help patients access safe places and learn to soothe themselves there. When necessary, we enter into fusional transferences with our patients. We help patients learn to identify and to have transitional experiences. We use an assortment of hypnotic renurturing techniques (Murray-Jobsis, 1990a, 1990b), and we frequently use the Inner Strength technique. Patients who are not able to utilize such techniques are not candidates for the Inner Love technique. We only use Inner Love after the patient has shown a facility with visual imagery, shown a capacity to access positive memory material of loving experiences and to respond to it with appropriate affect, and has had a meaningful response to the Inner Strength technique. We prefer that the patient be able to generate a positive hypnotic age progression before Inner Love is used. Inner Love is not intended to be used as a life-preserver technique, and it cannot give resources and hypnotic abilities to patients who do not already possess them (McNeal & Frederick, 1997).

Rather, Inner Love is a technique best employed to give patients another resource for soothing, self-love, and integration, and for a strength and organizing principle that many believe to be stronger than the strength that comes from our need for survival (McNeal & Frederick, 1997).

On the Path to the Transpersonal Self: Loving the Self and the Other

The Love of Oneself

The ability to love one's own self is the foundation of all relationships with others (Chodron, 1991; Gilligan, 1997; Spitz, 1965; Teilhard de Chardin, 1966/1973; Winnicott, 1962/1965). According to Gilligan (1997), the loving of the self can be promoted in a process of *sponsorship* within which one can work self-relationally. It is not enough to think abstractly of loving the self. When loving connections are not actively established within the self, Gilligan (1997) reminds us, and a model of self-love is only applied in an ideological sense, it becomes oppressive. Gilligan has recommended active ways in which the individual can sponsor her own love of self. These include such activities as centering and grounding as well as "opening within and beyond oneself" (p. 104). According to Gilligan, this dynamic process of self-love saves us from being reactive and allows us to be relational. For Teilhard de Chardin (1966/1973) as well, this is the First Stage of Love within a process. Gilligan (1997) emphasizes the necessity that the therapist be connected to herself in a loving way in therapy sessions. This is a precondition for the therapist's being able to accept the patient in her uniqueness.

For Gilligan (1997) love is a skill to which much work is devoted. It involves embracing one's own internal aspects or parts. Gilligan (1997) calls these aspects of self *complementary identities*. They need to be identified, experienced simultaneously, and honored for their differences. Although these differences may even represent opposing truths, these oppositions must be honored. This holding of the experience of aspects of self in all of their uniqueness and focusing on connecting these aspects closely resembles what is done in Ego State Therapy. It is also much like Teilhard de Chardin's (1966/1973) "unification of self within our own self" (p. 50). Gilligan's (1997) emphasis on loving one's own self as an ongoing process that both the therapist and the patient need to be involved with is another of his significant contributions in the field of psychotherapy.

> as any decent parent would emphasize the skill of love as the basis for effective parenting, therapists may acknowledge love and its corresponding principle of sponsorship as the basis for effective therapy.
>
> (Gilligan, 1997, p. 198)

It would be only redundant to term this active process *ego-strengthening*.

Love of Another

Love for the other is the essence of Teilhard de Chardin's (1966/1973) Second Stage of Happiness. It is a sign of growing maturity—one that will, as it continues, embrace humankind, the planet, and the cosmos. For many of our patients, the courage to reach out to another becomes an important step in strengthening the ego and a momentous move in the direction of developing the transpersonal self (see chap. 15). The promise of the heady effects of love may indeed seem like madness (Moore, 1992), and it can fail to prepare the lover for the downside of love, the failures that may accompany it, the emptinesses it cannot fill. Moore reminds us that Plato, in the *Symposium*, his great dialogue on love, "called love the child of fullness and emptiness" (p. 78). Moore (1992), like Gilligan (1997), emphasizes what love can do for the individual's own internal self. For it may lead to internal growth and deepening, a broader and more complex vision; it may be an act of initiation into new realizations of the self; it may lead to spiritual awareness.

Moore (1992) believes that Freud's view of love, an event that issues in transference, enriches the individual by ushering in "a whole community of people" (p. 79). He thinks of Freud as inviting us "to consider how love makes the soul fertile with memories and images" (Moore, 1992, p. 79). Within the atmosphere of love, new possibilities are experienced, as are new energies and a new consciousness.

Clinically, love appears to open a realm of possibilities that can lead the patient into a kind of strengthening that cannot otherwise be developed. We believe that therapists must remain aware of the potentialities for growth that may be released by the experience of love, even when failure and disappointment may ultimately enter the picture.

Case Example: Farley (Continued)

Farley made enough improvement from the symptoms of his eating disorder so that he was able to return to school in order to complete work for his bachelor's degree. He continued with therapy in his new location, but he missed many sessions, isolated himself, overworked, and lost a great deal of weight. In spite of this he was satisfied that his therapy had been productive.

Upon his return, he began to immerse himself in preparation for MCATS, tests he would take as part of his application to dental schools. It did not appear that Farley would have recovered sufficiently for him to enter dental school the following year.

This was discussed with him openly as was his need to carry an acceptable amount of weight. Farley decided that 190 to 195 pounds would be a healthy weight for him. At the time of this decision, he weighed 125 pounds.

As we proceeded with his therapy, Farley began to have many dreams that reflected a dark side. The ego states did not seem to know too much about this; however, it was a wonderful opportunity for me (CF) to discuss the possibility that Farley might be struggling with unacceptable wishes and impulses. Together we began to explore what these might be. During this time Farley's mind returned again and again to his early grammar school years. He revealed that he had either driven by his old grammar school in another city recently, or that he thought he had driven by. He was uncertain which was so.

Farley and I were able to explore further how very dissociated he was and how out of touch he was with his feelings as well as with the actual details of what went on when he regurgitated food. He continued to be preoccupied with his early grammar school years, which he reiterated had been characterized by quite positive experiences. He also began to speak a great deal about his now deceased grandfather who had been with the family when Farley was in the first few years of grammar school.

Farley's grandfather appeared to represent a positive resource. It was important for Farley to be able to go through some more of the grief process over his grandfather's death as he had felt quite depersonalized during his grandfather's terminal illness and shocked by his death. As he recalled his grandfather, he also remembered his grandfather's dog, Skinny, an Akita who had not been skinny at all, but had been just the right size.

One day Farley spoke longingly of the good times he had had with Skinny. I then asked him whether he had ever thought of having a dog of his own. The idea of it seemed to thrill him, and Farley began negotiations with his parents (in whose home he lived) to have a dog. He carefully thought about what kind of dog he might get. A Chow dog was one of the possibilities. "I already know what I'm going to call my dog," Farley told me. My grandfather called all dogs "Dizzy-Whizzy," and that's what I'll call my dog!!"

After careful consideration, Farley decided to get an Akita, and he found a beautiful puppy. He brought Dizzy-Whizzy to many of his sessions. From the time he decided to get the dog, Farley became noticeably more optimistic, and his weight gain accelerated. One day I learned that he had begun a telephone relationship with a woman who had been in high school with him. She was planning to return to the town in which Farley lived. At about the same time he began his relationship with Nan, he also started training as a bartender—an occupation he decided would allow him to continue with therapy and learn more about life.

After Farley had found the ideal job, he told me that he felt that he was, at last, beginning to have a life. The puppy had made a big difference. He spent a good deal of time and energy working with her, and he was quite clear that he did not want the puppy to regard his mother as her primary caregiver. "I have something to come home to after work ... I'm so happy I got her."

The case of Farley is continued in chapter 10.

The ability to reach out in love to the puppy, a creature who would require his commitment to her care and well-being, was a pivotal event in Farley's life.

His care of and for himself increased, and he was able to take the next steps by finding an interesting job and beginning a cautious relationship with a woman. The puppy was a particularly safe and auspicious beginning for Farley because of the associations to his grandfather. She also represented a healthy choice because she was the successor in the patient's history of another dog who had been "just the right size."

We can help our patients greatly whenever we allow ourselves to become aware of the value of appropriate love in their lives. One of our tasks is to identify the clues that point to such emerging resources and foster them:

Love feels no burden, regards not labors, strives toward more than it attains, argues not of impossibility, since it believes that it may and can do all things. Therefore it avails for all things, and fulfills and accomplishes much where one not a lover falls and lies helpless.

(à Kempis, 1471; pt. 3, ch. 6)

Chapter 9

Good Fences Make Good Neighbors

Internal Boundary Formation

Helping certain patients to form good intrapsychic and interpersonal boundaries is often a daunting challenge to the most competent and dedicated of therapists. The topic of boundary formation is inextricably tied up with the tasks of separation and individuation in human development. It is interesting that within a psychotherapy climate in which the terms *boundary*, *boundaries*, and *boundary development* have become commonplace, definitions of boundary development are not easily found. Brown and Fromm (1986) have located one of the few available definitions of boundary development, that of Blatt and Wild (1976), who define it as "the capacity to maintain a separation between independent objects and between representations of independent objects" (p. 6).

Our conceptualizations about boundary formation come from the fields of psychoanalysis, object relations, and self psychology. The work of Margaret Mahler is particularly relevant. Mahler (1968), a classical psychoanalyst, developed her theories from her "observations of children interacting with parents in a nontherapeutic environment" (St. Clair, 1986, p. 165). Mahler's "methodology rested on observations of the interactions of mothers and their babies. From these observations of repeated, overt behaviors in the child-mother interactions, Mahler inferred the preverbal psychological processes taking place within the child" (St. Clair, 1986, p. 105).

Separation-Individuation

Normal Symbiosis

Mahler (1968) believed that all successful human development proceeded from a universal stage of symbiosis between mother and child into a series of separation-individuation subphases. Mahler borrowed the term *symbiosis* from biology "while it is used to refer to a close functional association of two organisms to their mutual advantage" (Mahler, 1968, p. 7). Infants are not automatically symbiotic, according to Mahler (1968). They begin their lives in a state of *normal autism*, during which they constantly strive to achieve homeostasis and exist in

DOI:10.4324/9781003442585-9

a state of *absolute primary narcissism*. It is in the second month of the infant's existence that he begins to associate need satisfaction with the mother and to enter into a symbiotic unit with her. The term symbiosis needs to be understood as a metaphor (Angel, 1967) that is used to describe the situation in which the developing infant has not as yet learned to differentiate "I" from "not-I," nor what-is-inside from what-is-outside.

Other theorists have noted the pivotal position of the mother's role in the developmental sequence. Benedek (1949) described what she called the symbiotic phase of the mother–child dual unity. In this developmental stage the mother can be thought of as an auxiliary ego of the infant (Spitz, 1965). His *holding behavior* and his *primary maternal preoccupation* serve as the organizer of the symbiosis (Winnicott, 1960/1965). The good mother engages the child and directs him into an awareness of the environment that involves his senses. A shift occurs in the third or fourth week—from a focus on ways of relieving tension within the body, such as defecation or urination, to the periphery of the body and sensory awareness in the auditory, tactile, and other spheres (Mahler, Pine, & Bergman, 1975). It is interesting that the infant can be observed to display evidence of many ego states at the height of the symbiotic phase (Escalona, 1962; Wolff, 1959).

The Stage of Separation-Individuation

To develop an adult personality the infant must pass through the separation-individuation process. *Separation* means that the child has an intrapsychic representation of the self that is clearly distinct from that of the mother; he must differentiate, distance from, and disengage from the mother. Mahler relates *individuation* to the development of a sense of being, of psychic autonomy, of "I am." Later in the process, the child develops a sense of identity, "who I am" (Mahler, Pine, & Bergman, 1975).

Because separation and individuation are so completely enmeshed, Mahler (1968) uses the term *separation-individuation* to discuss their development. During this process necessary intrapsychic structures are formed by "a sequence of gratification and frustration" (St. Clair, 1986, p. 107) given by the mother who serves as an auxiliary ego. Her job is to permit frustration, but to keep the child from becoming overwhelmed with it. Mahler (1968) has noted several subphases in the separation-individuation process.

First Subphase: Differentiation and Body Image.[1] Mahler (1968) liked Freud's use of the metaphor of the hatching egg when he referred to human development. At about four to five months the infant begins to distance himself

---

1 The breakdown of Mahler's four subphases used here is adapted from St. Clair (1986, pp. 110–116).

physically from the mother. By eight months, continuing to check back with his mother, he expands his world, observing what is different and what is alike. Mahler (1968) has called this shift of attention from inside to the outside *hatching*.

Second Subphase: Practicing.   In the second subphase of separation-individuation the infant responds selectively to his mother's cues and begins to develop individuality and an identity. The process of separation-individuation is enhanced as the infant begins to express himself and to explore himself and the world with locomotion as a vital element in this developmental phase. He is, however, always checking his anchoring to his mother as he practices distancing and exploration. As he crawls and then walks away from his mother he develops stronger intrapsychic representation of the "I." By 10 to 18 months he is walking in an upright position and is intoxicated with the external world. The negativism of the anal phase is not far away.

Third Subphase: Rapprochement.   By the middle of the second year the infant has become transformed into a toddler who has independent locomotion, a number of ego states, an individualism, and a firm belief that he can do any-thing because he has limitless sharing of his mother's incredible magical power. The mother's task is to support the child's separating development all the while sustaining his support, nurturance, and soothing. The adventurous toddler still needs his mother to be there with him and to share each and every "new acquisi-tion of skill and experience" (Mahler, 1968, p. 25). The toddler has entered the stage of *rapprochement*. He can go away and discover, but he must return to put everything in place within him. The child is pulled between (realistically as well as psychically) needing his mother to meet his needs and his wish to be autonomous. *Rapprochement crises* may erupt as the child struggles to retain his autonomy while depending on his mother. In this subphase stranger anxiety, separation anxiety, conflicting wishes, and clinging behavior are evident. Tran-sitional objects assume great importance.

Fourth Subphase: Emotional Object Constancy and Individuality.   The fourth subphase begins and continues during the third year of life. During this subphase the child develops *object constancy*. He has successfully installed into his psychic architecture a loving, positive, comforting image of his mother that allows him to be able to perceive that the mother who frustrates him (the *bad mother*) is the same person as the one who comforts and delights him (the *good mother*). The good and the bad have become unified into a single recognizable and adequate internal object. This development is paralleled by the child's development of his own constant, unified self-image. Cognitive functions become increasingly complex, and verbal communication assumes primacy over other forms. There is increasing reality testing, and the reality principle has clear relevance.

Boundary Formation Pathology

Both the symbiotic phase and the subphases of separation-individuation may be subject to many vicissitudes, and development may go awry for a variety of reasons. Failures to form adequate boundaries in the stages of separation-individuation may burden the developing child so that serious emotional disturbances result.

Many patients present with pathology that reflects inadequate boundary formation. Some of these are schizophrenic, borderline, or narcissistic. These kinds of patients are commonly thought of as needing boundary formation, repair, and management. Psychotic patients have great difficulty distinguishing between the self and the other. Borderline patients tend to overdivide, or split their objects, so that there are good people and bad people. Those patients in the narcissistic range of development lack self-confidence, and, like borderlines, they have not achieved object and self-constancy.

Some patients with boundary problems have trauma-related developmental deficiencies (see chap. 13). The trauma may be catastrophic trauma, or it may be cumulative in nature (Khan, 1963). Many of these patients are able to function on their jobs, and have marriages and children. Their trauma may be concealed, even from themselves. Yet, their boundaries have been disrupted early in their development (see chap. 7). The inadequacy of their boundaries permeates all of their human relationships as well as their ability to separate, sort, and contain affect and impulse.

The Repair of Internal Boundaries

There currently exists a therapeutic basis for early developmental repair with individual patients (Baker, 1981; Fromm, 1984; Brown & Fromm, 1986). Both Baker (1983a, 1983b) and Fromm (1984) utilize these stages in their hypnotherapeutic work with borderline, narcissistic, and psychotic patients. These phases (related to Blatt & Wild, 1976) involve:

- Differentiating "me" from "not-me." Brown and Fromm (1986) call this "... articulation of the perceptual field or segregation of space" (p. 248).
- "Differentiation of inside and outside the perceived world" (Brown & Fromm, 1986, p. 248).
- Differentiating real from unreal. "Segregation of categories for developing concepts about the perceived world" (Brown & Fromm, 1986, p. 248).

Once the child has passed through these stages of boundary formation, he is able to develop further intellectually (Piaget, 1954) and emotionally (Jacobson, 1973; Kernberg, 1975, 1976; Mahler, 1968). Since internal self and object representations can only occur in the presence of boundaries, good boundaries are crucial to personality development. Equally important is the management of boundaries. They must be both flexible and permeable. However, if they are too flexible and too permeable, boundary diffusion occurs and a sense of self and others cannot be maintained, nor can there be adequate containment of affect and impulse (McNeal & Frederick, 1995).

We believe that these areas can be worked through successfully in long-term nonhypnotic psychodynamic psychotherapy, preferably done with an object relations or self-psychology oriented therapist. We espouse hypnotic interventions for boundary formation when possible, however, because work on helping patients to repair and learn to manage boundaries is labor intensive at best. Hypnotic techniques are not miraculous. However, when they are integrated with the rest of appropriately directed psychotherapy they can be helpful in shortening and effectively managing the treatment of many patients with boundary problems.

Hypnotic Techniques for the Formation of Internal Boundaries

Imagery Techniques That Rewrite the Past

Among the hypnotic techniques that have been demonstrated to be helpful with boundary formation and repair are those of Joan Murray-Jobsis (1984, 1985, 1990a, 1990b, 1990c; Scagnelli, 1976; Scagnelli-Jobsis, 1982). As we see in chapter 8, Murray-Jobsis (1990a) had developed visualization techniques for Creative Self-Mothering. She has also contributed imagery techniques for increased separation-individuation and boundary formation to her hypnotic renurturing techniques. The following scripts are from Murray-Jobsis (1990a) and are designed to be used with the patient who is in trance. These scripts can be used sequentially. Each script can be used a number of times until the therapist is satisfied that the patient has moved on to the next developmental stage. The scripts are intended to be integrated with the rest of the ongoing therapy. The first technique is a form of imaginary age regression whose purpose is to provide a corrective perception and experience.

Discovering the Physical Body and Boundaries

And it becomes easier, from this sense of wholeness and wellness and well-being, to move on to those later weeks and months when we begin to discover this physical body that contains the sense of self. We begin to discover the sense of boundaries and limits of this physical being, this body that we exist within. We begin to discover an awareness of the skin that contains this body, and the physical movement that defines our body. The fingers, and the toes, and the face, that set the boundaries of this body. We discover the sensations of the skin, the sensations of touch, and holding, and stroking, and caressing. And we discover the sensations of movement, of reaching and stretching, and rocking, all the good sensations of the body. And we begin to discover the sensations of the internal body, sensations of food going into the mouth, and down into the stomach, and feelings of satisfaction. We begin to know and identify the physical being, the physical body that contains our sense of self, whole, satisfied, well-being, being loved, loving, wanted, secure.

(Murray-Jobsis, 1990a, p. 326)

In the next script, the patient's horizon is broadened to include the external world. This represents a more developmentally advanced position than that which is being worked with in the preceding script.

Renurturing: Separation and Individuation

And then gradually we begin to understand and identify the boundaries and the limits containing this sense of self, and the separations between ourselves and that external environment. As we reach out and touch objects and let them go, we begin to discover the separateness between ourselves and those objects. And we begin to discover the separateness between ourselves and other physical beings. Discovering our physical being as separate from that other holding, protective, nurturing physical being, the holding, protective arms.

And even as we begin to discover a sense of separateness, of the boundaries and limits of our physical and emotional self, we also discover that our sense of separateness is experienced within an awareness of our earlier bonding and connectedness. And there is always an awareness and a memory of those early experiences of bonding and connnectedness, and of the well-being and the wholeness, loving and being loved and secure. Always an awareness of the bonding and connectedness, even as we begin to understand the separateness.

(Murray-Jobsis, 1990a, p. 327)

In the following script Murray-Jobsis (1990a) helps the patient deal with one of the themes that is central to all growth—that of dealing with loss and grief. This essential step in the reparative work can be overlooked.

Accepting the Imperfect World

But in the beginning, the awareness of that separateness can seem so painful. It can seem such a loss, and such an angry thing. Because it means the loss of that fantasy, the loss of the perfect, caring, nurturing parent, the symbiosis of being as if bound together, as if one. And it means the loss of the fantasy of the perfect world where all of our needs are met all of the time, whenever we need them, and where everything is exactly as we want it to be. And gradually we come to accept the loss of the fantasy, the loss of the perfect caretaker, nurturer. Gradually we come to accept the realities of the imperfect world, and the imperfect nurturing caretaker. We begin to accept the "good enough" nurturer, the "good enough" caretaker, and the "good enough" world that is the reality we are beginning to experience. A reality where enough of our needs are met, where there is enough care, enough protection, enough loving concern. And where our feelings of anger and sadness and loss are allowed expression in a holding, loving, supportive, accepting environment. And so we experience our feelings, absorb them, grow beyond them, come to accept the realities of the imperfect world, giving up the fantasy of that perfect union of perfect care, everything, every need being cared for and met.

(Murray-Jobsis, 1990a, p. 327)

The movement in the next script is from the painful affect that is dealt with in the previous script into the joy that comes with resolution of the sadness and mastery of the tasks associated with this aspect of growth. For certain patients this exercise could represent an age progression, as they may not have been able to completely move into this emotional position as yet.

Beginning to Enjoy Separateness

And gradually we begin to discover, perhaps to our surprise, that we may even begin to enjoy our sense of separateness. Perhaps we begin to discover that we may not really need that nurturing caretaker as much as we thought we did. We begin to develop capacities, competence, and mastery far beyond what we might have imagined. Because in the normal developmental process we seem to continuously grow and expand in our capabilities and mastery. And so we discover that we may not really need that nurturing parent quite as much as we once thought we did. And in similar fashion, we begin to discover, that perhaps we may not even *want* that nurturing parent as much as we once thought we did. We begin to discover that in our developmental growth and process of evolving, we begin to move toward curiosity and exploration, and challenge and growth, in ways that would have been so terribly limited by the old, fantasied, symbiotic union. A union so tight it would have prevented us from growing, and developing, and discovering all the potential of our individual identity. And in the normal course of development we begin to discover satisfactions in evolving and developing our own individual unique separateness. And we begin to discover strength from our experience of our original sense of connectedness and bonding. And the combination of strength and freedom that results from our bonding and the separateness begins to open a world of growth and satisfaction to us. And then it does begin to become satisfying to move into this "good enough" world with the "good enough" nurturing, caretaking parent. And we begin to grow in experience, and evolve into all of the satisfactions of developing into our own unique, very special human abilities, our own unique, special combination of abilities and capacities, and strengths and talents.

And gradually we begin to discover all sorts of adventures in that outside world. And we begin to discover other people, other children, other adults, who provide some of our needs and wants and care, alternative sources of solace and care and support. And alternative sources of interest and growth and excitement. And so we begin to move toward our natural evolution and development, discovering all the other possibilities of bonding in the outside world that go beyond that original nurturing caretaking, loving parent. And then things do seem to become easier, satisfying.

(Murray-Jobsis, 1990a, pp. 327–328)

Imagery Techniques of Formations and Movements in Space

According to Brown and Fromm (1986) the following hypnotic visualizations can facilitate boundary formation:

- Safe space imagery: The hypnotherapist helps the patient visualize repeatedly several safe spaces until it becomes easy for the patient to imagine himself contained in a safe place.
- Regulation of closeness and distance: The patient is encouraged to dynamically explore closeness and distance of varying degrees with the therapist in his imagination. In his stages of hypnotherapeutic work with patients with developmental deficits, Baker (1981) has the patient open his eyes during such a process to ascertain that the therapist actually exists as a separate entity with his own boundaries.
- Barrier imagery: The patient is encouraged to actively visualize boundaries about his own body. This could be anything the patient can comfortably visualize such as a shield of light, a bubble (Brown & Fromm, 1986), a safe place, or even a coat of armor.

Perhaps the most creative translation of object relations and self-psychology theory into hypnotic techniques that help with separation-individuation and boundary formation are those of Elgan Baker (1981). Baker, a psychoanalyst, "was the first hypnoanalyst to translate the theoretical insights of objects relations theory and self theory into a protocol of primary process language to be used with psychotic patients, so they can progress upward and forward again along the developmental line" (Fromm & Nash, 1997, p. 45). Baker's techniques are firmly based in the work of Mahler (1968). The patient is able to have a corrective experience when the therapist is both dependable and consistent and proceeds in such a way as not to arouse too much anxiety in the patient (Baker,

1981; Fromm & Nash, 1997). As with the work of Murray-Jobsis, the therapist is perceived as nurturing and protective; however, the imagery that Baker uses is not oriented to the past. Rather, its emphasis is on a new and different present. Fromm and Nash have called Baker's protocol "one of the most important innovations in the whole field of hypnotherapy" (p. 45).

Baker's Hypnotic Exercises for Boundary Development

Like those of Murray-Jobsis, Baker's exercises are presented to the patient as a sequential building process. Their purpose is to correct certain pathology that is developmental in nature. They were originally developed for psychotic patients, although subsequently they have been used with borderline and narcissistic patients (Fromm & Nash, 1997) and certain dissociative disorder patients (Phillips & Frederick, 1995). These are patients "who present with a poorly differentiated sense of self from the others" (Baker, 1981, p. 137). According to Baker (1981) these patients have several areas of structural pathology:

- They have unstable boundaries, and they are not able to differentiate the self from the object.
- Because the boundaries are unstable, the psychotic patient is confused about inner/outer, me/not me, and real/not real. This causes him to withdraw from the outer world. This withdrawal deprives him of the very consensual validation he needs to develop secondary process thinking.
- Such patients are unable to integrate what is *good* in their experiences with what is *bad*. This is a defensive use of primitive splitting (Volkan, 1976) that blocks the development of object constancy. The adaptive value of this defense is that it keeps the patient from being overwhelmed by the anxiety that would accompany his losing his good, nurturing objects.

The purpose of Baker's exercises is to help the patient experience the therapist as "a new whole object ... and to preserve the representation of the therapist from distorted and destructive externalizations of self and object images" (Baker, 1981, p. 140). They help the patient develop object permanence (Piaget, 1954) and object constancy (Mahler, 1968). The next step is for the patient to learn to undergo separation-individuation and develop good boundaries. Each one of Baker's exercises is made possible by the internal safety and security it provides the patient. Baker recommends that the patient be in a light to medium trance and that the therapist's voice be "calm and soothing."

First Hypnotic Exercise

In this exercise the patient is asked to develop a picture of himself, alone and engaged in a pleasant activity. The therapist encourages and supports the patient in this position, with direct suggestions of comfort, safety, and well-being. This exercise should be done repeatedly over a period of as many weeks as it appears that it evokes images of *narcissism*, a form of security that gratifies the patient and has the approval of the therapist. E. L. Baker (personal communication, 1995) has recommended that the therapist encourage the patient that he can evoke this image at any time he is experiencing psychic discomfort. The patient should be able to do this before moving into the next exercise.

Narcissism. Although the topic of narcissism is of vital import to clinicians, "narcissism has from the first been plagued by conceptual unclarity" (B. E. Moore, 1995, p. 229). *Narcissism* has been defined as "an investment or concentration of energy or interest in the self" (St. Clair, 1986, p. 189). Most psychoanalytic and structural theorists appear to agree that the term *primary narcissism* refers to the energy investment or love that the infant has invested in his symbiotic world. The energy that exists in this primary state must ultimately become invested in objects: internal representations of the self and of others. The energy investment that the infant eventually makes in his self-representation can be conceptualized as *secondary narcissism*.

There is no doubt that this exercise deals with a primitive and undeveloped self. This self that exists before the patient undertakes the exercise could be viewed as somehow representing the primary narcissistic state. Although the patient is inwardly gazing at an image of himself, it appears that the hypnotic state and the calming, reassuring, and soothing voice of the therapist may in some way join this image so as to mimic or even symbolize the primary narcissistic state in which the infant and the world are one. However, the narcissism that is fostered in Baker's first exercise is secondary narcissism. It could be argued that the patient who is so psychotic that he has regressed completely to a symbiotic sense of self might not be capable of engaging in this exercise because it presupposes some level of appreciation of the self as others.

Thomas Moore (1992) has considered the value of secondary narcissism, in which one regards the self as a love object, in his examination of the myth of Narcissus as found in Ovid's *Metamorphoses*. Moore emphasizes the positive value of the developmental move in which an individual is able to see himself as an object. This self, so viewed, is as strange and mysterious as the image that Narcissus beheld in the water. Moore believes that this new perception of the self, externalized, represents a deeper sense of the self. Narcissus fell into his self-image and lost his life because he could not move on. Yet, the evolution of healthy narcissism is essential for good intrapsychic development and is a key ingredient of self-esteem. The image that the patient is encouraged to hold in trance by the supportive, soothing therapist is much like the image Narcissus saw in the water. In the next exercise the patient's world of energy cathexis becomes expanded.

Second Hypnotic Exercise

In the second exercise the patient is asked to evoke the image of himself, alone and comfortable, and then open his eyes and look at the therapist. He then closes his eyes again and gazes inwardly at himself. This exercise is designed to help the patient expand his world to include a separate other. It also leads to the development of *object permanence*—a concept that comes from the work of Piaget (1954). *Object permanence* is the knowledge that the therapist still exists, even when the patient is not looking at him, and that the therapist he sees now is the same therapist he saw the last time he opened his eyes.

Third Hypnotic Exercise

The patient's next step is to visualize the therapist while he is relaxed and has a sense of well-being in trance. Some very disturbed patients are not able to do this. In these cases the patient is helped to produce a visualization of a less real and less threatening image of the therapist, such as the therapist's name on the office door, the therapist's initials, or some object in the therapist's office. This exercise helps with the continued development of object permanence (Piaget, 1954) as well as of *object constancy* (Mahler, 1968). With the development of object constancy the patient will become able to perceive the therapist he may experience as frustrating at one time to be the same therapist he senses as pacific and nurturing at others. Should the patient experience any discomfort during this exercise, he is helped to leave it and enter a deeper state of comfort and relaxation.

Fourth Hypnotic Exercise

By the time the patient has progressed to this exercise, he is able to produce images of himself and of the therapist and to use either one for relaxation. In this exercise the patient learns to alternate between images of himself and the therapist. Eventually, the therapist and the patient are brought together in some neutral activity. This may be difficult for some patients because of some of the kinds of transferences they may have for the therapist. For example, the patient's unconscious mind might be saying at first that closeness to the therapist is dangerous and could lead to engulfment. Fromm and Nash (1997) describe one of their patients finally taking the plunge into this exercise by placing himself high in the Rocky Mountains. From this perspective he could wave to the therapist whom he saw sitting on top of New York City's Empire State Building. In a variation of this exercise with the ego states of one of our patients (the case is described later in this chapter) different ego states took their places on different continents. The images of the therapist and the images of the patient are brought closer and closer through repeated use of this exercise in a hypnotic atmosphere of comfort and relaxation. We believe that one reason these exercises work so well is that the therapist's voice and suggestion to the hypnotized patient provide transitional experiences that permit him to become more autonomous. From the position of his increased autonomy, he is able to approach closeness.

Fifth Hypnotic Exercise

In this exercise several goals are achieved simultaneously. The exercise is one in which the patient learns to visualize himself and the therapist engaged in activities. At first these activities are parallel. Eventually they become mutual and involve interaction between the therapist and the patient. The therapist's role as a nurturer and caregiver are always featured in these hypnotic fantasies or dreams. The purpose of this exercise is to provide additional steps for installing the therapist as a separate, acceptable, and nurturing object within the patient's psychic structure. Because the fantasied interaction is an interpersonal one, it may reflect transference difficulties at times. These should neither be ignored nor allowed to dominate the exercise, whose purpose is to translate the totality of the patient's interpersonal interaction with the therapist in the therapeutic relationship into an intrapsychic change.

Case Example: Nelson

Nelson had been a victim of multiple childhood traumata, and he had been sexually abused by his mother. His adult functioning was quite split. As an oncologist he worked comfortably and creatively with patients, saving many who would not have survived with less up-to-date and dedicated treatment. In his personal life he felt neither comfortable nor in charge. He had a tendency to sexualize many personal interactions, and he could only achieve orgasm if he produced sadomasochistic fantasies in which he was being victimized. He had other difficulties with closeness. One was that he felt unable to resist people taking him over in personal relationships.

Nelson also had many referential thoughts, engaged in approach–avoidance maneuvers, and had great difficulties with separation. He appeared to be functioning at a narcissistic developmental level. I (CF) thought he would benefit from developmental work, and I (CF) discussed this with him. He progressed well with Baker's exercises (we started with the first exercise) until we arrived at the Fifth Exercise. In this exercise he was able to picture our working together in adjacent gardens, carefully tending the plants. When he visualized our working together in the same garden, he reported the intrusion of sexual fantasies about me.

This was a symbolic representation of his skewed relationship with his mother. Would I (CF) allow him to transgress our boundaries in fantasy as his mother had in reality? Instead of making transference interpretations, I directed Nelson to return to his own garden where he could work comfortably and see that I was working comfortably in mine. After Nelson had returned to his own garden, he was eventually able to entertain hypnotic fantasies in which we worked in the same garden, side by side, appreciating the profound significance of the care we administered to the tender plants.

Nelson's case material illustrates how Baker's exercise can be corrective for distortions and deprivations that come from negative, traumatic experiences as well as for deficits that are more connected with absence or neglect. Not only had Nelson achieved experiences of a good nonabusing mother in this exercise, but he had also developed a good self. These exercises proved profound opportunities for the introjection of a good mother and a good self.

Sixth Hypnotic Exercise

In this series of exercises the patient is encouraged to locate symbolic representations of distortions of his self-image as well as those of others, such as the bad parent. These bad or distorted qualities can be dealt with symbolically. For example, the patient could see himself shedding them as he grows a new skin, or he might destroy the externalized unwanted qualities. This is akin to what may happen in the dreams of certain patients in the integration stage of therapy (Morton & Frederick, 1997a, 1997b; Phillips & Frederick, 1995). We have found Stanton's (1989, 1990) Five Step ego-strengthening exercise to be helpful in this stage as less imaginative patients can use the structured disposal chute to get rid of unwanted and undesirable aspects of the self and objects as well as receive additional ego-strengthening before and after they make this courageous move.

Seventh Hypnotic Exercise

Although the various visualization exercises that precede this exercise are invaluable, there is always some negative remaining. Further and more importantly, the patient has been strengthened and is stable enough to move into integrating good and bad in interpersonal relationships.

Case Example: Blanca

Blanca, whose case has been described in detail elsewhere (Frederick, 1997), was diagnosed as having Dissociative Identity Disorder. Some of her very immature ego states functioned at the borderline level. This made it difficult for them to tolerate separation or understand that we were not glued together for life. In some hypnotic exercises Blanca learned to develop mental images of herself sitting in a chair in my (CF) office. She later learned that she could evoke these images for soothing and relaxation.

Next, Blanca was able to picture herself comfortable and alone and then open her eyes and look at me sitting across from her. Eventually she was able to produce images of me sitting in my chair. Later, Blanca was able to have images of the two of us engaged in a neutral activity. She could then open her eyes and see that, although I could be in her mind in separate images and in images in which she was as well, I was a separate person from her.

Hypnotic boundary work was also done with Blanca's ego states. The consistent use of these techniques helped Blanca develop much healthier boundaries. The formation of these boundaries then allowed Blanca to focus more on resolving apparent contradictions that came about because her therapist had boundaries too. Blanca had to reconcile the therapist who would not accept gratuitous faxes and phone calls with the equally real therapist who valued her and cared about her uniqueness and well-being.

In hypnotic exercises various visualizations of blending can be helpful. For example, a patient might be able to see blue and yellow blend into a lovely green color or could visualize many tributaries flowing into one river. The success of Baker's hypnotic work with borderline and seriously compromised dissociative patients has been reported by Phillips and Frederick (1995). They have suggested other hypnotic approaches that can be used to enhance boundary formation: (a) ideomotor signaling, (b) structured formal trance entrance and exit, and (c) careful titration of the uncovering work at the pace the patient can tolerate.

Ego-State Approaches to Boundary Development

Because the totality of affect and impulse that must be contained by the personality can be thought of as being held by the ego states, each of which has its own more or less permeable boundaries, ego-state approaches would seem to provide another avenue for helping patients establish more healthy boundaries.

It is crucial to understand that the word *boundary* is used in two quite different ways here. The reason for this is that two distinct theoretical frameworks are being considered in terms of how each might contribute to the others. The term *boundary* as it has appeared in the bulk of this chapter until now refers to developmental boundaries in the total personality and is an object relations and self psychology concept. When we apply the term *boundary* to ego states, it will at times have another quite different meaning. There is a concept in Ego State therapy that ego states are separated from one another by something like a semipermeable membrane. These metaphorical membranes are sometimes referred to as *boundaries*. The boundaries sought to be developed or strengthened by ego-state approaches are normal ego-state boundaries. By this we mean that correct boundary formation assistance will not cause a pathological ego-state boundary that is too thick or rigid to be formed. We believe that such boundaries are only created defensively in the face of trauma or overwhelming material that cannot otherwise be handled and may often be accompanied by inadequate parenting. In the same way individuals can develop healthy defense mechanisms rather than pathological ones unless they face certain stresses and/or deprivations. From the standpoint of Ego-State therapy, ego states do not lose their boundaries when they are in the normal state of integration. This concept of *merging* (Phillips & Frederick, 1995) differs from the concept of fusion (Kluft, 1993) which is held by many Dissociative Identity Disorder (Multiple Personality Disorder) therapists to be the norm for the healthy personality.

Safe Space Imagery.   Safe space imagery can be used with ego states to help them develop normal, semipermeable boundaries. As is seen, certain ego states whose boundaries are too thick can benefit from this approach, which eventually affords a bridge to other ego states with whom they can develop co-consciousness. We (McNeal & Frederick, 1994) have noted that the establishment of a safe place for an isolated ego state can prompt a focus on the existence of other ego states whose presences have heretofore been ignored. Within the safe place internal self-soothing occurs (McNeal & Frederick, 1994): this establishes a positive internal holding environment (Baker, 1981; Winnicott, 1960/1965) for the ego state.

At times ego states are not able to create safe place imagery initially. The therapist can intervene here by suggesting such imagery. This can be something connected to the therapist, such as the therapist's office, or it could be something that the therapist knows historically represents safety and security for the patient. Although the therapist is providing the ego state with a *transitional experience* (Baker, 1994) when he does this, it is our experience that ego states learn and grow so they are able to create other safe places for themselves, as Brown and Fromm (1986) recommend for the individual patient. At times the safe place may become an *intrapsychic transitional space* (Morton & Frederick, 1996) which is presented in detail in chapter 10.

Outside of trance and the therapy hour, patients have been able to embellish and further the ego state's safe place experiences by creating drawings and paintings of the imagery. This appears to be one way that other ego states are able to share in the boundary experience of an ego state. Thus a step in the direction of co-conscious has been taken when such productions occur, although we have no certainty which ego state (or how many of them) was involved in the creation of the art work.

As therapy progresses, we have found that ego states with adequate, but not pathological, membranes or boundaries are eventually able to share their safe places with other ego states. It is the adequate boundary formation/repair that makes these moves toward co-consciousness and integration possible. One of Helen Watkins' (personal communication, 1994) interventions in this direction is a general meeting of ego states within a safe room.

Regulation of Space and Time.   The use of imagery exercises for the regulation of closeness and distance allows the ego state to develop boundaries that protect it from damage, engulfment, and abandonment. Engulfment for an ego state is a situation in which it ceases to have boundaries, and its energy enters into the boundaries of another ego state. This is perceived correctly by ego states as death. It is true that some ego states elect to merge completely with other ego states during the integrative process. However, this is done by developed ego states and represents a deliberate choice for the greater good of the internal family. Other merging that resembles engulfment occurs when fragments or incomplete ego states are absorbed by complete ones.

Closeness and distance can be regulated from the safe place through sharing of that space, or by the use of other hypnotic interventions such as a telescope that can be used to inspect another ego state at a distance, using weaker and weaker lenses to produce closeness over time. A sports car for cruising through inner terrain could be employed, or even the development of another safe place.

Barrier Imagery.   Some of the most commonly used barrier imagery involves placing negatively charged ego states into protective custody into such places as jails, cages, and gunny sacks, and separating out and locking safely away overwhelming material (Kluft, 1989) into safes, safety deposit boxes, antique trunks, and so on. Other barrier imagery can involve direct protection or shielding with cloaks, armor, invisible shields of light, angels, protective animals, and so forth. The role of the therapist is to help the ego state develop this kind of imagery for boundary formation and transform and relinquish it as therapy progresses, boundaries are adequate, and frightening material is resolved and no longer threatening.

In the following cases the additional dimension of time is added. For example, allowing another ego state into one's safe place may be something that can only be done briefly at first. Incremental increases in the time may assist with boundary correction.

The Development of Affect Barriers.   Closeness and distance from therapist are significant issues that are usually managed in terms of emotional closeness and distance. Although trance-activated ego states may, at times, gaze at the therapist through open eyes (Baker, 1981), fears of engulfment and/or abandonment are usually communicated verbally or symbolically. In the case of nonverbal ego states that are in communication with the therapist, ideomotor signals may be invaluable (Frederick, 1994e).

Distancing from intense affect may be necessary because the stimulus barrier (Freud, 1920/1961) is inadequate. "According to Freud (1920/1961) internal stimuli are treated by this barrier as if they were external stimuli, and the stimulus barrier (Reitschutz) only permits fragments of the intensity of the original stimulus to be transmitted to the organism" (McNeal & Frederick, 1994, p. 5).

As mentioned earlier in this chapter as well as in chapter 7, Freud (1920/1961) thought the breaching of the stimulus barrier by trauma produces traumatic neurosis. Kluft (1984a, 1985) believes the disrupted stimulus barrier may be repaired by restorative experiences of soothing and nurturing. If ego states that are carrying traumatic memory material and affect do not receive satisfactory restorative experiences, the barrier may be inadequate, and ego-strengthening maneuvers, especially internal self-soothing (McNeal & Frederick, 1994), may be essential to its repair. Khan's (1963) concept of cumulative trauma also places the mother in the role of another shield for the infant/child. If he fails to function adequately in this regard, the child may develop as if he had sustained great trauma.

Closeness and distance from intense or overwhelming affect can also be modulated through the use of the *slow leak* (Kluft, 1989; Watkins, 1992), desensitization techniques, and careful pacing of the work. At times assisting an ego state to enter emotional withdrawal into restful, reenergizing sleep (Kluft, 1989) is another way of allowing it to find a useful barrier to affect.

There are several models of family therapy that illustrate the relevance of greater differentiation among individual members to more organic, holistic functioning (Kerr & Bowen, 1988; Satir, 1983) of the multi-member unit. In Bowen multigenerational family therapy (Kerr & Bowen, 1988), the family is thought of as possessing an *undifferentiated family ego* (Bowen, 1960). Pathology exists in this model whenever and wherever the members of the family fail to grow, individuate, and separate. It is only when these processes fail to occur that the family becomes closed, enmeshed, and dysfunctional. Family health or integration of the family system is always enhanced by the healthy differentiation of its members. We have observed that careful work with primitive ego states within the internal family of selves, like family therapy (Frederick, 1995e), may yield significant therapeutic results.

Case Example: Lotti (Continued)

Some aspects of the case of Lotti were described in a previous paper (McNeal & Frederick, 1994). Lotti has a diagnosis of Dissociative Identity Disorder (DID), although most of her friends, acquaintances, and business associates would be surprised to hear it. Several of Lotti's ego states created their own individual safe places.

During the course of treatment, what can only be called the safe place wars occurred. Morgan, while allowing no one into her safe place, made raiding parties in which she attempted to take over other parts' safe places. Eventually parts were able to talk about their senses of safety in their own places, and their reluctance and fear about sharing them. As treatment progressed, three goals concerning safe places were shared by the parts and me. One was for them to feel increasingly safe and protected there; another was to begin to allow other parts to visit the safe place for limited periods of time that could be extended gradually; finally, parts would ask permission to enter the safe places of other parts for limited periods of time.

This arrangement became one of the things we discussed regularly in the hypnotherapy sessions. As parts felt more comfortable, traumatic material was revealed, and ego states were able to begin to visit one another in their respective safe places. The holdout was Morgan, who insisted she had to stay in his room a little longer. Fifteen months after he had taken over Lotti's safe place, Morgan was able to leave it to visit others. My (CF) hypnotic discussions with the parts about safe places included several elements. One was a reminder of how comfortable and soothing safe places could be; another had to do with barrier imagery: safe places were safe, and no one could harm anyone there. I also talked about the joys of exploring new places that one could discover were also safe. Finally, I discussed boundary manners—how one should not enter another's safe place without permission.

The concept that the parts were all members of the internal family who wanted to help Lotti was frequently mentioned. Integration as a goal of therapy was openly discussed despite a number of objections to this as a goal, especially if it involved a part named Thirteen who was initially perceived as malevolent by the other ego states.

Eventually, I found all the ego states lying side by side in the warm sun of the south of France. They told me that they felt very close and had come to love one another, and that they frequently visited the other safe places. In time now, because they felt so much stronger, they would be able to reveal to Lotti, a little bit at a time, the rest of the trauma material that needed to be acknowledged and worked through. Lotti was about to take her first long airplane trip to several Caribbean Islands. Because Lotti and the ego states feared flying, we worked on turning the airplanes they would be traveling on into safe places that could be enjoyed instead of feared.

Case Example: Tim

Tim, a 35-year-old male, sought treatment with me (SM) for his social phobias. Although he was living in a house with three roommates, he spent most of his time isolated in his room reading and doing art work. He found any social interaction highly anxiety-provoking, always feeling obliged to please the other person and subordinate his own feelings and needs. He wanted to feel more comfortable socially, especially to meet women and date. In years of previous insight-oriented therapy, he had learned of many family dynamics and historical events that contributed to the inhibition of his social and sexual development. Strong feelings often produced psychosomatic symptoms, usually gastrointestinal pain and distress, so he had become highly intellectualized avoiding any situations that might evoke emotion and suppressing whatever emotions did occur.

He was highly hypnotizable and readily responded to Ego State therapy. Several ego states consistently emerged in relation to his fears of social interactions and his tendency to get sick. One was an immature, angry male—the introjected abuser, and another was Hoodlum, a crippled male who carried a gun to protect himself. A female state, Desire, contained the longing for emotional and positive physical contact with others, while a very helpful ego state, Wise Man, served as an inner advisor. Ranger was an authoritarian, rigid ego state who kept Tim in protective custody (i.e., kept him in his room). Any of these ego states could cause him to become ill if he did not keep his feeling and impulses in check.

Although some of the ego states could tolerate each other, their ability to interact with one another only changed after the introduction of a safe room where they could meet. Here a robot installed a security system around the perimeter to ensure safety, and this system kept the ego states safe with one another and from the outside world as well.

During their first meeting there a new ego state, the Well of Pain, emerged. Tim learned that if he could allow his strong feelings to be present in the Well of Pain, he did not have to experience them as somatic symptoms. Next he discovered that he could lower a bucket into the well and retrieve his feelings a little bit at a time. This allowed him to handle them carefully over time and kept him from becoming overwhelmed.

As the ego-state work continues, Hoodlum became more understandable. The other ego states began to show him some compassion based on their new understanding that he carries a gun because he has no other form of self-defense. They believed it would only be a matter of time before he could turn in his gun because he would realize that he could protect himself in other ways and rely on other ego states to help protect him.

Tim started to set more limits, become more assertive, and experiment with new behaviors in social settings. He is now dating successfully.

The ego-state therapist can play an important role in helping immature ego states with inadequate or defensively hypertrophied boundaries regulate their boundaries in ways that facilitate integration. In the case of Lotti we have demonstrated the use of safe place imagery by several ego states as steps in the formation of adequate boundaries that were precursors to and vehicles of integrative momentum. Her ego states' safe places were used for internal self-soothing

(McNeal & Frederick, 1994) as well as for distancing and closeness imagery in both space and time which allowed them to experience one another without engulfment or abandonment. The presence of many safe places inherently contributed to boundary formation (Brown & Fromm, 1986) through an expansion of repertoire. Barrier imagery was implied semantically through the use of suggestive phrases such as "no one can hurt you there."

Lotti's ego states worked together to present traumatic material at only the rate they believed Lotti could tolerate; this also strengthened boundaries (Phillips & Frederick, 1995). The use of these maneuvers required the development of a great deal of mastery by the ego states. We believe that this mastery was another contribution to internal boundary formation.

In the case of Tim time was introduced as a factor in creating an affective barrier. The Well of Pain represents a container (Baker, 1981; Winnicott, 1960/1965) whose existence has been a manifestation of early boundary formation in Tim's therapy. The ego state named Hoodlum needed to carry a gun as his protective barrier until he learned to say "no" to express anger appropriately and become more assertive.

The barrier imagery represented by the security system around the safe room (Watkins, 1990) allowed the ego states to feel even safer because it kept out intruders and permitted a sense of privacy. The level of fear present in Tim's ego states made it especially important for defenses to be strengthened so that they could feel truly safe. Containing pain within the family of selves inside the safe room became a way to (a) retrieve dissociated affect, (b) deal with it over time, (c) prevent psychosomatic symptoms, and (d) reassociate the affect with new behaviors in the external world.

Healthy differentiation of ego states appears to parallel that of healthy differentiation within the family system. Boundary issues can never be ignored in family therapy. Adequate boundary formation occurs naturally in healthy families. In family therapy certain family members may require work to help them form healthy boundaries. There is also a need for family members to learn to respect each other's boundaries. Based on our work with many cases, we believe that, when needed, adequate boundary formation and containment in ego states are necessary precursors to integration. We believe that those who would criticize such work as increasing dissociation are probably among those who similarly criticize Ego-State therapy. These criticisms do not appear to be based on what Ego-State therapy really is or how it really works. The proof of the pudding is in the tasting. If helping ego states to form and repair boundaries contributed to further dissociation, integration could not follow.

Chapter 10

Other Projective/Evocative Techniques

Ideodynamic Healing

The term *ideodynamic* has been used "to designate all the relationships between ideas and the dynamic physiological responses of the body" (Rossi & Cheek, 1988, p. 3). It reflects a shift from the dualism that dominated science since the time of Descartes. Western science is only just beginning to release itself from the grip of Descartes' (1596–1650) division of the human being into a mind and a body. The only point of intimate connection between the two for Descartes was the pineal gland. There, like strangers, they could meet in some undefined and presumably insignificant way. The real mind–body connection, Descartes believed, was effected by God. The function of the body was to house the mind and give it some access to the external world through sense perception and motor functions.

Descartes' dualism continued to prevail in the following century, although public healings became a conspicuous part of the Western culture. Some were performed by clerics, of whom Johann Joseph Gassner (1727–1799) is an outstanding example (Ellenberger, 1970). Gassner allowed that there were diseases that belonged strictly to the body and whose causation was exclusively natural; their province was that of the physician. Gassner also believed that some natural diseases had preternatural causes that involved possession by the devil or sorcery (Ellenberger, 1970). Gassner conducted many exorcisms and produced a number of healings.

Franz Anton Mesmer (1734–1815) vigorously opposed Gassner. His explanation for his own equally dramatic healings was physical. They had been produced by an invisible fluid that passed from the healer into the sufferer. He had called this powerful substance *animal magnetism* (Ellenberger, 1970).

The Cartesian separation of mind and body that Gassner and Mesmer strove so energetically to maintain is unusual in terms of what history tells us about the connection between words and ideas with the responses of the body. Rossi and Cheek (1988) remind us that ideodynamic—or mind–body—healing existed long before Descartes. Evidence of such healings can be found in the Ebers

DOI:10.4324/9781003442585-10

papyrus, in the ruins of the temples of Isis Serapis, Apollo, and Asclepius. The royal touch of kings was observed to be healing, and as medicine developed, some of the most renowned physicians of their time, such as Paracelsus, mixed physical medicine with prayer, incantation, and arcane practices (Ellenberger, 1970; Rossi & Cheek, 1988).

Gassner was also performing ideodynamic healings, albeit unwittingly, as was Mesmer. The subsequent experiences of clinicians with hypnosis pointed again and again in the direction of there being an intimate connection between the mind and the body. The discoveries of Chevreul (1833, 1854) were significant in this respect. Chevreul was a French chemist who published *De la Baquette Divinitoire* in 1854. In it he critiqued ancient healing practices and described his own experiments with the use of the pendulum on pregnant women to determine the sex of their unborn children. Chevreul suspended a pendulum over the abdomens of these pregnant women. If the pendulum swung in one particular direction, the presence of a male fetus was indicated; if in the other, that of a female. Chevreul was able to demonstrate that the movements of the pendulum were most often successful in accurately predicting the sex of the unborn child. Cherveul believed that the movements of the pendulum were the result of the influence of the "unconscious knowledge and belief ..." (Rossi & Cheek, 1988, p. 4) of the mother on the small muscles in her fingers

James Braid used the word *psychophysiological* as a general term for hypnosis. His observations had led him to believe that the mind and the body had a reciprocal influence on one another. Another pioneer, Bernheim, regarded all hypnosis as an ideodynamic (mind–body) process. He thought that, in trance, various types of mind–body *excitabilities* became increased in the brain. He believed this to take place on a level that we would call *unconscious* today. He described the process as one in which the higher centers of the brain would not be able to interfere with or to stop the process. This is strangely reminiscent of Erickson's thinking (see chap. 3).

Rossi and Cheek (1988) have developed a comprehensive approach to ideodynamic healing. In *Mind–Body Therapy: Methods of Ideodynamic Healing in Hypnosis* they explain their view of ideodynamic healing as a utilization approach to healing that capitalizes on state-bound material (see chap. 2).

The State-Bound Perspective

State-bound material is information, usually processed and stored on a psychophysiological level, that was acquired during a particular course of events. It is stored on a deeply unconscious level and contains not only the problem situation, but also the resources that can help resolve the problem (see chap. 2).

Another way to view state-bound material is in terms of psychophysiology and biochemistry. In human events, especially those related to difficulty, trauma, and survival, the body is flooded with informational substances, millions of messenger molecules (Pert, Ruff, Weber, & Herkenham, 1985) that communicate with the cells. A unique chemical outpouring of hormones such as epinephrine-norepinephrine, adrenal cortical hormones, and endorphins occurs. Information is processed and retained within the physiological and chemical substrate of the state in which the individual is at that time. Because it is a unique portal to the inner world, hypnosis can allow the individual to have access to state-bound material and other inner resources (Rossi, 1993; van der Kolk, 1996a). In the example given in chapter 2, a man who has had a bicycle accident is not able to recall the experience very clearly until he accesses the state-bound material connected with the accident hypnotically.

The Utilization Perspective

From the standpoint of ideodynamic healing the individual has, on an unconscious level, much, if not all, of what she needs to solve certain problems. A question that must be answered about ideodynamic healing is how it accesses relevant material and allows it to be worked with therapeutically on an unconscious level.

Erickson (1961) began his experimentation with ideomotor signals in the 1920s. He noted that they could be used for trance induction and could appear spontaneously as well. Ideomotor signals with their emphasis on the wisdom of deeper levels of mind were also developed as tools for uncovering material held within those deeper levels of mind (LeCron, 1954, 1963). They became premier tools in hypnoanalysis; they also found their way into emergency medicine, pain control, psychosomatic medicine, and a host of other clinical applications (Rossi & Cheek, 1988).

Ideodynamic healing always begins with a basic accessing question such as: Would it be alright for (here the patient is named) to go within so that her inner mind can focus on the problem of why she is having headaches? And resolve that problem? The basic accessing question is intentionally broad and nondirective. It simply states the general problem and asks for help. The therapist can get some indication of the level of cooperation by hand or finger movements whose meanings have been agreed upon previously. The open secret of ideodynamic healing lies in the therapist using the signals as a ritual that begins the procedure of activating the patient's unconscious mind to reach and resolve the problem. Not every therapist can be as skillful as Milton Erickson in devising utilization techniques (Erickson & Rossi, 1976). Ideodynamic healing takes the mystery out of utilization by openly asking the unconscious to utilize and resolve.

Ideodynamic healing can be of particular value with patients who are resistant to hypnosis as well as with patients who are frightened of bringing painful material, such as trauma, into consciousness. There is less pressure on the patient to come up with specific information and experiences or to feel that she must produce detailed and correct answers. It is also most helpful with patients who are resistant to classic hypnosis. It can be combined with other therapeutic and hypnotherapeutic techniques in a number of creative ways.

Rossi and Cheek (1988) discovered ideodynamic healing's "useful generalizability to almost any therapeutic situation" (p. 35). The theoretical orientation of the therapist is not particularly significant. "The most useful common denominator that ideodynamic signaling provides for healers of all persuasions is that a convincing, overt behavioral signal is generated by the patient whenever a useful bit of therapeutic progress has been experienced" (Rossi & Cheek, 1988, p. 35). Moreover, Rossi has stated that it is not necessary to assume that ideodynamic healing is truly hypnotic in nature. He reminds us that a valid empirical method for discovering or measuring the presence of an altered state does not exist today.

Although ideodynamic healing is often done with ideodynamic finger signals, the ideodynamic signals could instead involve parts of the body or even other kinds of behavior. For example, the hypnotherapist could establish such signaling with the hands and how they attract or repel one another, the height or heaviness of the hands, whether the patient's eyes are open or closed, or even whether the patient wishes to remain in trance or feels herself awakening.

Frederick and Morton (1998) have found ideodynamic healing to be quite helpful in Ego State Therapy. Ego states are all part of a greater personality and reside within the unconscious. Like the greater personality, they may not have all the answers. They may need to turn to deeper levels of mind for additional resources and the benefits of unconscious learning. In Ego State Therapy ideodynamic healing has an integrating capability that has often been overlooked. The following material from the case of Farley has been described in Frederick and Morton (1998).

Case Example: Farley (Continued)

Farley's decision to get his puppy, Dizzy-Whizzy, was one he did not regret. His attention was directed to the life he was beginning to have; however, his continued weight gain was very slow. In therapy sessions we noted that although the ego states were happy to be activated, they really didn't seem to know what they wanted to do. They would engage in any ego-strengthening hypnotic work I (CF) suggested. For example, they loved the transitional experience of taking a trip to the daisy pond (see chap. 7). However, they did not appear to be able to access any trauma material; they seemed rather passive, and they lacked initiative in the treatment process.

I discussed with Farley my sense that we might help the ego states along by activating even deeper levels of mind commonly associated with a plenum of resources. We would do so in such a way that these aspects of mind could even assume responsibility for some of the healing process. Farley was intrigued and eager to do whatever might be helpful. We set up his trance induction. In the induction Farley held his hands about 6 inches apart from one another. They faced one another, and Farley was able to become aware of the sensation of there being a magnetic current between them.

I posed the basic accessing question in this way: "If Farley's inner mind, or much, much deeper levels of mind would like Farley to enter trance so that they can do healing work on the eating disorder, the current that Farley feels between his hands will draw them together, very slowly. If, on the other hand, these deep levels of mind do not wish for this to happen today, then the current will cause his hands to be repelled, one from another."

For about 90 seconds, there was no visible movement of Farley's hands. Then they slowly began to move closer to one another. The movements were so slow that they occurred over a 5-minute period. When Farley's hands came together and touched one another, I gave a second time-bound instruction: "And, when ... Inner Mind ... deeper levels of mind ... whoever ... you feel that a significant degree of resolution has been reached today, then Farley's hands will begin to drift, possibly down into his lap ... perhaps one hand will drift into his lap and the other will move in some other direction ... but somehow there will be a very noticeable hand movement."

Farley's left hand drifted into his lap. The right hand followed shortly after. I then said, "And when these deep healing levels of mind feel that just the right amount of work has been done today, then Farley's eyes will open, and he will return to the external world in an alert and refreshed condition."

Upon re-alerting, Farley reported that he had seen the word RESOLU-TION in letters that ran clockwise in a circle. Neon-lighted arrows pointed to this word, and below the circle were many puppies just like Dizzy-Whizzy. They were looking at the circular word and barking excitedly.

After this session, Farley began to have a sense that he was nearly out of his danger period. He was enjoying his job as a bartender tremendously. He was also seeing Nan regularly as she began to travel to her parents' home, which was near his own. He became very busy with his dental school applications, and his weight shot up by 10 pounds within two and a half weeks. He looked physically different because he was filling out. In a session in which we accessed the ego states, he noted that the fat ego state seemed to have trimmed down, while the skinny ego state had put on a nice amount of weight and looked very good. When we attempted to locate the ego state, Slime, which caused the regurgitation, he was nowhere to be found. The other ego states did not know what had happened to him. Farley and I speculated that he may have surrendered his energy to the rest of the system.

In a subsequent session we decided that we would use the ideodynamic healing again. Farley spoke to me while he was in trance during this experience. He said, "I can see myself lying on a table, like in a doctor's office. My body's tingling ... I know that, and I can feel it in my hands right now ... Now I see the word RESOLUTION again ... It's surrounded by exclamation marks." After the experience had been completed, Farley had several things to report. "You know, that wasn't a doctor's table. It was an autopsy table." Farley looked shocked. "Now why would I see an autopsy table?"

I reminded him that his body had been tingling while it was on the autopsy table. Farley said, "I think it means I've just come back from the dead!" We agreed that he had been in a dangerous medical condition and that he had not been really living. From the viewpoint of his greatly changed life, Farley could see that previously he had been moving through life like a dead man.

Farley was profoundly moved. He added, "I also could see that we will have to go deeper, but that will happen when it's time." Farley was moving out of his previously compartmentalized, defended, and fragmented way of life, and he wondered with me what it had all been about. This, he realized, would become another important part of his therapy as well as an important part of his discovering who he really was. At this point his weight had gone up to 155 pounds.

Ideodynamic healing in Farley's case affected his body and supplied him with rich symbolism for the incredible changes that were taking place in both his social and inner life. We were both curious to see how the various parts of Farley's personality were reacting to the additional help they were receiving from deeper unconscious levels of mind.

Case Report: Farley (continued)

Farley appeared for the next session wearing a T-shirt. This was the first time I had seen him when he had not been concealing his body with voluminous jackets and sweat shirts. I (CF) remarked on this, and Farley replied "I was hot. Now I have something to make me warmer!" He was consciously referring to the fact that he now had some body fat.

In trance the ego states were activated. When they were asked for comments or information on how they regarded what had been happening with Farley, they supplied two words. One was good, and the other was weird. Through ideomotor signaling they indicated that they were now ready to work on the weird or dark material. We had some dialogue about the necessity for this. It was wonderful that Farley was so much better. However, the work needed to be completed so that Farley would not be in danger of relapses.

Ideodynamic healing is a powerful projective/evocative ego-strengthening technique that can be used in hypnotic and nonhypnotic therapy. It is evocative because it activates a network of inner resources; it is projective because the visible and palpable signs of body responses tell the patient and the therapist something about what is going on with the patient. It is ego-strengthening because it (a) expands conscious–unconscious complementarity, (b) increases unconscious mastery, and (c) promotes integration. It can be used to enhance the patient conscious–unconscious complementarity, and it mixes well with Ego State Therapy.

There will always be those who question the clinical reliability of ideomotor signaling and ideodynamic healing. They ask whether ideomotor signals are reliable, whether there is such a thing as an unconscious mind, and whether it knows all it should know. These processes and rituals can be considered as metaphorical. There is no apodictic reliability to be found anywhere within the field of psychotherapy. Ideodynamic processes, when used by properly trained therapists, are significantly helpful in the processes of extending the range and complexity of the therapeutic alliance, in ego-strengthening, and in information gathering.

Active Imagination

According to Jung (1958/1967) there is a mental activity that allows the reasoning of the conscious mind to cooperate with the information held within the unconscious mind. Jung (1958/1967) called this activity the *transcendent function*. Clearly, Jung believed that the relationship between the conscious and unconscious minds was extremely important (see chap. 13), and described a therapeutic method for exploring and transforming that relationship (Cwik, 1991). He called that method *active imagination* and felt it was the most effective way to understand material that was residing within the unconscious. Jung wrote about the active imagination in a number of papers, beginning with his famous paper, "The Transcendent Function" (Jung, 1916/1971).

Active imagination can be best understood when the importance of the symbol within Jungian thought is grasped. For Jung the symbol was a locus where the conscious and the unconscious could join in a harmonious way. Many of the imaginal figures that inhabit the Jungian unconscious are archetypes or transpersonal figures that belong to the collective unconscious. They often struggle to become known by the rest of the personality just as the *complexes* do. Jung believed that the unconscious mind holds a plenum of resources, such as the transpersonal archetypes, which are available for the regulation of the psyche and the establishment of internal harmony:

The unconscious, then, gives us all the encouragement and help that bountiful nature can shower upon man. It holds possibilities which are locked away from the conscious mind. For it has at its disposal all subliminal psychic contents, all those things which have been forgotten or overlooked, as well as the wisdom and experience of uncounted centuries which are laid down in its archetypal organs ... For these reasons the unconscious could serve man as an inner guide.

(Jung 1926/1966, p. 126)

The issue that the technique of active imagination addresses is just how the richness of the unconscious can be presented to the conscious mind in a way that will allow the transcendent function to establish the desired harmony. Active imagination is often referred to as a process in which the patient focuses on internal imagery. However this process of self-reflection is usually multimodal in nature. Jung (1916/1971) suggested that an emotional state could be a valuable starting point for the procedure. The patient was to make herself as conscious as possible of a particular mood and to follow the associations that ensued:

sinking himself in it without reserve and noting down on paper all the fantasies and other associations that come up. Fantasy must be allowed the freest possible play, yet not in such a manner that it leaves the orbit of its object, namely the affect, by setting off a kind of chain reaction association process.

(Jung, 1916/1971, p. 289)

Jung recommended that critical attention should be eliminated. The patient need only wait and expect an image to occur. It would appear as a visual image, words, or for some, an inner voice that might be a critic or judge. Out of this kind of absorption, Jung believed, "there comes a more or less complete expression of the mood" (Jung, 1916/1971, p. 289) revealing the contents of the mood either concretely or symbolically. He stated that, "The whole procedure is a kind of enrichment and clarification of the affect, whereby the affect and its contents are brought nearer to consciousness, becoming at the same time more impressive and more understandable" (Jung, 1916/1971, p. 289).

Jung believed that it was important for the patient to give the emotional state experienced in active imagination a visible shape through drawing, painting, or sculpture. This expression of what had been experienced was thought to be an important part of active imagination as it furthered the task of joining unconscious content with conscious activity. Active imagination, then, is a therapeutic technique that facilitates the actions of the transcendent function, thereby promoting collaboration between the conscious and unconscious parts of the mind. It is the most important way the transcendent function can be brought into play in psychotherapy. Active imagination is a process not dissimilar to Freud's elucidation of *free association*; yet it is, for all of that, quite different.

In terms of what can be done with the material obtained through active imagination, Jung (1916/1971) postulated two main tendencies or principles: *creative formulation* and *understanding*. *Creative formulation* is a principle that refers to the making and perception of symbols, the subjective way in which the patient receives information via the transcendent function. It always involves a "condensation of motifs into more or less stereotyped symbols" (Jung, 1916/1971, p. 291). Thus, it produces a creative, aesthetic, and artistic formulation. When the principle of *understanding* predominates, "... there is an intensive struggle to understand the meaning of the unconscious product" (Jung, 1916/1971, p. 291).

Creative formulation is basically the creation of an image, while *understanding* gives meaning to the image. Both these tendencies have their dangers. One is the diversion of the imagination from the transcendent function into problems of subjectivity, such as artistic expression. Another that could occur, in the case of understanding, is that the content could be intellectually analyzed and interpreted to the degree that its symbolic character is lost. Jung's two principles are like Kant's (1781/1929) version of percepts and concepts. "Thoughts without contents are empty; intuitions without concepts are blind" (p. 61). The transcendent function also appears to bear some resemblance to Kant's transcendental unity of apperception. Jung believed that one tendency is the regulating principle of the other, and that they are "bound together in a compensatory relationship (Jung, 1916/1971, p. 293). They supplement each other to form the transcendent function.

The second part of the procedure known as active imagination, according to Jung, has to do with the relationship of the ego to the new material formed during the process. "When the unconscious content has been given form and the meaning of the formulation is understood, the question arises as to how the ego will relate to this position, and how the ego and the unconscious are to come to terms" (Jung 1916/1971, p. 295). This entails the bringing together of opposites for the production of the transcendent function. "The ego takes the lead, but the unconscious must be allowed to have its say too" (Jung, 1916/1971, p. 296). The capacity for inner dialogue marks the process by which the ego and the unconscious consider each other's views and arguments. Comparing and discussing, they thereby modify the conflict. It is not necessary that the confrontation become totally conscious, but rather that the feelings that appear in consciousness are valuable. Consciousness in this way is continually expanded on the part of the patient, through her own process, rather than through dependence on the therapist. There can be no doubt that the reverie that Jung felt was necessary for engagement in the process of active imagination is a trance state and that active imagination is a form of hypnotically facilitated psychotherapy (see chap. 2).

We could say that use of the active imagination can be ego-strengthening because it helps to crystallize the relationships between the ego and unconscious, so that these relationships can be understood and transformed in the direction of healing. When some of the archetypes of the unconscious become conscious, they can be utilized in psychotherapy in creative ways, as the following sections will indicate.

Other Imagery and Imagination Techniques

There is a plethora of imagery techniques that are ego-strengthening. Some have been derived from Jung's active imagination. Others are outgrowths of experiences that clinicians have had while working with dissociative patients and appear to rely on certain ways of looking at Ego State Therapy. We have included several of these techniques, but we caution the reader not to become swept away by overtheorizing. Although we know many of these techniques are useful, it is not at all clear why this is so.

We do not agree with all of the theoretical explanations given by the creators of every technique described after. For example, we do not think that a deep unifying aspect of self (commonly called the Center, the Center Core, etc.) is an ego state or that it is synonymous with the safe place. What we do endorse is the general helpfulness and ego-strengthening qualities of the techniques described below. For the sake of faithfulness to the material of their creators, we attempt to explain how they view their techniques theoretically.

Many think an experimental basis for these concepts can be found in Hilgard's (1984) hidden observer phenomena. Hilgard (1984) made hypnotic suggestions for anaesthesia to subjects who were being subjected to painful stimuli. Upon testing then he discovered that they had, indeed, become insensitive to pain. He inquired of his anaesthetized subjects whether there was an awareness of the painful stimuli at any level of consciousness. This is how he discovered that in many subjects there was a hidden observer that could experience pain while the experimental subject did not react to painful stimuli.

Other studies have demonstrated hidden observer phenomena in college students and in patients (Lynn, Mare, Kvaal, Segal, & Sivec, 1994; Watkins & Watkins, 1979–1980). Lynn and his associates (1994) do not believe the hidden observer is a personality structure, but rather a therapeutic metaphor. Lynn et al. conducted a series of studies of hidden observer phenomena in regard to hypnotic dreams and age regression. They concluded that, "hidden observer instructions can be used to secure personally meaningful information from both hypnotized and non-hypnotized subjects in a variety of test conditions and situations" (Lynn et al., 1994, p. 135). They state that,

> Clinically, hidden observer suggestions can be used to facilitate interpretation of events, experiences, and motives; to encourage clients to adopt multiple

perspectives about their feelings and behaviors; to foster distance and dissociation from painful thoughts and feelings; and to facilitate hypnotic amnesia
(e.g., the hidden part can remain hidden.

(Lynn et al., 1994, p. 135)

The Inner Advisor

The concept of inner guidance is certainly not a new one. It is a central tenet of
most religions. For example, many Christians are taught that they have a guard-
ian angel whom they can call upon in times of crisis. In Native American cultures, young men engage in fasting and rituals to evoke images of guiding spirits
that would exert strong influence over the rest of their lives. It is part of the
human condition to want a source of guidance and that guidance can take many
forms depending on one's religion or other belief system. Common phrases such
as *a little birdie told me, that still, small voice within,* or *to thine own self be true*
are expressions of the concepts of wisdom within oneself.

In his brilliant book about the discovery of the unconscious, Ellenberger
(1970) traced the development of the unconscious as the source of inner truth.
Among the pioneers of psychiatry, Jung (1954/1971) was the main one to view
the unconscious mind as a source of wisdom extending beyond earlier conceptualizations of the unconscious as a repository of repressed instincts, thoughts, or
wishes. Psychoanalytic writers developed the concept of an observing ego which
is a part of the ego that "like a detached spectator, watched the hubbub of illusion
go past" (Freud, 1940/1964a, pp. 201–202). Greenson (1967) believed it was
important for the patient to have an observing ego to form a working relationship
with the therapist (see chap. 1).

Inner Guides and Hypnosis

Within the hypnotic tradition, concepts of inner guidance have been developed most
extensively by clinicians working with patients with Dissociative Identity Disorder
(DID; Beahrs, 1986; Bliss, 1984; Kluft, 1989; Putnam, 1989; Ross, 1989). Hilgard
(1977) performed experiments demonstrating hidden observers that have been regarded as ego states by John and Helen Watkins (1997; see chap. 4).

Many different variations of the use of inner guides have been discussed in
the hypnosis literature, and scripts have been developed to assist in accessing
these parts of the conscious or unconscious mind. The script included in this
section (Rossman, 1987) is an example of how the *inner advisor* can be accessed
in the clinical hour.

The inner advisor technique was originally developed by physicians who
were part of the early group of pioneers who were interested in using imagery
techniques with serious illnesses. Martin Rossman (1987) expanded on the technique that he had learned from Oyle (1975). Oyle, in turn, had been influenced

by Simonton, Matthews-Simonton, and Creighton's (1978) work with cancer patients and by the writings of Carl Jung. The inner advisor technique can be utilized to access and develop a part of the personality that can become like a cotherapist in therapy or an ever-present guide in the individual's life.

According to Rossman (1987) the inner advisor is a source of understanding, comfort, and support. The inner advisor is compassionate and has one's best interests in mind. Inner advisors appear in many guises. Although they often appear as images of a wise old man or wise old woman, they take on many other forms, including animals, plants, trees, and/or religious figures. They could also appear as characters from books or movies, or sometimes as light, energy, or invisible spirits. In whatever form the inner advisor occurs, the task is to welcome it, get to know it, and form a relationship with it.

Rossman (1987) has created a script for meeting your inner advisor:

Meeting Your Inner Advisor

Begin to relax by taking a comfortable position loosening any restricting clothing, and making arrangements for thirty minutes of unrestricted time ... take a few deep breaths and begin to let go of tension as you release each breath ... allow yourself a few to relax more deeply, allowing your body to let go and your mind to become quiet and still....

Imagine yourself descending the ten stairs that take you deeper to your quiet inner place ... 10 ... 9 ... deeper and more relaxed ... 8 ... 7 ... easily and naturally ... 6 ... 5 ... deeper and more comfortably relaxed ... 4 ... your mind quiet and still, but alert ... 3 ... 2 ... deeper and more comfortably at ease ... and 1 ....

As you relax more deeply, imagine yourself in that special place of beauty and serenity you found as you did the previous imagery exercises ... take a few minutes to experience the peacefulness and tranquillity you find in this place ....

When you are ready, invite your inner advisor to join you in this special place ... just allow an image to form that represents your inner advisor, a wise, kind figure who knows you well ... let it appear in any way that comes and accept it as it is for now ... it may come in many forms—a wise old man or woman, a friendly animal or bird, a ball of light, a friend or relative, a religious figure. You may not have a visual image at all, but a sense of peacefulness and kindness instead ....

Accept your inner advisor as it appears, as long as it seems wise, kind, and compassionate ... you will be able to sense its caring for you and its wisdom ... invite it to be comfortable there with you, and ask it its name ... accept what comes ... when you are ready, tell it about your problem ... ask any questions you have concerning this situation ... take all the time you need to do this ....

Now listen carefully to your advisor's response ... as you would to a wise and respected teacher ... you may imagine your advisor talking with you or you may simply have a direct sense of its message in some other way ... allow it to communicate with you in whatever way seems natural ... if you are uncertain about the meaning of its advice or if there are other questions you want to ask, continue the conversation until you feel you have learned all you can at this time ... ask questions, be open to the responses that come back, and consider them carefully ....

As you consider what your advisor has told you, imagine what your life would be like if you took the advice you have received and put it into action ... do you see any problems or obstacles standing in the way of doing this? ... if so, what are they, and how might you deal with them in a healthy, constructive way? ... if you need some help here, ask your advisor, who is still there with you ... when it seems right, thank your advisor for meeting with you, and ask it to tell you the easiest, surest method for getting back in touch with it ... realize that you can call another meeting with your advisor whenever you feel the need ....

Say good-bye for now in whatever way seems appropriate, and allow yourself to come back to waking consciousness by walking the stairs and counting upwards from one to ten, as you have before. When you reach ten, come wide-awake, refreshed and alert, and remembering what was significant or important to you about this meeting.

(p. 102)

Rossman (1987) suggests that the person then write down what happened in her meeting with the inner advisor, including a description of the inner advisor, what was asked, what the response was, and what has been learned. He suggests recording what obstacles might be encountered in taking the inner advisor's advice and whether other people would be affected by this advice.

At times people have reported that no inner advisor appears. When that happens, Rossman advises the person to have patience and to continue to go the quiet place daily until the advisor shows up. He suggests, "Just wait in your inner place, as if you were waiting for a bus. There's nothing you can do to make it come sooner" (Rossman, 1987, p. 110). The problem may be one of difficulty relaxing and remaining receptive. Other methods that can be used if the inner advisor is not there are to: (a) imagine what the inner advisor might be like, (b) draw or sculpt the inner advisor, (c) imagine having a talk with a close friend, (d) think of a historical or mythological figure, or (e) write a letter to one's wisest self. These exercises can stimulate the imagination and result in the inner advisor's showing up.

If a critical and hostile inner advisor appears, it is probably not the inner advisor, but rather an internalized representation of a judgmental parent or authority figure from one's external life. Rossman (1987) advises confronting a critical or hostile inner advisor, and letting it know that you will not tolerate criticism that isn't constructive. He also suggests that you ask for feedback that will lead toward health and healing. Rossman (1987) reports that the advisor may change when confronted in this way. He recommends listening to this inner critic but not taking it seriously. This will result in its beginning to sound repetitious and recognizable. If the image that comes is a frightening one, Rossman proposes that a way be found to befriend it. It is also possible to have that "critic" refer one to another inner advisor that is more appropriate for her.

You may recognize in this conceptualization of the inner advisor similarities to ego-state concepts (see chap. 4) and other theories about parts of the personality. The inner advisor could be considered to be a resource part, and, depending on how it appears, it may or may not be from the conflict-free sphere of the ego. There are also similarities to the experiences some individuals have when they meet Inner Strength (see chap. 6). The kinds of images that emerge could correspond to Jung's archetypes, especially those of the *wise old man* or the *wise old woman*, who could also be viewed as the animus and anima.

The ego-strengthening aspects of meeting the inner advisor are evident in that the experiences validate a wise and loving inner part that is there to provide comfort, support, and wisdom. It is encouraging to feel that the part is available and can be called on for guidance at any time. It can become a selfobject for calming and soothing (see chap. 7) and an expression of objective thinking.

Case Example: Judy

Judy, a 35-year-old woman, had entered therapy to explore her relationships with men in an attempt to understand why she had a pattern of choosing partners who ultimately were inappropriate and incompatible with her. She was interested in hypnosis, readily entered trance and has talents for vivid visual imagery. I (SM) introduced the script for meeting the inner advisor. From the frown and pained expression on her face, it was evident she was displeased by the image that came up for her. She described a middle-aged woman with dyed red hair who was dressed flamboyantly in billowing, brightly colored clothing. She wore heavy makeup and costume jewelry in "poor taste," Judy reported. The woman had the appearance that one could imagine might be characteristic of a madam in a house of ill repute, or perhaps a medium, or a gypsy fortune teller. Judy confronted this image of her inner advisor and exclaimed, "I never thought my inner advisor would look like you."

The inner advisor responded, "That is your problem, dear, you can be deceived by appearances." As it happened, once Judy accepted this inner advisor in the form that she appeared, she found this image to indeed be wise, compassionate, and a source of objective advise. This experience was also very helpful in provoking Judy to examine her biases in how she evaluated other people in her life.

Utilization of the Internal Self Helper or Core Personality

Inner or Internal Self Helpers

As described in chapter 7, Allison (1974) spoke of the Internal Self Helper (ISH) in patients with Dissociative Identity Disorder (DID). He saw them as an aspect of the personality, much like the inner advisor, that could help to guide treatment. Allison (1974) thought of it as an internal resource or helper part of the personality that was a source of wisdom and understanding, free from the conflicts involved with other parts.

Allison had been influenced by Assagioli (1965), who had founded psychosynthesis (see chap. 4). According to Assagioli, the personality consists of sub-personalities, or parts that influence the whole person. One of these parts, he hypothesized, is the *higher self*, the center of the psyche or the true self; it is very similar to Allison's (1974 Internal Self Helper (ISH).

Comstock (1991) elaborated on this concept by developing the idea of "a structure or force within the multiple [personality disorder patient] that was stronger, wiser, and connected to all parts of the person" (p. 169), that she called the *center*. She believed this part differed from Allison's concept in that she viewed the *center* as less spiritual and mystical than Allison's Internal Self Helper. She thought it was able to demonstrate the whole range of human emotions in contrast with Allison's Internal Self Helper which was described as being pure intellect.

Another function of the Internal Self Helper, according to Beahrs (1986), is to act as a central unifying force—the force that provides a person with his sense of unity in spite of the different ego states he believes we all possess. Beahrs (1982b, 1986) views the Internal Self Helper as a healthy and creative part of the unconscious.

Comstock (1991) pointed out certain controversies surrounding the Internal Self Helper. The skeptics posed the same arguments as those commonly made to negate the existence of Dissociative Identity Disorder (DID) as a valid clinical syndrome, that the Internal Self Helper is iatrogenic, unprovable, and the creation of narcissistic therapists. These arguments illustrate the ongoing debates between those who study the phenomena in the laboratory and the clinicians who observe and utilize conceptualizations. Differences in perception of the Internal Self Helper also involve variances in belief systems, especially those concerning spirituality. Allison and Schwarz (1980) believed the Internal Self Helper could be the expression of God. Although some of Comstock's reported Internal Self Helpers may believe in God, others may be atheists, or may even be angry at a God who causes them suffering. Comstock (1991) describes many ways in which the Internal Self Helper can be contributive, especially in dealing with dissociative patients. An Internal Self Helper can (a) provide information and clarity during the processing of abreactions, (b) influence dreams, (c) blend or integrate alters, and (d) assist in the postintegration process.

The Center Core

In working with Dissociative Identity Disorder (DID) patients, Torem and Gainer (1995) posited the existence of a center core, the part of the personality that is also an inner advisor and the safe place. According to Gainer and Torem (1993) the center core is an aspect of the patient that thinks logically and rationally and has access to knowledge of the whole person. This part can be interpreted as a symbolic representation of the patient's ego strength and/or as an introject of the therapist (Gainer & Torem, 1993, p. 260). It is "experienced as a distinct ego state, the function of which is to preserve logical, rational, mature and objective thinking" (Gainer & Torem, 1993, p. 260).

Gainer and Torem (1993) use the designation of *center core* because they view the resources experienced by the patient while in this ego state to be an "aspect of the patient's own core personality or innermost, central self" (p. 260). Gainer and Torem believe that when the patient is in this ego state, he can provide an overview of the specific areas of conflict and can identify "hidden agendas that affect the therapy through subtle or covert difficulties of conflicting ego states" (Gainer & Torem, 1993, p. 260) as well as predicting and averting crises.

Torem and Gainer (1995) have taken the position that the resources experienced by the patient while in the *center core* ego state encourage the experience of mastery while discouraging the tendency, particularly in dependent patients, of disowning or externalizing therapeutic gains. They believe that, in addition to providing rational, logical thinking and self-observation, the *center core* serves a deeper purpose—of striving toward the experience of unity and wholeness. This sense of unity is impaired when an individual has been traumatized, or when there is chronic dissociation. In this respect, Torem and Gainer (1995) have taken a page from Beahrs (1986) in their vision of resources residing deep within the patient.

Torem and Gainer (1995) propose that the experience of unity is an ongoing function of consciousness and that "… by strengthening the dissociated patient's reliance on, and experience of the Center Core, the perception of self as a unified whole is facilitated" (p. 127). They characterize this ego state, the *center core*, as the *unifying* self and have developed imagery for enhancing this function.

When the *center core* is experienced as an ego-state, it can be accessed hypnotically and enter into dialogue with the therapist as the patient's internal consultant. It can enter into alliances with other ego states to affect therapeutic changes. According to Torem and Gainer (1995), sometimes the *center core* is experienced as a part of the self, different from other ego-states, but can communicate through other ego states. It need not be personified, but rather it is a metaphorical representation of the patient's strengths and resources. It may be experienced as a place, usually with imagery of a dwelling, a garden, meadow, cavern, or whatever imagery is symbolic for the patient of a peaceful, tranquil interior place. When the *center core* is experienced as a place, the patient may experience the influence of this place across a variety of ego states. For example, a patient might experience his *center core* as his safe place—a meadow where all the other ego-states can assemble (see chap. 7). Some patients experience their *center core* as a thing, an energy, or light. These patients can then imagine accessing their resources through use of this object or force-field (Torem & Gainer, 1995).

The Center Core can be accessed hypnotically or nonhypnotically. The therapist may only need to give instructions to certain patients that they sit quietly, close their eyes, and follow the suggestions of the therapist. With other patients, a formal hypnotic induction followed by a script for accessing the Center Core can be used. Torem (1990) has developed a specific script for accessing the Center Core—a script similar to the one by Rossman (1987) for accessing the inner advisor. Another script (Torem & Gainer, 1995) is elaborated and amplified for use with patients who resist the idea of the Center Core as part of the self (Torem & Gainer, 1995).

Torem and Gainer (1995) also address the issue of iatrogenic creation of a dissociated ego state. They agree that an ego state of this nature may be created, but argue that it seems unlikely that the therapist could suggest the presence of ego strength where none exists in the patient. They believe that "the use of the Center Core allows the patient to become more aware of his/her own capacity for healing and recovery, by making those capacities clearly accessible to the patient" (Torem & Gainer, 1995, p. 131). Over the course of psychotherapy the Center Core may undergo transformation, especially in Dissociative Identity Disorder (DID) patients as the process of integration progresses. In this sense it provides the unifying function necessary for integration and formation of a new identity.

Concepts of Core Personality

All of these techniques assume a part of the personality or self exists that is objective and apart from internal conflict. This part can be conceived as the observing ego and ego state or some other part of the whole person, which may be conscious or unconscious. When this part is viewed as an ego state, it can be accessed through imagery, either hypnotically or nonhypnotically, and can be experience as person, place, or thing. As an ego state, the part can be personified and imagined as a wise person with knowledge to share who can enter into alliance with the therapist, as a cotherapist, and can function as a helper ego state in the internal system. In addition to appearing in human form, the ego state could also be an animal or a mythological creature.

As a place, this inner part can be visualized or experienced kinesthetically as a calm, serene place where the individual can find peace. She can retreat to it when she feels overwhelmed by internal or external conflicts. When this part is experienced as a thing, it can be a source of mystical or spiritual guidance.

The inner advisor (Rossman, 1987) can take any of these forms as can the Internal Self Helper (ISH; Allison, 1974). The theorists who work with patients with dissociative disorders and who are familiar with ego-state theory or other parts theories are most likely to think of the source of inner guidance as an ego state that is usually and can be accessed through hypnosis. Other theoreticians conceptualize this objective part of the ego or self as more or less conscious; they call it the *observing ego*, an *archetype*, a *selfobject*, or the *higher self*, the *natural self*, or the *real self*. It may be considered to be part of psychic structure or to be dynamic energy or a unifying force. The concept of Inner Strength (see chap. 6) embodies many of these possibilities, but is also conceived to be even more fundamental in that it represents the survival instinct—the force for growth, change, healing, and life itself.

Active imagination, guided imagery, and visualization techniques are all ways in which this source of inner guidance can be accessed. Accessing and utilizing conflict-free spheres of the ego as represented in the Internal Self Helper (ISH), Center Core, and other conceptualizations can have many applications in psychotherapy. These include strengthening the therapeutic alliance and providing information from deeper layers of the mind, usually thought of as unconscious. Center Core and other inner guidance activations can also facilitate exploration and further insight, access resources for control and mastery, and allow the patient to become more self-reliant. All of these functions are ultimately ego-strengthening.

There are patients who do not easily access these kinds of resources. There are many possibilities for why this might be the case. Trauma always offers the possibility for complicating clinical responses. Additionally, emotions such as fear or anxiety or clinical conditions such as depression or obsessionalism can interfere. At times the patient may simply be overwhelmed.

Finally, there are always patients who have a great fear of the unknown. They can be just as fearful of discovering powerful, unknown internal forces as they would be should they have to explore unknown external forces. A patient's failure to access Internal Self Helpers, *inner wisdom*, or other types of archetypal selfobjects should never be permitted to develop significant anxiety over this. We tell patients who are successful in these arenas that this simply gives us more information about what kind of strengthening techniques will be best for them. Sometimes, we explain, a process of elimination has to be experienced.

Patients' inability to access these kinds of experience is usually a signal that other kinds of ego-strengthening are more relevant. It could also indicate that the patients need direct ego-strengthening and a secure holding environment as well as the interplay of transitional phenomena (see chap. 7).

Chapter 11

Ego-Strengthening in the Treatment of Performance Anxiety

It is of great value to have a working model for formulating what is troubling our patients. Such a model can help us understand what kinds of interventions will be most helpful. It can also motivate us further into discerning as much about our patients' psyches as we can; this is another way of discovering even more of what is unique (see chap. 3) about the patient. There is nothing completely fixed or sacred about any theory. This belief is based on the nature of theory. It is important to remember that theories are simply ways of sorting and understanding observable phenomena called data. Of necessity, theories change over time. Those that do not may simply end up being dismissed. Freud had the courage to discard a number of his major theories over a period of time because he believed they could not account for some of the important data he was observing. There is no dearth of explanations for the causation of diagnostic entities from a number of theoretical standpoints. However, a comprehensive and more universal approach can be quite useful in helping the clinician understand how ego-strengthening can be advantageous for the patent.

Freud (1917/1964) proposed a model for understanding the theoretical basis for psychoanalysis. He called this model *metapsychology* and believed that it provided "the theoretical assumptions on which a psycho-analytic system could be founded" (p. 222). Freud's metapsychology attempted to objectify what the analyst observed subjectively and, from this objectification, to derive a lawful (as opposed to random) psychic determinism. Freud's metapsychology examined the patient's psychic structures from psychodynamic (instincts, defenses), structural (id, ego, and superego), and economic (libidinal energies and aggressive energies) perspectives. Rapaport and Gill (1959/1967) expanded what was implicit in Freud's metapsychology to include interpretations that were also *genetic* (psychological origins and development) and *adaptive* (interrelationships with the environment) as well. This model has been modified greatly by various schools of thought into several contemporary versions (Frank, 1990).

It is not surprising that Freud, a confirmed maker of theories, would construct a framework for his new science of psychoanalysis that was in step with how Western science tended to sort data. The most commonly agreed upon logical

DOI:10.4324/9781003442585-11

basis for Western science is Aristotelian in nature. In his examination of the nature of objects and events, occurrences, and outcomes in nature and in human behavior, Aristotle believed that the thinking observer could discover lawful principles at work. He demonstrated that the observer could always determine four causes:

1. *The material cause.* The *material cause* constituted the underlying *matter* that was the substratum or essence of anything. In Aristotelian and Scholastic use, *matter* is defined as that which is undifferentiated and formless and which, as the subject of change and development, receives form and becomes substance and experience. The form could be atomic structure, molecular structure, genetic code, or matter conceived of in other terms. The word *matter* comes from the Latin *materia*—a rough equivalent of the Greek word meaning timber. Timber is the material cause of a wooden ship.
2. *The efficient cause.* The *efficient cause* introduces the notion of *energy* or *motion* into the field of causation. It also contains the concept of time. The efficient cause of a wooden ship would be the actual physical construction by the ship builders, the sawing of the wood, the fitting of proper lengths, and the pounding of the nails.
3. *The formal cause.* The *formal cause* is the underlying plan, structure, or framework of the object or event. The formal cause of the wooden ship would be the plan or blueprint for the ship.
4. *The final cause.* The *final cause* is the reason or purpose for the existence of an object or event. The final cause for the wooden ship is to navigate the waters.

These causes can be applied to psychological and somatic events. For example, the material cause of Obsessive Compulsive Disorder (OCD) is the genetic and biochemical substratum. The efficient cause is the series of events that triggers the symptoms, for example, a stressor such as the birth of a child into the family. The formal cause would be found in the personality type of the patient, which can be described psychodynamically. The formal cause of Obsessive Compulsive Disorder (OCD) is the adaptive behavior of the disorder, the avoidance of harm to the self and to others, and the control of internal chaos.

The Stress-Diathesis Model

These basic Aristotelian principles of causation can be applied to clinical syndromes in a convenient way with the use of a *stress-diathesis model* (see Figure 11.1). This model appears to emphasize the material and efficient causes, thus reflecting the tendency of modern science to follow the advice of Hobbes, Locke, Berkeley, and Hume to deal only with what is observable (Wallace, 1974). However, there is ample opportunity to include the formal cause (the

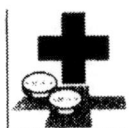 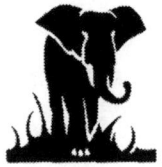 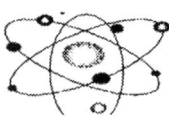

DIATHESIS	UNRESOLVED UNCONSCIOUS CONFLICTS	STRESS
Infectious	Object Relations	Physical
Genetic	Psychosocial	Social
Idiopathic	Psychosexual	Interpersonal
End Organ Damage	Traumatic	Intrapsychic

HYPNOTIC AND OTHER INTERVENTIONS

Hypno-Imagery	Uncovering	Psychosocial Rx
Symptomatic Relief	Hypnoanalysis	Life Style Changes
Behavioral Programs	Ego State Therapy	Family Therapy
Ego-Strengthening	Ego-Strengthening	Explore/Change
Ideodynamic Healing	Ideodynamic Healing/	Belief Systems/
Internal Resources	Internal Resources	Values
Medication		Ego-Strengthening
Chemotherapy, Radiation		Behavior Modification
Other Therapies		Ideodynamic Healing/
		Internal Resources
		Symptom Management
		Stress Management

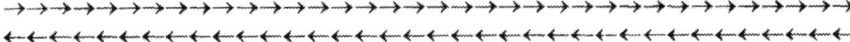

Figure 11.1 The stress-diathesis model.

character structure and other psychodynamic factors) into an explanation of this model, just as there is latitude for the clinician to include teleological explanations based on a final cause such as the adaptive nature of the clinical syndrome, should he wish. This can also be described as giving *meaning* to the illness.

The word *diathesis* refers to a hereditary disposition of the body to disease. It could be a disposition or tendency to manifest a single disease or a group of diseases or to produce such bodily reactions as allergies, or any other kind of genetically driven disorder. Within the realm of psychopathology, a number of clinical syndromes have become associated with data that suggest significant hereditary influences. As therapists we cannot afford to ignore the individual's genetic self. In terms of causation, the diathesis is the *material cause* of the illness.

The stress-diathesis model (Figure 11.1) provides a dynamic way of viewing any clinical syndrome in terms of all the forces at play. It helps us understand the patient's identity, individuality, and uniqueness. It allows us to transmit to the patient a more comprehensive view of his illness. We would be remiss were we to ignore the genetic and psychodynamic factors as well as the precipitating stresses in our patients' lives. We can use the model to clarify for the patient, as well, the wisdom of his mind–body in producing the symptoms in order to insist he look at the deeper meaning of his situation.

The clinician who uses this model may find it easier to grasp the nature of his patient's total situation and understand where and what kind of ego-strengthening can be particularly helpful. When we introduce this model to patients, we emphasize the *efficient cause*—stress. We usually begin by telling them that when anyone is stressed too much, he will develop something (i.e., the diathesis will become manifest). We explain that the stress-precipitated disorder could be something like an anxiety disorder or depression, that some people display psychosomatic problems such as hypertension or ulcers, and that in extreme cases it is thought by many that some cancers are stress-related illnesses. We find that patients accept this kind of thinking well. Indeed, it is even ego-strengthening in that it normalizes the patient's symptoms and conveys to the patient that we are considering many factors in his illness. The introduction of a final causation such as adaptation also helps take the burden of blame for his own illness off the patient's shoulders and, in many instances, allow him to look beyond the discomfort of the disorder into the direction of whatever greater good may be gained from it.

We use the concept of *hidden childhood trauma* as part of the succession of events (when it applies) that constitute the efficient cause of the illness. Much of the material described in this chapter displays a rich interplay of causes and a multitude of opportunities for ego-strengthening.

Anxiety

The philology of the word *anxiety* reveals much about its nature. It comes from the Latin noun, *anxieta*, which is related to the adjective, *anxius*, meaning *anxious*. The Latin adjective, *anxius*, is in turn derived from what is perhaps an older Latin verb, *angere*, which means *to torment*. The term *anxiety* has been in use for over 500 years (Goodwin, 1986); for many who suffer from the symptoms of anxiety, it is a torment indeed.

Subjectively, anxiety is, with one exception, identical with fear. Unlike fear, it lacks an external focus or precipitant. The danger that triggers the anxiety reaction is purely internal and its nature is often unknown to the sufferer. It may be experienced as a sense of loss of control, pervading or impending doom, or extreme agitation. Since the same physiological mechanisms are activated by anxiety as by fear, the person who is experiencing anxiety is in the midst of a physiological fight-or-flight reaction. Thus, it is frequently accompanied by such phenomena as dry mouth, accelerated respiration rate, rapid heartbeat, sweating, muscle tension, and enlargement of the pupils.

Anxiety may have profound behavioral and psychological effects. The sufferer may indeed feel that he is in a torment of apprehension. It can also produce muscular and cardiorespiratory distress. Some individuals who are experiencing anxiety reactions feel depersonalized or detached. When the anxiety is severe in its manifestations, the sufferer often fears that he may be going mad. Psychodynamically, anxiety can be thought of as that which underlies all repression and all of the defense mechanisms. Whenever the defenses fail, anxiety becomes a conscious phenomenon. The *DSM–IV* (American Psychiatric Association, 1994) lists 11 kinds of anxiety disorders. Among these are disorders such as generalized anxiety disorders, specific phobias, Panic Disorder with and without agoraphobia, Obsessive Compulsive Disorder (OCD), and Posttraumatic Stress Disorder (PTSD). Many clinicians believe that posttraumatic stress disorder, although it may have strong anxiety components, should be classified with the dissociative disorders.

Anxiety can profoundly affect human behavior. It can interfere with one's ability to conduct oneself in the world, perform, express oneself, or act effectively. It can also prompt the victim to seek relief from its torments with alcohol and/or drugs or with other behaviors that are able to reduce the anxiety, such as eating or sexuality.

We recommend a wide range of ego-strengthening maneuvers with all the anxiety disorders. However, we believe that all interventions should be preceded by careful history-taking, which will permit the therapist to know something about the nature of the anxiety, its meaning in the patient's life, and what psychodynamics may be involved. Further, the importance of a complete physical examination and appropriate medical work-up for patients with anxiety disorders cannot be overemphasized. Certain medical conditions such as that caused by a secreting tumor of the adrenal medulla or hypoglycemia can produce anxiety symptoms that need medical and/or surgical correction. Some specific treatment techniques for several of these anxiety disorders are described in the sections below.

Performance Anxiety

Performance anxiety is a broad term that is generally used to describe anxiety connected with one's performance. The accompanying fear is that the outcome will possibly, or even probably, be a negative one. Any kind of performance can become the subject of this kind of anxiety, and fear of the performance is often classified as a specific phobia. Performance anxiety is commonly associated with a variety of activities ranging from test-taking to artistic performance, including such activities as singing, instrumentalism, acting, public speaking, and athletic performance. Psychodynamically, performance anxiety can be driven by a number of significant and unresolved intrapsychic and interpersonal issues. Consequently, we find among them such themes as fear of failure or a need to fail, fear of success in competition, fear of achieving the maturational role completion that the successful performance would mark, and fear of exceeding the levels of accomplishment in the family of origin as well as those of the subculture and social class. Performance anxiety can be treated from a cognitive-behavioral perspective, and psychotherapeutic uncovering of the root causes of the anxiety can also be effective.

There are several hypnotic approaches to the treatment of performance anxiety. Some of them are based on the learning paradigm. Kroger and Fezler (1976) worked within this framework to reduce anxiety through a conditioning model. They used counterconditioning and operant conditioning. In counterconditioning, phobic reactions to performance situations were systematically desensitized with either relaxation or active coping imagery. In operant conditioning, covert reinforcement techniques were used.

Hypnotherapists have successfully used hypnosis to influence such learning process variables as achievement, motivation, concentration, coping, memory, recall, confidence in ability, and so forth (Frederick & Kim, 1993). Fowler (1961) discovered that hypnosis had a positive effect on concentration. Subjects in hypnosis could concentrate more deeply for longer periods of time than subjects who were not hypnotized.

Krippner (1963) reported obtaining better study habits, relaxation during tests, and motivation for studies in university students after hypnotic suggestions had been made for their improvement. Erickson (1965a) noted that he had successfully treated patients who developed panic either during or immediately before examinations. He believed the hypnotherapy had been successful because it improved the motivation of the candidates, eliminated anxiety and tension, and built up mental ease and confidence. A more recent application of the hypnobehavioral approach is in the area of sports performance. The ideas of self-hypnotic mental training (Unestahl, 1983) and "mental rehearsal" as well as posthypnotic suggestions and cues (to create a specific positive response and winning feeling before and during play) are typically utilized to help athletes achieve their optimal performance levels (Unestahl, 1983; Zilbergeld & Lazarus, 1987).

A quite different approach utilizes hypnoanalytic techniques for the performance anxiety state (Crasilneck & Hall, 1975). Psychodynamically based, it seeks underlying causes. Many therapists typically incorporate various forms of ego-strengthening into the treatment of performance anxiety. As we have often noted, it increases one's confidence and problem-solving ability. Hypnoanalytic, ego-strengthening, and cognitive behavioral approaches can often be successfully combined within the treatment of the same patient (Brown & Fromm, 1986; Frederick, 1993b).

Public Speakers, Opera Singers, Musicians, and Others

It is doubtful whether anyone who has ever given a speech or performed in public in any way has not at some time experienced performance anxiety or "stage fright." The desire to perform well and please others is so strong that fear of failure can be equally intense. The anticipation of failure has the potential for creating such apprehension and dread that the resultant anxiety can definitely inhibit and interfere with actual performance. Public speakers and performers may seek out therapists to help them overcome performance anxiety as well as enhance their performance. Performance enhancement or peak performance has been discussed in the literature primarily with regard to athletic performance, and sports psychology has become a whole new field of study. However, much less has been written about performance anxiety as it affects public speaking and performing, although public speaking has been identified in surveys as the major fear experienced by the most people. Even less has been written about the stress and anxiety experienced by musicians whether they are soloists or ensemble players.

The desire to decrease anxiety has led some performers to seek prescriptions for beta blockers such as propranolol marketed under the name Inderal (Mar, 1997). These drugs compete with hormones for receptor sites and block the effects of the hormones involved in stress. Initially beta blockers were developed to be used for the treatment of high blood pressure, heart disease, and sometimes migraine headaches. Many physicians seem to feel that occasional use of these drugs has no negative effects. However, one never knows at any given time the effects of Inderal, so an element of risk is always involved. Too much Inderal can produce spacey feelings and difficulty in concentration. In addition, there are side effects such as sleep disturbances, fatigue, depression, and cold hands and feet (Mar, 1997). Certain individuals will seek out therapists because they wish to give up beta blockers and learn other methods of coping with anxiety.

Hypnosis is especially useful in dealing with individuals who experience performance anxiety. Salmon and Meyer (1992) have developed a clinic for musicians to help them cope with stress and anxiety. It is interesting to note that the methods they recommend focus on relaxation techniques, cognitive restructuring, and mental rehearsal involving imagery. Ristad (1982), who wrote specifically about singers, strongly emphasized the use of visualization techniques. These techniques can be utilized during a hypnotic trance to increase their potency. The addition of ego-strengthening suggestions can further increase the effectiveness of these methods.

Evaluation of Performance Anxiety

Initially, it is important to do thorough history-taking and examine what factors contribute to the anxiety the individual is experiencing. A person with performance anxiety experiences an array of physical symptoms. They usually include rapid heartbeat, hyperventilation, dry mouth, profuse sweating, trembling, and the urge to urinate (Mar, 1997; Salmon & Meyer, 1992). These symptoms are produced by the release of hormones from the adrenal gland when a stressful stimulus triggers the fight-or-flight response. The interpretation of or reaction to experiencing these symptoms is also part of the anxiety response. One person might expect a catastrophe, while another person, perhaps a more mature or experienced performer, might tolerate these symptoms and accept them as an inevitable fact of life. Anticipation of the onset of anxiety symptoms can create anxiety and panic as well.

There are at least three dimensions of anxiety: degree of arousal, cognitive appraisal of the situation, and escape and avoidance behaviors. These are important to consider in assessing how a particular individual experiences performance anxiety. We can evaluate behavior, affect, sensation, imagery, cognitions, interpersonal relationships, and physiological factors, which comprise the BASIC-ID model of Lazarus (1989) adapted by Salmon and Meyer (1992). This model includes multimodal aspects of the experience. For example, *behaviorally*, the anxious performer may procrastinate and avoid practicing. Emotionally, he might experience alternating anxiety and depression. Anxiety may be signaled by the *sensations* of sweaty palms, pounding heart, and shaking hands, along with imagery of being laughed at or becoming faint and falling off the piano stool. *Thoughts* might be catastrophic as well, more typically: "I must play this perfectly or I'm a failure and will never have another chance." *Interpersonal* factors can contribute, such as relationships with teachers, conductors, spouses, parents, and so on. It is important to evaluate who the performer is trying to please and where the sources of support and/or criticism might be. Finally, any limits imposed by physiological conditions must be considered. Is the person medicating anxiety with alcohol or drugs? The combination of contributing factors can be complex and the problems involved can be complicated, sometimes necessitating the therapist's teaching the individual to self-monitor before an accurate report can be obtained.

A collaborative relationship between therapist and performer needs to be established. Otherwise, the therapist may become, transferentially, too much like the teacher or the jury who will judge the performance of the patient. It can be helpful to emphasize to the patient that "we will work together to find solutions, and create hypnotic suggestions that are specifically most useful to you."

Although it is necessary to carefully evaluate each individual, there do seem to be certain issues that frequently occur in individuals who seek therapy for performance anxiety. These are:

• Fear of criticism and harsh judgment from teachers, peers, and listeners;
• Fear of becoming overwhelmed by anxiety that can lead to forgetting what to do;

- Fear of being unable to perform;
- Expectation of perfection;
- Catastrophic thinking (i.e., expecting the worst);
- Self-consciousness, or thinking about the act of performing rather than being caught up in the activity;
- Irrational beliefs about what one *must* or *should* do; and
- Fear of the body failing in some way, such as through coughing, aphonia, paralysis, tremor, or even fainting.

Hypnotically Enhanced Ego-Strengthening With Musicians and Performers

Inducing a trance for relaxation can facilitate overall relaxation as well as help the patient to begin to learn a series of tasks such as how to retrain specific muscle groups, how to breathe properly, or how to be attentive to cues. The induction can involve attention to breathing, progressive muscle relaxation, and relaxing imagery. Auditory and tactile imagery should be used as well as visual. The first induction for relaxation is instructive, as the patient's responses give information about hypnotizability and about what kinds of suggestions are most helpful and which may be superfluous. Asking for feedback about the patient's subjective experience also promotes the atmosphere of collaboration and strengthens the therapeutic alliance.

The next time the patient experiences the hypnotic induction for relaxation, the therapist can utilize the feedback obtained in the previous trance session to create suggestions that will uniquely work for the patient. These will facilitate an even more relaxed state in which various aspects of breathing, muscle relaxation, and imagery are emphasized. It is also necessary to help the patient learn how to self-monitor his subjective experiences, physical sensations, cognitions, and imagery. This will later assist in the creation of suggestions for relaxation and often feels empowering to the patient. This second session can be taped for the performer to take home and use for practicing relaxation.

We strongly favor the use of self-hypnosis methods (see chap. 7) for performers with anxiety. This helps to ego-strengthen by increasing control and mastery over the trance experience. Learning that it is possible to relax and be in charge of that procedure is experienced as ego-strengthening.

The next phase of the process involves obtaining information in as much detail as possible about the kind and degree of preparation needed for the upcoming speech, musical, or theatrical performance. None of the stress management techniques is helpful if the performer is not adequately prepared. The speaker must have a command of the material to be presented, and the musician must have learned and rehearsed the music. We recommend overpreparation. There are some important factors to consider about how and when one practices music (Salmon & Meyer, 1992). We have found hypnosis useful in the preparation phase. The patient is instructed how to use self-hypnosis for going into an altered state of consciousness during each day's practice of the material (singing, instrumentalism, speech making). This trance is a light trance of the awake-alert type (see chap. 10). In this awake-alert trance state, the patient can utilize suggestions about being able to focus, concentrate, screen out distractions, and experience time distortion (in which the subjective impression is such that much can be accomplished in a short period of time). It can be hypnotically suggested to the patient that he can enter a light trance state with his eyes open. The patient can also be taught to enter deep trance and, on alerting, to remain in a light eyes-open trance. He can attend to whatever stimuli from the environment are important. However, he will discover that he can become so completely absorbed in the task before him that he will be unaware of the passing of time until his bodily sensations inform him that he needs to take a break.

Rossi (1993) employs the notion of *ultradian rhythms*—natural rhythms of the body characterized by the ebbing and flowing of one's energy level and alertness. According to Rossi, the body has approximately 90-minute natural psychobiological rhythms. With this in mind, the therapist can design suggestions such as, "You can allow yourself an hour and a half or two hours of clock time to be fully absorbed in your preparation." The musical performer can be taught to mentally rehearse the performance, and the speaker can visualize himself speaking in a relaxed and animated fashion to the audience.

We can think of the tendency to worry or dwell on worst-case scenarios as forms of negative hypnosis. The challenge, then, is to teach the performer to think of best-case scenarios and of how the performance could go well. Again, the therapist can obtain detailed information on the circumstances of the performance—the location, the time of day, the order of events, and as much detail as possible about the nature of the actual performance. Salmon and Meyer (1992) have listed the conditions that enhance the effectiveness of mental rehearsal for a musical performance:

- Accuracy of the mental rehearsal, which is a description of the closest resemblance possible
- Inclusion of positive statements
- Perspective of realistic optimism as opposed to expectations of perfection
- Focus on performing rather than the reactions of the audience
- Mental rehearsal carried out under tranquil conditions

Salmon and Meyer (1992) do not mention hypnosis, but we can assume that when mental rehearsal is done with the patient in a state of relaxation, it is the hypnotic state that supplies the tranquility.

Given that sensitivity to criticism and expectations of perfection are so characteristic of performers, especially of musicians, we need to carefully craft suggestions that reflect helpful and realistic cognitions. Assessing the performer's self-talk will indicate what attitudes and beliefs might be contributing to performance anxiety. The cognitive restructuring discussed by Salmon and Meyer (1992) involves encouraging and helping the performer to self-monitor and identify thoughts and feelings associated with performing, changing, and reframing the dysfunctional attitudes. By the same mechanisms that allow negative thoughts to produce anxiety, positive thoughts seem to contribute to a feeling of increased confidence. The goals of treatment are to help the performer to accept his stress and anxiety rather than ignore or deny it and to integrate positive feelings, thoughts, and imagery with the sensations and technicalities of playing music, singing, or giving a speech.

Test-Taking

Test-taking can be viewed as another form of performance anxiety, and much of the material in the prior section on public speaking and musical performing also applies here. Almost everyone at one time or another has experienced test anxiety. The *examination dream* is universally experienced as that dream wherein the individual realizes that he has a test coming up that he has not studied for. Perhaps he has not been to class, or he does not remember until too late that he registered for the class and is not prepared at all. The examination dream is the quintessential anxiety dream experienced by many people when they are anxious about myriad other concerns. It is symbolic of the kind of panic and anticipatory anxiety that exams evoke.

As previously mentioned, studies of the effects of hypnosis on examination performance have shown that hypnosis can enhance concentration (Fowler, 1961); improve motivation, relaxation, and study habits (Krippner, 1963); and increase mental ease and confidence (Erickson, 1965b). Palan and Chandwani (1989) reported studies using hypnosis to increase learning skills in grade-school children.

Stanton (1993b) reviewed studies of test anxiety, most of which used a combination of systematic desensitization and relaxation techniques. Stanton used only two 50-minute sessions of hypnosis training designed to increase confidence in the ability to handle anxiety in 11 medical practitioners who had previously failed examinations. These subjects all attributed their lack of success in previous exams to anxiety rather than lack of knowledge or failure to study or adequately prepare. In the first session the practitioners were introduced to Stanton's five-step ego-strengthening procedure (Stanton, 1989) involving relaxation, imagery, and suggestions. They were also asked to imagine a success scenario of taking the exam, and writing the answers fluently and effortlessly. For an oral exam, they were to imagine speaking articulately, feeling confident, and thinking clearly. In the second session Stanton introduced Stein's (1963) clenched-fist technique. (With this technique the subject is able to condition positive feelings and associations to his clenched fist. The test anxiety is conditioned to the nondominant fist. It is then suggested that the subject can open his non-dominant fist and allow the negative feelings to flow away and be replaced by the positive feelings in the dominant fist.) They were also provided with ego-strengthening metaphors: a cloud into which they could put all the contributions to their anxiety, and a pyramid from which they could access their inner strength and powers. Nine out of the 11 practitioners passed their tests and reported decreased levels of anxiety.

In contrast to Stanton's (1993b) results, a controlled experimental study (Palan & Chandwani, 1989) of 56 medical students in three groups balanced for number of subjects, hypnotizability, and performance at last examination showed no change in performance on examinations. The hypnosis group attended eight weekly group sessions where they received ego-strengthening and specific suggestions for study habits, with a ninth session of mental rehearsal and age progression. They were to practice self-hypnosis with positive ego-strengthening suggestions daily. The second group was the same with the exception that hypnosis was not used. Rather, they were instructed to sit quietly with eyes closed and practice self-suggestions each day. In the third group, passive relaxation for the same period of time was used along with instructions to practice relaxation daily. The hypnosis group improved significantly in coping with examination anxiety even though there were no significant differences in test scores among the three groups. The authors felt that the lack of individualized procedure may have affected the lack of significant differences in test scores. Needless to say, other factors (such as command of the material) also could have affected the actual examination performance.

We believe that individualizing ego-strengthening suggestions that can be presented in a hypnotic trance is an effective method for treating examination anxiety. The following discussion shows how that can be done.

Evaluation of Test Anxiety

Evaluation in each specific case should involve careful questioning about the factors affecting examination performance. Often an individual will seek therapy and be particularly interested in hypnosis because he has failed an important exam and is needing to take it again. Licensing exams such as the bar exams, medical boards, and licensing exams required to practice one's profession are particularly fraught with anxiety. Fear of failure is extremely strong, especially when failure has occurred previously. The anticipation of another failure can produce negative self-hypnosis, which only increases the anxiety. The *thought patterns* are important to assess along with accompanying *behaviors* such as degree of procrastination. *Affect* and *bodily sensations* are significant. Often the individual will say he feels blocked or paralyzed. What physiological symptoms of anxiety are experienced? Are there other people the person feels he may let down, or are there relationships that interfere with exam preparation? What concerns does the person have about how his life will change if he fails the test? Are there other escape and avoidance behaviors involved?

Hypnosis and Ego-Strengthening for Test-Taking

An approach that combines hypnosis for relaxation, mental rehearsal during trance, creating ego-strengthening suggestions, teaching self-hypnosis, and use of audiotapes is described next. The procedure is similar to that described for musicians and public speakers. The goals are to prepare the person in such a way as to (a) facilitate a positive anticipation of taking the examination in a relaxed manner, (b) to enhance concentration, to increase motivation to adequately prepare, and (c) to maximize the possibility of passing the test.

Case Example: Roger

Roger came to see me (SM) specifically to explore whether hypnosis would help him study and pass his medical boards in anesthesiology. He was particularly worried about the written exam, which consisted of all multiple-choice items. He had taken the test before and almost passed. This time he was determined to pass, but felt very anxious about it. He was so busy in his residency at the hospital that he had little time to study and felt he did not use his time efficiently. He tended to procrastinate and rationalize that he needed to socialize and relax in his free time such that studying was often deferred. Yet, he was having difficulty sleeping and often woke up in the middle of the night worrying about the exam.

He was especially concerned about the multiple-choice items, because he believed he was very bad at those kind of items, where choices were often dependent on the wording. He was afraid that his anxiety would interfere with his concentration, and he would misread the items and answer incorrectly. He believed he could easily be tripped up by misinterpreting the intent of the question and misreading double negatives or other convoluted wording.

After evaluation of his situation, we discussed the nature of hypnosis and how it might be helpful to him. He was interested and was able to readily go into trance. Initially, suggestions for relaxation were given: focusing on his breathing, letting go of tightness and tension in his muscles, creating a safe place, and remembering relaxing experiences. When he was brought out of trance, he exclaimed that he had not felt so relaxed in a long time. I obtained feedback from him about his subjective experience in trance and what suggestions felt most useful to him.

In the next session I utilized his feedback from the previous session and induced a trance where I made suggestions for relaxation and then suggested he allow an image to form of the place where he studies and imagine himself there. I suggested that when he settled into his chair to study, he could put himself into an awake-alert trance where he could respond to anything in his environment that he needed to, but otherwise he could concentrate fully on the task before him. I presented ego-strengthening suggestions about experiencing his mind as calm, clear, and fully absorbed in the material in front of him. I suggested that he could experience time distortion, in the sense of being unaware of the passing of time, until his body's natural rhythms had signaled to him that it was time to take a break. The session was tape-recorded so that he would have a tape of the suggestions to play at home. I also taught him a rapid method of self-hypnosis, the Spiegel eye roll technique, which he was able to rehearse in the session.

The following week he reported that he was able to study much more effectively. He had used self-hypnosis to go into a light trance when he settled into his chair to begin studying. Each day he listened to the tape for reinforcement of the suggestion, and to help him go back to sleep whenever he awakened. His sleep had been more restful and the nightly disturbances were happening less frequently.

We next focused on using hypnosis for mental rehearsal of taking the exam. While Roger was in trance, I suggested that he could go forward in time in his imagination to the night before the exam, when he could do something relaxing and then go to bed and sleep well. I made suggestions about waking the day of the exam feeling perhaps some excitement, but also calm and clear-headed. When he arrived at the location where the exam would take place, I suggested he could go into a light trance, an awake-alert trance, where he would be able to concentrate fully while remaining calm and focused. I then guided him through a mental rehearsal of the exam process.

I mentioned that if, at any time, he felt a little anxiety, he would be able to quickly and easily calm himself with one of the self-hypnotic techniques he had learned. One of those techniques had been to give his anxiety a color and then change the color to a serene, calm, cool color. I included suggestions about the multiple-choice items, as well as how he could concentrate very well, draw upon all the knowledge he had gained, and let his intuition guide him. I made suggestions about time distortion: "Before you know it, it will be time to break for lunch" and "You will be able to find a comfortable place where you have all the time you need to finish the items in the time allowed." A tape was also made of this session.

For the last few weeks before the test, he played the tape of this session each night before he went to sleep. He told me that he often went to sleep before the tape finished playing, but that he felt it must be working because he was sleeping much better, and felt generally more relaxed and optimistic. When Roger later received the results from the exam, he called to tell me he had passed.

The Awake-Alert Trance

Banyai and Hilgard (1976) described a method of inducing trance whereby a hypnotic state could be achieved while the subject was riding a stationary bicycle with his eyes open. While the subject was riding the bicycle, suggestions were given to enhance alertness, attentiveness, and a feeling of freshness. This induction produced an altered state of consciousness where susceptibility to hypnotic suggestions was essentially the same as that following a relaxation induction. Banyai (1980) investigated a variety of hypnotic phenomena and found both similarities and differences between traditional inductions and the awake-alert induction. Both inductions are similar. They involve: (a) relinquishment of planning functions, (b) lack of reality testing, and (c) heightened attention. As opposed to the traditional induction, the awake-alert induction produced: (a) a higher degree of alertness, (b) a more positive mood state, and (c) a higher activity level. Banyai believes this type of induction is particularly useful for people who are control oriented because they can experience mastery and success. As they pedal for approximately 45 minutes they experience an increase in tension followed by relaxation. Banyai utilizes this trance state for providing suggestions for remembering, feeling, and experiencing these sensations and feelings again. She feels this type of induction can be very ego-strengthening. The results of her studies suggest that,

> altered states of consciousness may be produced by a wide variety of agents or maneuvers which interfere with the normal inflow of sensory and proprioceptive stimuli and the normal outflow of motor impulses. There seems to be an optimal range of exteroceptive stimulation and activity level necessary for the maintenance of normal, waking consciousness. Levels of stimulation and activity either below or above this range might produce an altered state of consciousness.
>
> (Banyai, 1980, p. 270)

It seems unlikely that practicing clinicians in many Western countries will install bicycles in their offices. However, it may be useful to consider having one available for inpatient units of hospitals. Research needs to be done to study whether a subject could *imagine* riding a bicycle or performing other strenuous activities. Testing could be done to determine whether some of the same hypnotic phenomena were occurring.

Others have reported on the use of similar awake-alert trance states for learning, concentration, comprehension, and test-taking. Their ways of achieving awake-alert trance states are different from Banyai's, however. Oetting's (1964, 1990) subject entered trance by gazing at his desk. The only material that was allowed on the desk was the material to be learned. He continued to gaze at the desk and the material as he seated himself before it. Then Oetting had the subject become aware of parts of the body while continuing to gaze at the desk and material. The subject relaxed as he got more in touch with points of reference for relaxation in his body and was able to concentrate further on the material.

Oetting (1964, 1990) had the subject attend almost simultaneously to varied stimuli. This induced a flexibility of focus and attention that culminated in greatly heightened attention to the work at hand. He called this *concentration* and used a cue for the subject to turn the concentration on when needed.

Wark (1990a, 1990b, 1996) has described a useful technique for awake-alert trance called the *Lever*. It is so named "because you lift your mind to a state of sharp focus and relax your body while holding your mind's tension. Then you lever up your mental focus a bit higher, and again relax your body. And then a third time, you raise your mental focus and relax your body" (Wark, 1990b, p. 449).

We have found that an awake-alert trance can be induced by using standard induction techniques to induce a light trance combined with posthypnotic suggestions for experiencing a trance state. Subsequently, this light trance state can be induced by a conditioned cue. The suggestion is that the subject can feel fully alert, calm, clear-headed, and able to concentrate fully on the task before him. Patients dealing with examination anxiety are taught to use self-hypnosis to induce an alert-awake trance before beginning to study or starting to take a test. Many variations are possible, limited only by the imaginations of therapist and patient.

Case Example: Brie (Continued)

Brie (whose case is discussed in chap. 3) made great strides in her therapy and in her life. One day she discussed her test anxiety with me with me (CF). We decided that hypnosis could be helpful for this. Brie was a good hypnotic subject, and she leaned self-hypnosis easily. I (CF) decided that I would include the active-alert trance state as one of the techniques that could help Brie with her test-taking.

While Brie was in trance I (CF) said to her: "In a moment I will count to three. At the count of three you will open your eyes. You will still be in trance, an active-alert, or eyes-open trance. You will remain in that state for sixty seconds of clock time. Then you will return to a state in which you are completely awake, alertness, and oriented to the outer world." I then counted to three.

Brie opened her eyes. She had a dreamy look. I said to her, "You are in an active alert trance state. In this state you can live in two worlds at the same time. Look, Brie, look around the office." Brie looked around my office.

"Now, Brie, look within, at your place of relaxation ... Can you see it?"

Brie smiled and nodded yes. She was able to alternate between a focus on my office and one on her inner world. Then the 60 seconds was up, and Brie became more alert. We discussed how she would use this technique in test-taking. Brie was very happy. "I've got some good new stuff to use."

Awake-alert trance would be able to help Brie take her tests.

The Creation of Helpful Ego States for the Management of Performance Anxiety

"Heidi and the Little Girl"

Cognitive and behavioral strategies often used in the treatment of performance anxiety tend to be oriented to the present and to a future that is artificially structured. They "can be limited in their abilities to draw motivation and strength from past experience as well as from future identifications. Practicing hypnotic and other therapeutic techniques is not merely a matter of 'doing it'" (Frederick & Kim, 1993, p. 50). "Feeling and acting on the motivation felt is closer to the heart of the matter. In our view the integration of motivational and other dynamic factors geared to success and change into the therapeutic work is crucial" (Frederick & Kim, 1993, p. 51).

Frederick and Kim (1993) found it useful and helpful to incorporate the patient's past resources together with his future potential in their work with performance anxiety. They became interested in using the ego-state perspective in a creative way. This interest led them to the work of the 19th- and early 20th-century French psychologist, Binet (1890/1977, 1896/1977), who is best known to us for his work with Simon in developing tests to measure human intelligence (Ellenberger, 1970). Binet was also a clinician who worked with dissociative disorders; in the course of his work he became aware of something in the human mind that compares with what we think of ego states today. Binet believed not only that consciousness was divided, but also that he could experimentally create alters in highly hypnotizable subjects.

Since Binet's discovery there have been further experiments in this century that have shown that some manifestations of alter behavior can be created experimentally (Harriman, 1942a, 1942b, 1943; Kampman, 1976; Leavitt, 1947; Spanos, Weekes, & Bertrand, 1985; Spanos et al., 1986). Within the clinical realm the ongoing production of alters as a continuation of the dissociative defense process is not only observed in certain Dissociative Identity Disorder (DID; formerly known as Multiple Personality Disorder) patients, but can also constitute a genuine therapeutic issue in their management. At times contracts to discontinue this method of dealing with stress and conflict by producing new alters is essential to continued treatment with such patients, because the continued use of this defense does not allow the resolution of conflict. Although Federn (1952) believed that ego states could only be formed in early childhood, both current clinical (Watkins & Watkins, 1997) and experimental evidence seems to show that such formation can occur much later in life. In view of their observances of this kind of pliability within the human personality, Frederick and Kim (1993) wondered whether helpful ego states could be created in the therapeutic process as well as activated. Such new ego states could then become the vehicles for certain kinds of corrective emotional experiences.

The Corrective Emotional Experience

Frederick and Kim's (1993) work involved another important mainstream within the hypnotic literature: Milton Erickson's work, *February Man: Facilitating New Identity in Hypnotherapy* (Erickson & Rossi, 1989). Chapter 3 reviewed the case described by Erickson in terms of his February Man hypnotic renurturing technique. Deliberate attempts to symbolically renurture patients hypnotically have also been described as *renurturing* (Murray-Jobsis, 1990a) and *creative self-mothering* (Murray-Jobsis, 1990b; McMahon, 1986; see chap. 9).

Frederick and Kim (1993) wondered what the effect of renurturing techniques might have on the structure of the internal family of ego states. How might they modify personal identity? Did these techniques of renurturing ever create new ego states, or did they rather modify or even activate ego states that were already present but perhaps inactive or dormant? They worked with several patients with severe, crippling performance anxiety and used various hypnotic techniques, including age regression, age progression, and ego-strengthening. In each case an important ego state was symbolized by a specific visual image. In one case the image was that of Heidi, a dog; in the second, that of a little girl. The symbolic representation of these ego states was presented in heterohypnosis while the patient was experiencing hypnotic age regression. Later, the ego states were projected into the future through hypnotic age progression. The future-projected ego states had specific assignments or roles there that were given to them by the therapist.

Visual imagery is important to this technique as is self-hypnosis, which is used for reinforcement. The utilization of self-hypnosis and the permissive, gentle ways in which the helpful ego states are presented are ego-strengthening because they place so much involvement and control of the activation and/or creation of the helpful ego states into the hands of the patient. The following case examples are found in Frederick and Kim (1993).

Case Example: Heidi

Stan was a married Caucasian man who was in his mid-20s. He had good academic potential, but he had become disillusioned with his studies when

*he was in high school. There he had developed poor study habits of procras-
tination and cramming. Although he had attended a reputable university,
his academic work had been mediocre. He had always loved animals and
wanted to become a veterinarian. After his graduation he applied to several
veterinary schools, and while waiting for acceptance, he married. Soon
afterward he was accepted by a school in England. He left his new wife
to attend this school. As a student in his new school he reported "hating
being there." His study habits were poor, he missed his wife, the weather
was "dreadful," the teaching methods were different, and he experienced
a strong bias against American students. In fact, "none of the American
students passed the exam" that determined whether they were to stay at the
school beyond the first year. It was these examinations that Stan also failed.
He sought hypnotherapy during his summer vacation because if he did not
pass his examinations in the fall, he would lose his opportunity to realize
his dream of becoming a veterinarian.*

*At the time Stan sought therapy he was demoralized, anxious, apprehen-
sive, ambivalent, and depressed. His ambivalence seemed to involve the
conflict over his reluctance to be successful as this would result in his leaving his home and his wife again. His attitude was filled with self doubt and
his emotional stance was one of, "I cannot."*

*Stan was treated hypnotherapeutically for 10 sessions. Age regression work
revealed and allowed him to reexperience his desire to be an animal doctor.
This had been the only goal of his life since he was 5. He also reexperienced
his affection and attachment to Heidi, a companion dog he had come to love.
Heidi had died a few years earlier, and Stan recalled how helpless he had
felt when she died and how he had wanted to be an animal doctor to help
Heidi live.*

*In further hypnotic work Stan had an encounter with Heidi in which he
experienced her absolute faith and trust in his ability to become the animal
doctor. It was suggested that Heidi be called upon as a guiding spirit, that,
like light from a lighthouse, beckoned him to become the animal doctor.
In other trance sessions Stan entered hypnotic age progressions in which
he was able to experiment and to experience himself fitting into and then
becoming the animal doctor. In these age progressions he lived the reality
of the animal doctor in its various facets, all with the help of Heidi. These
experiences evoked powerful emotions in Stan, and Heidi helped to focus
his emotions toward his becoming the animal doctor.*

*Stan also practiced other hypnotic techniques to help him have success
experiences with test-taking (e.g., imaginal modifications of past examination situations and rehearsal of upcoming examination situations under the
condition of peak performance state). Heterohypnosis and self-hypnosis*

were also used to do a great deal of ego-strengthening. The self-hypnotic exercises done at home began with the invocation of Heidi, and the patient's experiencing powerful emotions.

At the termination of treatment the therapist (S. K.) gave Stan a gift of a framed photograph of Heidi with instructions to keep it next to his bed when he slept and upon his desk when he studied and to continue this in England until the day of his examination. The picture of Heidi and the awareness were posthypnotic triggers for powerful and focalized emotion to become the animal doctor. In his final letter Stan wrote that he had not only passed his examination but also had passed every paper individually. He knew that he was, "... back on the right track!" What was "rekindled within" him was "not only my desire to become a vet, but my need to succeed."

Case Example: The Little Girl

Ann was a 42-year-old woman who was experiencing some major changes in her life. She and her husband were living apart and involved in divorce proceedings. At the time of her first session she revealed that she had recently become a buyer for a foreign based chain of stores. After she had begun her new job, she discovered that an important aspect of it involved her giving presentations to both large and small groups. The very thought of doing any public speaking filled her with terror. She recalled that she had done quite poorly with the public speaking course which had been required at her college. She had fallen to pieces in the first exercise which was a demonstration, and she recalled that even speaking up in a college English class was troublesome. "If I would just get past the initial panic, I'd be O.K. But I can't catch my breath ... I can't organize my thoughts!" She recalled having had a panic attack once when she was giving routine information at a hospital. For 10 or 15 seconds she felt that she had made an error and that there was no way out. In a previous job as a store manager she dreaded the routine of having to speak to her employees every Saturday. When she discovered she would be expected to address larger audiences, she quit the job. "I can make myself sick just thinking about it." In another, more prestigious job she had been asked to make a presentation. "To get out of it I thought I'd have myself hospitalized ... my hands were numb, and I told them I had a disc ... I'm not kidding! ... I put myself in the hospital so I wouldn't have to make another speech." The patient's first speech in her new position was scheduled 13 days from the time of her initial interview.

The patient had been raised on the east coast. Her father was 30 years older than her mother. When the patient was 12, her mother died of alcohol *poisoning. However, the patient was told her mother had died of cancer, and she did not discover the truth about her mother's death until 3 years prior to her coming for help with her public speaking.*

After her mother's death the patient was sent to a religious boarding school. There her anxiety began to interfere with her performance in reading aloud. Neither the nuns in the school nor her father could tolerate her making a mistake. The warm, nurturing figures in her life were the family servants, Samuel and Agnes, who had died several years earlier.

The patient found it very interesting that in spite of her history, that there had been a time in her life when she had been able to speak in public without any difficulty. She had taken a creative writing class on a ship, and she talked to the whole class. "It was different ... I was with a friend ... maybe I felt I had control. I felt people were interested in what I was writing." This memory led to another of herself as a little girl before her mother died. This little girl had no public speaking phobia whatsoever. She was able to stand up in class, make presentations, ask questions, and give invited comments with great confidence.

The patient made it clear that she had limited time to work on her problem, that she needed results, and that she had little or no interest in psychodynamic exploration. The therapist (CF) held the impression that Ann was afraid of opening Pandora's box. Her sister had a serious connective tissue disease, and her brother's behavior as described by the patient was compatible with that of a serious dissociative disorder. The patient was seen in two individual sessions after the initial history taking.

In the first session the patient was helped to enter trance. She was then invited to look into the future to a time when the problem for which she sought help had been resolved. She was asked to notice where she was, with whom she was, and what she was doing, and she was told that she would be able to remember everything. Of this hypnotic progression the patient later reported: "What I saw was ... in the future ... I don't know where I was, but the president of the company was there and also the president from Hong Kong ... I was at ease, and everyone liked me ... they liked me, and they would be interested in what I had to say. I was informing ... No one was hostile."

The patient was taken from her progressive experience into a hypnotic regression, the end of which she identified ideomotorically. She was asked to return to grammar school at a time when her mother was alive and to observe and experience herself as the little girl who was comfortable speaking in the presence of others, who spoke clearly and with confidence. She was then invited (when she signaled ideomotorically that this was happening) to pretend that she could put on the little girl's head right over her own like a sock or a ski mask. She was then invited to give her upcoming speech from the stage of an imaginary theater to an audience of one person: the little girl she had once been and whose mask she now wore upon the stage. With the help of ideomotor signaling by the patient the therapist was able to introduce more and more people into the theater: First, a good friend, then other friends, acquaintances, and eventually strangers until the theater was filled with people. At any point of anxiety she could throw as many people as she wished out. This session was audiotaped, and the tape was given to the patient for practice.

In the following session an exploration was made in trance of the patient's connection with her dead mother. She perceived her as cold and distant, and she could not visualize her in any idealized way. Inasmuch as the internal mother was not an available source of strength or nurturance, more trance work was done utilizing the little girl. The suggestion was made that the patient could experience the little girl with or without the mask as it was right for her by simply touching the tip of the thumb of her right hand to its little finger. She was asked to imagine herself speaking to groups with and without the mask of the little girl.

At the end of this session the patient felt she had tools to solve her public speaking problem. She reviewed the family pathology which was extensive, and a strong recommendation for future psychotherapy to help her understand and resolve her early life situation was made by the therapist (CF). In a follow-up the patient revealed that she had been able to make presentations in public without difficulty. Although she was quite satisfied with this aspect of her treatment, she chose not to do further uncovering therapy.

In both cases the therapists used ego-strengthening maneuvers that were integrated into the trance inductions and deepening; in both cases the patients were helped to experience hypnotic age progressions. The animal doctor's progression was structured in nature; he was to see himself in the future performing successfully. The little girl's hypnotic age progression was unstructured and seemed to indicate resources within that believed her difficulty could be resolved. In each case the patient had a successful hypnotic age progression. This was followed by the patient being introduced to a powerful ego-state activator from childhood. It appeared that the picture of the faithful, loving dog, Heidi, was able to activate a forceful ego state in the animal doctor. This ego state was capable of totally allying itself with the trust and confidence that the dog, Heidi, had in the animal doctor to care for her.

However, this was probably not just an ego state from the past that had merely undergone activation. "This Heidi was a symbol and the promise of growth and responsibility, and in this sense was new, different. The triggers and reinforcers for this nurturing, strengthening ego state (now called Heidi) resided in the autohypnotic work and in the termination gift of the framed photograph of Heidi" (Frederick & Kim, 1993, p. 55).

The little girl, the ego state who represented the child the patient remembered, was competent and confident. She assumed strengthening and nurturing roles in the hypnotic work. She became Ann's supportive, encouraging companion or alter ego. This ego state had been modified by the hypnotic work. She no longer seemed to be only a state from the past. Instead, she had been projected into a successful future that could only have been accomplished through the power of her caretaker qualities. This ego state, like that of Heidi in the case of the animal doctor, was reinforced by autohypnosis and a trigger mechanism.

The technique used by Frederick and Kim (1993) is characterized by the use of progressions to establish the capacity for the mental experience of success. The second element of the technique is an image that can activate an ego state from the past and that can help the patient to experience it in the present as well. Finally, the ego state is modified into a helper state that is re-projected into the future. Frederick and Kim wondered whether they had tapped a process in which new ego states had been created, or whether old states were merely activated, given new tasks to perform, and pressed into service.

They believed the question was possibly philosophic, or even semantic. In Ego State Therapy ego states are constantly changing, and everyone involved in the successful treatment of Dissociative Identity Disorder (DID) has had the opportunity to observe how ego states grow and mature in their advancement on the road toward integration. The classic psychoanalytic concept of the ego is also one that conceptualizes the ego as continuing to grow and change as conflicts are resolved (A. Freud, 1936; S. Freud, 1932; Hartmann, 1965).

Frederick and Kim (1993) have suggested that such changes may occur only because new ego states are created through the modification of old ego states. They suggested that the helper states created by the sequence of age progression, age regression, assignment of a new role, age progression, and reinforcement by self-hypnosis, "like other kinds of hypnotic productions (Phillips & Frederick, 1990) are distillates of past, present, and future, and that in this sense they are 'new' and have become integrated into the personality with new and different significance" (Frederick & Kim, 1993, p. 56).

Chapter 12

Ego-Strengthening in the Treatment of Complex Clinical Syndromes

The most uncomplicated hypnotic treatment of anxiety is that of direct suggestion (Hammond, 1990a). There are other hypnotic approaches that have strong ego-strengthening components and give the patient a sense of mastery and control. Among them are the learning of relaxation skills that can be reinforced in self-hypnosis, reframing and utilization of anxiety (Gilligan, 1987; Gurgevich, 1990; Yapko; 1990), dissociation of the anxiety, systematic desensitization in trance, mental rehearsal, and posthypnotic suggestion (Hammond, 1990a).

The ability to experience deep muscle relaxation and to soothe and calm oneself (see chap. 7) can play a vital ego-strengthening role in the treatment of anxiety disorders. This kind of experience should not be limited to the therapist's office. The patient needs to come to view it as an ordinary part of his life. For this reason it is important that he learn to use self-hypnosis to produce relaxation and internal self-soothing as part of his regime for conquering anxiety. Such rich scripts as Hammond's (1990b) "Serenity Place" or Stanton's (1993b) elaboration of it can be most helpful. Another estimable source of scripts is Hunter's (1994) *Creative Scripts for Hypnotherapy*.

Scripts that are more specifically aimed at ego-strengthening, such as Stanton's (1989) Five Step approach, are also helpful with anxiety. Projective/evocative ego-strengthening can be extremely powerful with the anxiety disorders. For example, Inner Strength has particular value here inasmuch as it addresses the issue of becoming fearless.

Hypnotic techniques can often be combined with one another and with nonhypnotic techniques in the treatment of many disorders. Thus, it is not uncommon for anxiety disorders to be the subject of psychodynamic, nonhypnotic uncovering and hypnotic uncovering techniques such as ideomotor exploration of unconscious material (Hammond & Cheek, 1988), hypnotic age regression (Crasilneck & Hall, 1975), and Ego State Therapy which are combined with systematic desensitization in trance.

DOI:10.4324/9781003442585-12

Panic Disorder With and Without Agoraphobia

The individual who suffers from a panic attack faces a catastrophic event. What begins with a somatic sensation such as dizziness or palpitations rather swiftly becomes an overwhelming situation often misinterpreted as a heart attack or some other serious physical harbinger of death or insanity (Gelder, 1990).

The diagnosis of Panic Disorder carries with it implications for serious health and social consequences (Markowitz, Weissman, Oulette, Lish, & Klerman, 1989). Sufferers are at risk for alcohol and drug abuse (Cowley, 1992), a higher likelihood of suicide attempts, serious disturbances in marital functioning, social impairment, and financial dependency. There is also a greatly increased risk of overuse of minor tranquilizers as well as of co-morbidity with major depression (Gorman & Coplan, 1996), agoraphobia, and drug and alcohol abuse (Markowitz et al., 1989). Approximately 9% of the population will experience at least one panic attack during the course of their lives, and more than 3% will have them on a recurrent basis (Markowitz et al., 1989). Panic attacks are often linked with agoraphobia of which they are often thought to be a major component (Winter, 1986).

Noyes et al. (1986) have reported a 14% to 15% incidence of panic disorder in first degree relatives of patients with this disorder, and a small unpublished twin study has revealed a 31% concordance rate among monozygomatic twins. These findings suggest of a genetic disorder (Torgersen, 1983). More recent research, including functional imaging studies, pharmacologic challenge paradigms, and clinical observations, have produced confirming evidence for an anatomical basis for panic disorder that is currently conceptualized with a "network model" of neuronal system deregulation (Krystal, Deutsch, & Charney, 1996). The etiology of panic disorder is often considered in terms of its heredity, pathophysiology, and neuroanatomy (Ballenger, Burrows, & Dupont, 1988; Gorman, Liebowitz, Fryer, & Stein, 1989; National Institutes of Health, 1991).

The Consensus Development Conference on the Treatment of Panic Disorder (National Institutes of Health, 1991) has recommended an 8- to 12-week course of treatment consisting of behavioral and cognitive therapy in conjunction with the use of psychopharmacologic alagents. Currently, anxiolytics such as the benzodiazepenes, selective serotonin reuptake inhibitors, tricyclic antidepressants, and monamine oxidase inhibitors are used for symptom control. It is interesting that no recommendation for insight-oriented treatment was made.

It is possible that the efforts of the Consensus Conference have resulted in a more orderly treatment approach to the symptoms of the disorder and a higher incidence of recognition of comorbidity problems and other risks for many sufferers. However, within a few short years, data have emerged that show that short-term treatment does not free over half the panic disorder sufferers treated with the recommended combination of cognitive-behavioral therapy and drug therapy. "Despite pharmacologic and cognitive behavioral treatment, panic disorder often remains chronic" (Rosenbaum, Pollack, & Pollack, 1996, p. 44).

Indeed, panic disorder is becoming more widely viewed as chronic and relapsing (Marshall, Pollack, & Otto, 1997).

One of many questions that remain is whether cognitive-behavioral therapy and medication are the best kind of help for everyone and whether the symptoms of panic disorder in certain individuals represent a deep communication from within that deserves to be understood rather than be drugged or trained into quiescence. Do they, in many patients, have a final cause, or meaning that needs to be understood?

Nonhypnotic Psychological Treatments

The greatest difficulty in evaluating treatments for panic disorder has to do with the fact that panic disorder has been separated into its own diagnostic category for less than 20 years (American Psychiatric Association, 1987). Consequently, reports concerning the efficacies of various kinds of treatments for this disorder can be found under categories of *agoraphobia, phobias, anxiety disorders*, and *obsessionalism*. Other salient difficulties in evaluation are the complex dimensions of the treatment of panic disorder as well as the lack of controlled empirical studies concerning the efficacy of certain kinds of treatment (Straface, 1994).

Cognitive therapies (Barlow, 1997; Barlow & Cerny, 1988; Beck & Emery, 1985) have been found quite useful in dealing with avoidant behaviors, and behavioral therapies have been successful in eliminating symptoms and improving the quality of life. Among these therapies is systematic desensitization, which involves the use of anxiety hierarchies, identification of triggers, relaxation training, and the use of mental imagery with relaxation (Emmelkamp, 1979; Wolpe & Lazarus, 1966). Psychoanalysis also has been used effectively in the treatment of anxiety disorders and agoraphobias (Nemiah, 1981).

Hypnotic Treatments

Hypnobehavioral therapy (Clarke & Jackson, 1983) and hypnotic systematic desensitization (Thorpe & Burns, 1983) have been shown to be useful with panic disorders and agoraphobia. Brown and Fromm (1986) have noted that such treatments may reach a plateau and "it may be necessary to use dynamic hypnotherapy to uncover unconscious conflicts associated with the agoraphobia. More contemporary psychoanalytic studies suggest conflicts associated with separation-individuation" (p. 238). Hypnoanalytic work with an agoraphobic patient has been described by Gruenewald (1971). Goldstein and Chambless (1978) have reported on the combination of psychodynamic and behavioral principles in the therapy of panic disorder. The successful braiding of several kinds of hypnotherapeutic interventions with cognitive-behavioral therapy, insight-oriented psychotherapy, and medication has been described by Straface (1994).

Work in the field of dissociation (see chap. 13) has cast further light upon reasons why hypnotherapeutic interventions may be particularly useful with panic disorder. The symptoms of panic disorder and phobias have been as reported as sequelae of incest (Fine, 1990), and panic attacks are common in Dissociative Identity Disorder (formerly known as Multiple Personality Disorder) patients (Bliss, 1984; Putnam, 1989; Putnam et al., 1986; Ross, 1989). Certain situations may trigger switches of alters or ignite posttraumatic flashbacks with resultant phobic or panic symptoms (Putnam, 1988, 1989). Nevertheless, panic disorder and agoraphobia are not usually described as dissociative in nature in the literature. This is the case even though symptoms that are frankly dissociative (such as derealization, depersonalization, and dizziness) have been reported as part and parcel of the clinical picture in approximately 90% of cases (Grunhaus, 1988). Making the diagnosis of a dissociative problem when one is present is extremely important, especially if it appears to be ego-state driven. The prognosis for appropriately treated ego-state driven panic disorder with or without agoraphobia is usually quite good, and the changes frequently affect other aspects of the personality positively (Frederick, 1993c).

The clinical case presented next has been described previously (Frederick, 1993c) but in less detail. It is one that illustrates the multiple factors that contribute to the formation of the symptoms of Panic Disorder (genetic, structural, learned, dissociative, ego-state driven) and shows how the essential ingredient of ego-strengthening can be woven with other techniques into the patient's treatment.

Case Example: Craig

Craig was a 38-year-old consulting engineer. When I (CF) first saw him, he denied any previous history of phobias or anxieties. He told me that he had been an avid skier all of his adult life. Craig sought treatment because he had become overwhelmed by a panic attack when he was in a chair lift. The lift stopped suddenly while it was very high in the air, and it did not move for a considerable period of time. Craig became aware, at first, of feeling strange. Then he developed an adrenaline rush, sweating palms, and terrible chest pain. "I felt stuck, really stuck!" He thought he might be having a heart attack.

Craig had grown up in a turbulent and dysfunctional alcoholic family; his father was harsh and constantly expected perfection of Craig. In his late latency and adolescent years Craig often feared that he would lose his mind. He sometimes felt like he was drifting away.

Craig was anxious about whether he could be helped. I (CF) assured him that if we worked together, we could do the job. I explained to him that I had worked with a number of other patients with panic disorder and that, in my experience, he would be able to feel much better. I explained the stress-diathesis model to him and wondered with him whether anyone in his family might also have panic attacks. I also invited him to speculate about what was really stressing him in his present life. A few minutes later, and almost as an aside, he described that he was a distant father to his children. He was frequently hypercritical, and the children often irritated him. He saw his father in himself at these times, and it concerned him.

In the second session Craig was able to recall felling similarly stuck in a freeway jam when he was 18. He also remembered yet another panic episode while he was exploring some caves. "Part of me said, 'Run down that tunnel!!' The other part said, 'This will be embarrassing.'" The rest of the session was focused on ego-strengthening. The patient was taught to establish a safe place, a deep zone of relaxation to which he could retreat should he experience any signs of an impending panic attack. It was also suggested that he would find it most desirable to visit this place for relaxation and stress reduction. He was given an audiotape of the hypnotic exercise with which to practice. In this session Craig was able to generate a positive hypnotic age progression (Phillips & Frederick, 1992). In it Craig was able to picture himself both having a pleasant flight in an airplane and skiing happily on the mountain.

In the third therapy session Ego-State Therapy was begun. An ego state, Death, revealed that he had come to protect Craig. This ego state stated that it had emerged very early in the patient's life. It described helping at a time when the patient had nearly drowned. Death agreed to participate in a hypnotic age regression, and was able to recall, with Craig, memory material of an episode in which Craig had nearly drowned when he was 3.

After the patient had several sessions of consistent work in and out of trance, the symptoms were still present. I suspected that we may not have completed our knowledge of all Death's helpful work, and Death was somewhat reluctant to explore matters further. Craig was helped to have the Inner Strength experience, and Death was invited to join him. After this experience, Death was asked to help us understand more about Craig's panic attacks.

Death was feeling stronger because he had participated in the Inner Strength experience, and he was willing to undergo even further hypnotic age regression. This time Death traveled to an earlier time of difficulty that had threatened the patient's life: Craig's "birth experience." In the memory material that was produced the patient said that he could only interpret his experience as one of being stuck in his mother's birth canal and being removed, eventually, with the assistance of forceps. Death said that this experience was also connected with the patient's chair lift experience of being stuck. Death's menacing symptoms had been attempts to help the patient survive by becoming aware of the danger of being stuck. Death agreed that it would be acceptable now to clear the circuits for this experience as he realized that Craig was not really in life or death danger anymore.

In the following session the patient reported: "In the past couple of days I feel like I've dumped a bunch of stuff ... I've lightened up ... I'm having fun. I'm grateful for my family." The patient was reminded that the imagery of the birth canal could well be related to his delivering himself of a new self. Craig and I were able to discuss further the frightening "birth experience" that had been taking place in his current life. A new identity as a good and nurturing father, different from his own father, was in the process of being born. We agreed that this could well be the stressor that had precipitated the panic attack. After a period of reprocessing and integration of the hypnoanalytic and other material, the patient was discharged free of symptoms. He felt that the quality of his life had greatly improved, and he was able to use ski lifts again without difficulties. He had been seen for 12 sessions. No medication was used with this patient at any time; he has been symptom free for 4 years. Approximately 6 months after the termination of his treatment Craig's wife telephoned me to thank me for the remarkable improvement that had taken place in Craig's relationship with her and their children.

The clinical manifestations of Panic Disorder are the result of a combination of many causes: genetic predisposition, current stress, and, in many instances, unresolved unconscious problems. They may be expressive of the patient's approaching a critical new era or important task in his life; in this final cause the true meaning of his sufferings may be discovered. This places them with many other psychological difficulties into the general category of the stress-diathesis syndromes. We maintain that education that is aimed at normalizing such a complex disorder and a firm therapeutic alliance are ego-strengthening essentials in the treatment of panic disorders. A wide variety of ego-strengthening maneuvers that emphasize inner resources can help the patient achieve mastery over symptoms and prepare the way for necessary uncovering work. Ego-strengthening is of assistance in the areas of both the stress and the diathesis as well.

As psychotherapists who frequently use hypnosis, we do not encounter "birth experiences" with any frequency. Indeed, they are uncommon for us. Within the hypnosis field there is much debate about the meaning of such experiences; opinions range from absolute concrete belief that these kinds of occurrences are accurate representations of what actually transpired during the patient's birth to rational denial that such material could be anything other than the result of the patient meeting the therapist's unspoken demands and expectations (Watkins &

Watkins, 1997). We view such experiences in therapy as simply more grist for the mill. Like all memory experiences or memory material (see chap. 13) they need to be dealt with in terms of what their meaning is in the patient's life. We believe that these experiences may be metaphorical in nature and that they should be interpreted (as are dreams and hypnotic dreams) in terms of their unique meaning within the psychodynamics of the patient's life. Ultimately, it is only the patient who can make this kind of determination for himself as he searches for his own truth (Phillips & Frederick, 1995). We explore the topics of memory and traumatic memory more thoroughly in chapter 13. However, it is important to recall the viewpoints of Spence (1982) and Ganaway (1989) in distinguishing between *narrative truth* and *historical truth*. Narrative truth may be totally false from a historical point of view, or, it may be a combination of facts, fantasy, and/or symbolic material.

It may be of some interest to note that the author (CF) is currently working with another panic disorder patient, Sheila, who has brought up a great deal of primitive memory material including some that has appeared to be representative of her passage through the birth canal. Like Craig, Sheila is on the verge of making a major identity change and giving birth to a new, much more adult self.

Obsessive Compulsive Disorder, as is seen next, is another of the stress-diathesis syndromes that exists in a spectrum from the most biologically to the most psychologically determined.

Obsessive Compulsive Disorders

Obsessive Compulsive Disorder (OCD) has been described traditionally as "a relatively rare extremely debilitating condition which is highly refractory to treatment" (Turner, Bidel, & Nathan, 1985). A persistent feature of this disorder is its ego-dystonia. It has been noted that, although the purpose of the symptoms appears to be the relief of anxiety, the ego-dystonic nature of the thoughts produces anxiety in and of itself—an anxiety that is a consistent characteristic of the disorder.

It is also characteristic of the disorder that the sufferer believes that he lacks voluntary control over the symptoms despite his knowledge that the thoughts he entertains and the acts that he must perform are unreasonable and may even be preposterous (Salzman & Thaler, 1981). Epidemiological data suggest that obsessive compulsive disorders and related disorders may be much more widespread than previously believed (Rasmussen, Eisen, & Pato, 1993; Turner, 1985).

As with many psychiatric disorders, the treatment of Obsessive Compulsive Disorder (OCD) has varied considerably according to the fashions of the time. During the considerable period of time that psychodynamic psychiatry reigned, OCD was thought to be a symptomatic manifestation of psychodynamic conflict, and the treatments of choice included psychoanalysis and psychodynamic psychotherapy. Behavioral therapy and hypnosis were also used (Tan,

Marks, & Marsett, 1971). In recent times a search for biological factors in OCD has become quite prominent (Turner, Bidel, & Nathan, 1985), and OCD has come to be widely accepted as a model neuropsychiatric illness.

It is perhaps a testimony to the stubbornness of the symptoms of OCD that a panoply of treatments has been leveled at the disorder. These have included physical therapies such as drugs, electroconvulsive therapies, insulin therapy, and psychosurgery, including leucotomy. In the 1980s particular attention was focused on the investigation of a newly released antidepressant medication, clomipramine (Anafranil), which was shown to produce marked improvement in obsessive compulsive symptoms in 35% to 42% of the cases treated (Thoren, Asberg, & Bertilsson, 1988). Other serotonin reuptake inhibitors such as fluoxetine (Prozac), sertaline (Zoloft), and paroxetine (Paxil) have now been shown to offer alleviation of OCD symptoms (Goodman, McDougle, & Price, 1992).

Historically, OCD was originally related to demon possession (Ross, 1989)—a manifestation of dissociation. A resemblance of certain aspects of Dissociative Identity Disorder symptoms and the manifest symptoms of OCD was noted by Beahrs (1982b). He suggested a link with dissociation: "Obsessive compulsive symptoms certainly bear a resemblance to a subject's carrying out a post-hypnotic suggestion" (Beahrs, 1986, p. 46).

The dissociative origins of some specific OCD cases were reported by Ross and Anderson (1988). Through the use of amytal interviews in two refractory OCD patients, Ross and Anderson were able to activate states that have been described as "alterpersonalitylike" by Ross (1989). Ross and Anderson found that the scores of a number of their patients more closely resembled Dissociative Identity Disorder patients' scores on the Dissociative Disorders Interview Schedule (DDIS), the Dissociative Experiences Scale (DES), the Anxiety Disorder Interview Schedule, SCL-90, and the Lynfield inventory for obsessive compulsive disorder. Ross questioned the appropriateness of listing OCD with the anxiety disorders. He felt that: "A minority of obsessive-compulsive patients appear to have a freestanding disorder limited to the obsessions and compulsions" (p. 165). He also suggested that those patients who had posttraumatic symptoms as well as the symptoms of OCD should be placed into a new category of disorders: *trauma disorders*. Ross felt that obsessions and compulsions in DID patients could be compared with the Schneiderian symptoms and that the therapist should always be ready to investigate their origins.

Frederick (1990) proposed that the etiology of OCD should be viewed from the frame of reference that a stress-diathesis model could provide: Certain individuals constitutionally disposed to develop OCD would develop such symptoms when their stress levels were high enough to trigger them. Frederick also called attention to the hidden stressor of unresolved childhood conflict—trauma that had been dissociated in certain patients.

New medication discoveries, together with the current emphasis on managed care (and what amounts to a rationing of treatment for many individuals), have helped the pendulum swing far from psychodynamic approaches. As with panic disorder, combinations of medications and behavior therapy (Baer, 1993) are now in vogue. A therapist set on being in the mainstream of neuropsychiatry when considering appropriate treatment for his OCD patients may even elect to use decision upon which to base his therapeutic judgment (Greist, 1992). (A decision tree is a mechanistic decision-making device that leads the clinician to ultimate treatment decisions about patients based on specific information signs, symptoms, and responses to various medications.) Currently, the satisfactory resolution of treatment-resistant OCD is commonly considered from a biological standpoint alone (Goodman, McDougle, Barr, Aronson, & Price, 1993).

The Hypnotic Treatment of Obsessive Compulsive Disorder

Several hypnotic techniques have been reported as successful with obsessive compulsive disorder. They fall into three categories. The first is the hypnoimagery approach of Kroger and Fezler (1976), which utilizes hypnotic desensitization. Kroger and Fezler also recommended hypnosis for deep relaxation because in certain cases this appeared to neutralize anxiety-ridden obsessions. Difficulties with the use of behavioral techniques and hypnosis arise when no triggering situation or stimuli can be discerned. Without them a behavioral program cannot be set up (Marks, 1981).

A second category of hypnoimagery intervention involves the use of a variety of ego-enhancing techniques that are initially structured for the patient by the therapist. Johnson and Hallenbeck (1985) worked with a young woman who was plagued with a number of obsessional fears. Her 8-year history of fearfulness had been accompanied by hand washing and undoing rituals. They used hypnosis as the facilitator for mastery techniques (Dimond, 1981; Gardner, 1976) as well as for ego-enhancing hypnotic age progressions. The patient was asked to imagine herself several years in the future in a fashion structured by the therapists. In a subsequent session, the progression was extended to the time when the patient as an old woman would look back on a life full of accomplishments.

The third approach is the use of hypnotherapeutic techniques that are generally thought of as hypnoanalytic. These deal with the ideology and psychodynamics of the symptoms (Crasilneck & Hall, 1975). A classic case in the hypnotic literature is that of the treatment of an obsessional neurosis by Milton Erickson (Erickson & Kubie, 1939/1980). Erickson was aware of the adaptive nature of dissociation in many patients. He (Erickson & Kubie, 1939/1980) worked therapeutically with a young woman, Miss Damon, who suffered from a severe case of obsessive compulsive disorder (OCD). She attempted, often successfully, to conceal this disorder from her friends and coworkers. (For a detailed description of this case, see chap. 4.)

Miss Damon decided to volunteer as a subject in some experiments in hypnotism. As a result of the hypnotic interventions, a second personality, Miss Brown, emerged via the medium of automatic writing. Miss Damon had been completely unaware of this other personality, and only deduced her existence from the evidence of the handwriting. Miss Brown became quite helpful to Miss Damon and eventually specified exactly when certain insights would be given to her. She also guided Miss Damon in the recollection of a traumatic incident that had taken place when she was 3. The memory, involving her grandfather, may have been a screen memory. Nevertheless, it appeared to explain the phobias and compulsions and the experimental hypnotherapeutic process resulted in the permanent cure of Miss Damon's obsessional phobia.

A fourth approach to the treatment of OCD is Ego-State Therapy (Watkins, 1993; Watkins & Watkins, 1991, 1997; Watkins, 1992). In 1990 Frederick reported a case in which the symptoms of OCD had been removed quite rapidly with the use of Ego State Therapy. The treatment extended over a 2½-month period. Memory experiences of severe childhood trauma surfaced, and the patient, with one exception, remained free of his symptoms for a year and a half. The exception was a recurrence of the symptoms for a 24-hour period when the patient was ill with pneumonia.

The case material presented next is from Frederick's (1996c) review of the stress-diathesis syndrome in some clinical cases of OCD. In each of these cases (one treated without success) ego-strengthening techniques were used in combination with various other treatment modalities.

Case Example: Jodie

Jodie entered treatment because she was depressed. However, almost immediately she revealed that her real problems were the obsessions that plagued her and the compulsions that drove her and her husband nearly mad. Jodie was happy with her husband but unhappy with her own failure to find work that had any great meaning to her. She was embarrassed to reveal that she, now in her early 40s, had developed an overwhelming desire to learn to ride horses and perhaps in time to work with them. Her husband repeatedly told her that this was unrealistic.

Jodie had a big desire to change and a limited budget. Her family history revealed that several members of her family of origin had also displayed signs of compulsive behavior. I discussed the treatment possibilities that were available for her. She decided that she would like to come to therapy sessions every 2 weeks and take medication for her depression.

I (CF) started Jodie on fluoxetine (Prozac). It helped the depressive symptoms and improved her focus. I moved into trance work with her, emphasizing ego-strengthening. In time, we used Ego State Therapy and worked with ego states that had originally appeared to help the patient with trauma in childhood. Helping these ego states to strengthen, mature, and cooperate was the major focus of our work with them. Such ego-strengthening techniques as *Inner Strength* (Frederick & McNeal, 1993) and hypnotic age progressions (Phillips & Frederick, 1992) were used frequently with immature ego states. Eventually, the traumatic memory material was renegotiated internally by these ego states, which had now become much stronger and more developed. Jodie reported to me that she was at last really learning to ride and she had made a deal at a stable whereby she could ride the horses and get some instruction in exchange for her doing heavy stable cleaning work. She also reported that her husband thought she was nuts to do this and suspected that I also was nuts inasmuch as I had not stopped her.

With the resolution of the patient's ego-state problems her symptoms began to fall away: both the depression and the obsessions and compulsion. Eventually, she discontinued the fluoxetine and decided to terminate her treatment which she felt had been successful.

Jodie called me two and a half years later. She was successfully completing a 2-year course as a veterinarian's assistant for which she had had to commute to a university some distance away. She was now looking forward to work in her new profession and was happy and proud of herself. Her husband was delighted with what had come out of what he had thought was just another of Jodie's obsessions. She told me she thought the Prozac had been quite helpful to her in the beginning, but that she had nothing to complain of now.

Case Example: Helen

Helen wanted relief of her compulsive worrying and housecleaning. She was motivated by the unhappiness and the fatigue they brought her. Her symptoms had begun during interpersonal conflict with her husband by whom she felt neglected. He was a quite domineering man, and it appeared that it was only through her symptoms that she controlled him. Her own father had also been quite domineering, had displayed an abusive temper constantly, and had even beaten her mother.

From the beginning, Helen was interested in the easy way out. She wanted a miracle cure from one of the medications she had been reading about. I (CF) agreed to medication if she would become involved with the rest of what I felt was indicated. Helen consented to attend therapy sessions. We began with work on the therapeutic alliance and slowly moved into other forms of ego-strengthening. Ideomotor signals were not helpful, however. Despite of her protestations to the contrary, I thought the patient was deliberately controlling her finger signals. I had serious doubts about her motivations and level of sincerity with me in the sessions. It appeared that trust in the therapeutic process would be interpreted by the patient as a loss of control. Whenever this was gently interpreted to her, she vigorously denied it.

Helen made some improvements. She lessened her focus on control through cleanliness sufficiently to buy a puppy who grew into a quite large dog. Then she began to reduce the frequency of her sessions, employing money as her reason. I refused to see her on a medications only basis and referred her to an excellent counseling service that had a sliding scale. I would continue to medicate her if she was truly in ongoing therapy. Her new therapist noted Helen's refusal to participate in any behavioral program. Although Helen was seen conjointly with her husband, and it appeared to be helpful, Helen denied the efficacy of any of her treatment. When her counselor moved out of the area, she rejected the new therapist, a colleague with excellent training and clinical abilities, and she attempted again a "medications only" arrangement with me. I declined, gave her my reasons for so doing, and gave her the names of some other treatment resources.

Case Example: Ted (a 7-Year Follow-Up)

Ted was seen in individual psychotherapy for a year after his OCD symptoms had been resolved with the use of Ego State Therapy (Frederick, 1990). He had lived in a great deal of social isolation and needed therapy to help him adjust to the outside world. Eventually, he went into a design business with a cousin who had decided to move to the area.

Ted noticed that when he was under stress, he could keep his OCD symptoms from recurring, but he found that it required some effort on his part. His wife continued to espouse the chemical theory of OCD, and prevailed upon Ted not to return to treatment with me but to seek medication from a psychiatrist in another geographic location. Ted was started on Prozac, and he noticed that he simply felt more comfortable on the medication.

Although the Prozac helped Ted's comfort level, it did not teach him how to cope with life's problems. Ted returned to see me 4 years after his original treatment and after a series of debacles had befallen him. He was planning to move to Chicago. His marriage had broken up, and the woman for whom he had left his wife had rejected him. His wife would not take him back in spite of the fact that he had made a serious suicide attempt in a bid for her attention. Now he sought help for the complications of his life and the consequences of his difficulties with the girlfriend who had helped finish off his marriage. When I discovered that Prozac had been so helpful to Ted, I agreed with his suggestion that he continue on it.

Ego-state exploration revealed that the childlike ego state, Ted, had been behind the suicide attempt. It also revealed that all the parts liked the Prozac very much. A review of Ted's life history over the past 7 years made me suspect that he suffered from Dissociative Identity Disorder (DID). I (CF) expressed to Ted my concerns about the suicide attempt and the lack of integration I thought it represented. Our work in the 2 months we met this time was devoted to ego-strengthening of both the parts and the greater personality so that Ted could actually carry out his scheduled move to another geographical area. This was necessary, because it afforded him a chance to support himself in the new occupation he had trained for over the past several years. He agreed to get into therapy in his new location.

The Stress-Diathesis Syndrome, OCD, and Ego-Strengthening

The approaches described in these cases are illustrative of treatment that is based on an appreciation of the symptoms of OCD as manifestations of a stress-diathesis syndrome. There is not a unitary profile for the OCD patient. The tendencies to the syndrome may simply lie dormant and unexpressed unless the stress component of the model is also present in sufficient strength to ignite them into clinical expression. Not all stress is obvious, recent, or situational. In some individuals, unresolved childhood conflicts and/or failure of adequate psychic structures to develop may constitute hidden stress that must be attended if progress is to be maintained. The case material illustrates how the therapist's understanding can be widened by this multifactorial concept of illness. It also demonstrates the limitations of psychotherapeutic approaches in patients whose OCD is heavily driven by the inborn or genetic components, or whose family dynamics and life realities impinge upon the meaning of their symptoms. The case material also illustrates the importance of weaving ego-strengthening with all of the treatment modalities to enhance the treatment of Obsessive Compulsive Disorder. Although it would be tempting to say that the case of Helen was not successful because it is illustrative of OCD that is most biologically determined, the author (CF) suspects that this is not the case at all. The failure seems to lie somewhere in the combination of the patient's lack of motivation for uncovering therapy and the therapist's inability to engage her into a working alliance.

Ego-Strengthening and Complex Cases

Because complex cases challenge us in so many ways, it is invaluable to keep possibilities for ego-strengthening in mind as we work with their many facets. When we look at the "stress" side of the stress-diathesis model, we realize how important ego-strengthening can be for stress management and the institution of lifestyle changes. For example, it is not unusual for individuals to develop OCD after the birth of a child. The call to parenthood appears to be the stress that triggers the diathesis into manifestation. With certain patients the simple use of daily self-hypnosis with internal self-soothing could greatly mitigate the symptoms, while others might improve when they expand and strengthen their egos by taking parenting classes and making lifestyle changes. On the diathesis side of the model, we can locate interventions aimed at reducing the effects of the diathesis. For example, hypnoimagery and behavioral approaches with the symptoms of OCD, panic disorder, or eating disorders can bring a sense of mastery to many patients. Ego-strengthening is essential for the working out of the unresolved childhood conflicts, particularly because only a strengthened ego can come to tolerate facing what lies beyond the defenses.

Depression

Depression is one of the most common diagnostic categories seen in clinical settings. Symptoms of depression have been reported to accompany up to 36% of medical conditions (Goodnick, 1997) and occur in 4% of the general population. In the *Diagnostic and Statistical Manual of Mental Disorders* (4th ed. [*DSM–IV*]; American Psychiatric Association, 1994) the incidence is reported to be 2.3% for men and 4.5% to 9.3% for women (Goodnick, 1997).

In *DSM–IV* there are two major categories of mood disorders: Depressive Disorders and Bipolar Disorders. The depressive disorders, Major Depressive Disorder, Dysthymic Disorder. and Depressive Disorder NOS, are those most likely to be seen in an outpatient practice. Under Bipolar Disorders (commonly called *manic-depressive*) are Bipolar I Disorders, Bipolar 11 Disorder, Cyclothymic Disorder, and Bipolar Disorder NOS. In addition, there are mood disorders due to general medical conditions, substance-induced mood disorders, and mood disorders NOS. The bipolar disorders have a strong biological component and usually require treatment with mood levelers such as divalproex (Depakote) or lithium carbonate. More recently, with the advent of the SSRI medication, almost all forms of depression, especially major depressive disorder, will improve somewhat with these medications. However, often what psychotherapists see in their offices are individuals with comorbidity, that is, presenting with both depression and anxiety, or depression superimposed on a personality disorder (Torem, 1987b).

Symptoms characteristically reported are depressed mood, sadness, crying spells, and aches and pains such as headaches, stomach aches, or backaches. Depression can also be manifested by insomnia or hypersomnia, loss of appetite with weight loss, binge eating and weight gain, psychomotor agitation or retardation, fatigue or low energy, neglect of appearance and hygiene, difficulty making decisions, feelings of worthlessness and low self-esteem, pessimism, difficulty concentrating, and the inability to experience happiness or anhedonia. Sometimes depression is experienced mainly through physical pain and illness or through pervasive negativism. There may be suicidal rumination with or without a plan to commit suicide. It can be important to distinguish bereavement caused by loss of a loved one or other significant loss; and from drug-induced depression or depression resulting from other medical conditions.

The stress-diathesis model of causation can be applied to depression. Here the material cause involves the biochemical make-up of the individual and whether inherited predisposition exists. This is the area where evaluation for appropriate medications is very important. Determining the efficient cause leads us to look for those events in the patient's life that triggered the onset of symptoms and are maintaining them now. The formal cause would involve looking at the underlying personality structure, while consideration of the final cause motivates us to explore what is the meaning or purpose of the symptoms for the patient. As psychotherapists, we need to attend to all of these causes, but the major focus is usually on the efficient cause. We know that stress can produce symptoms of depression in individuals who are predisposed in that direction. These stressors can be external and/or internal, and include the stress caused by accumulative or hidden childhood trauma.

Treatment of Depression

According to the type and severity of the depression, it can be treated on an inpatient or outpatient basis and with a combination of medication and psychotherapy, medication alone, or psychotherapy alone. The focus of psychotherapy depends on what theoretical orientation or model of treatment is chosen. Cognitive-behavioral and psychodynamic treatment models have proven successful in treating depression. The former approach is favored by managed care health plans because it is usually touted to be short term and substantiated by outcome studies, and because it is easiest to describe studies that objectify and measure. However, the cognitive-behavioral model can only deal with what symptoms can be observed and what the patient can consciously report. A psychodynamic model provides much more to work with in that patients and therapists can consider the unconscious factors that underlie the symptoms as well. Clinical hypnosis can be particularly useful here and is applicable in a multitude of ways.

Hypnosis in the Treatment of Depression

Torem (1987b) has listed major underlying dynamics of depression for which hypnotic interventions can be useful:

- *An unconscious sense of guilt*: Pain and suffering can be a way of atoning for unconscious guilt such as survivor's guilt. Torem gave an example of a patient who suffered intense chronic physical pain with no organic cause. Use of a hypnotic age regression technique, the affect bridge, revealed a trauma. The patient had lost a twin brother at the age of 5; he had died from a blow to the head by a swing on which both brothers had been playing (Torem, 1987b).
- *Masochism*: Torem (1987b) characterizes masochism as a symptom of depression associated with interpersonal relationships. There the repetition of misery and suffering represents a bid for affection from a parental figure who has been neglectful or abusive.

• *Reenactment of childhood traumata*: Depressive character structure, Torem (1987b) believes, has its roots in an unhappy childhood filled with traumatic experiences (p. 290). This dynamic causes the patient to reenact the original trauma by unconsciously living in self-inflicted misery. Unless this comes into consciousness, the patient may engage in self-destructive behavior should there be symptom relief without resolution of the underlying pathology. Hypnosis can be useful in uncovering dynamics of this nature.

• *Identification with the aggressor*: Here the patient unconsciously identifies with an introjected rejecting and abusive parent. The patient turns the abuse of an introjected object against herself. Ego-state therapy can be useful in identifying this introjected object. It can manifest as an ego state that can be worked with and ultimately transformed into a positive ego state (see chap. 4). The same principle would apply in working with hidden, persecutory ego states.

• *Unresolved grief and anniversary reactions*: Unresolved grief or incomplete mourning may underlie depression. This can be triggered by the approach of a date at which a significant death or loss occurred. Hypnosis may be useful in uncovering the dynamics associated with this kind of depression.

Many hypnotic techniques may be useful in dealing with various manifestations of depression. Torem (1987b) mentions exploratory tools that include the affect bridge, movie/TV screen imaging, the crystal ball technique, age regression, ideomotor signalling, and dream induction. Hypnotic techniques are useful for abreaction and working through traumatic material, as well.

Ego State Therapy for Refractory, Intermittent Depression

Ego-state therapy can be especially valuable in working with problems of intermittent depression. Frederick (1993b) reported two case studies using Ego State Therapy with patients who had completed therapy but periodically experienced the return of depressive symptoms. The case of Felicia was also reported in greater detail in Phillips and Frederick (1995).

Case Example: Joan

Joan, age 58, had had Freudian psychoanalysis and other kinds of psychotherapy and body therapy. However, in spite of a great deal of therapy she continued to fall into a pool of sadness. This depressive symptom appeared periodically.

Joan revealed that her parents had been busy professional people and that her rearing had been turned over to a nurse maid, Katya. When she was 3, her little sister was born and Katya was discharged from service with the family. Joan did not remember Katya's leaving. In the second session

Joan was helped to enter trance and ideomotor signals were established. Through the signals, contact was made with a part of Joan's personality that had never gotten over the terror and grief of Katya's departure. Joan sobbed like "an extremely distressed pre-verbal or non-verbal child" (Frederick, 1993b, p. 223). When she was able to calm down, Joan was able to mentally hold and rock this child ego state. She promised that she would never leave her and agreed to continue this renurturing on a daily basis until the need for it no longer existed. In a follow-up appointment, Joan was free of her symptom and confident that it had been resolved.

Case Example: Felicia

Felicia had recovered from a significant depression and was in recovery from alcohol addiction. However, she returned to therapy to report that she had become aware of welling of sadness. She reported that she had had these all her life. They were unpredictable and accompanied by crying. Ego State Therapy was initiated and a child ego state who was experiencing intense terror was activated. As the details of the situation were unclear, I (CF) helped Felicia leave this scene and enter the Inner Strength experience.

The strong part of Felicia was instructed in trance to help Felicia remember the source of her fear at her pace. After this session, Felicia had spontaneously recalled a scene in which her alcoholic mother had burned her hand on a floor grate. This memory was accompanied by a strong sense. The depressive symptom, the wellings, vanished. I continue to hear from Felicia over the years. She is now, 5 years later, still doing well.

Frederick (1993b) discussed these cases in terms of the clues that indicate ego-state pathology (see chap. 4). The pools and wellings that were affect-laden occurrences were *ego-dystonic* with the patient's normal everyday functioning. Frederick also focused on the importance of ego-strengthening in ego-state therapy. When a trauma that is overwhelming to a part is recalled, ego-strengthening techniques can provide rest, strengthening, integration of the previous work, and the confidence to continue the exploration and cope with the trauma.

Newey (1986) discussed utilizing ego-state therapy with depression. He theorized that unconscious fears are often the basis of unremitting depression. He used ideomotor signalling to communicate with the patient in trance and to access frightened aspects of personality. They are usually child parts with fears of rejection and punishment. In Newey's model the frightened parts are identified and their fears explored. Then the assistance of a *strong part* is enlisted to separate them from an internally abusing parent and take them to a safe place. Newey (1986) conceptualizes the strong part, which he has utilized for ego-strengthening, as "… an innate, universal dimension of self which has to do with the capacity for clarity and directness of response" (Newey, 1986, p. 199). Newey (1986) has defined that part as both fearless and present from birth. He states that, "In the depressed person, the Strong Part will inevitably be bound to be prevented from acting freely and openly" (Newey, 1986, p. 199). He believes the strong part may be angry because of what has happened, and that it is necessary to work with the part to resolve the anger, before it can proceed most effectively to help with the frightened parts. This concept of a Strong Part is another illustration of how ego-strengthening and ego-state therapy can work together in psychotherapy—not only in the treatment of depression, but with many other syndromes and diagnoses as well. This strong part of Newey (1986) bears some resemblance to aspects of the Inner Strength concept (McNeal & Frederick, 1993).

A cognitive-behavioral brief therapy approach to treating depression has been proposed by Yapko (1996). Yapko identifies patterns that cause and maintain depression, such as the depressed person's "present temporal orientation" (Yapko, 1992), an orientation to the immediacy of one's experience at the expense of long-range planning, and consideration of behavioral consequences. According to Yapko (1996), other patterns underlying depression are low frustration tolerance, internal orientation, low compartmentalization, and diffuse attentional style (Yapko, 1996). Yapko believes hypnosis is useful in focusing attention on the skills the depressed patient needs to develop to manage her life. According to Yapko, useful techniques include the use of future age-projection work to develop future long-term goals orientation and greater frustration tolerance. He believes hypnosis to also be useful in anxiety reduction and accessing inner resources for increased impulse control.

Other goals of treatment that can be enhanced through hypnosis involve recognizing the possibility of change, and shifting from a reactive to a proactive position for responding to life's external circumstances and internal perceptions and attitudes. Yapko lists six reasons why hypnosis is useful in psychotherapy and for the treatment of depression in particular:

- Hypnosis can amplify portions of subjective experience making it easier to identify patterns of maladaptive thinking and behavior.
- Hypnosis can be a method of pattern interruption.
- Hypnosis can facilitate experiential learning.
- Hypnosis helps to associate and generalize desired responses.
- Hypnosis models flexibility and variety.
- Hypnosis is helpful in focusing.

Yapko (1992, 1996) uses both formal and informal trance as well as Ericksonian methods of direct and indirect suggestions, metaphors, and posthypnotic suggestions.

In the past the use of hypnosis for treatment of depression was controversial. Many clinicians believed that hypnosis could be dangerous with depressed patients because of the risk of suicide (see chap. 5). It was thought that hypnosis might weaken the patient's defenses against suicide and increase the possibility that the patient might actually act on her impulses. It is important to evaluate the nature and severity of depression before considering hypnotic interventions. Hypnotic progression can be quite helpful in the evaluation (see chap. 5) because of its prognostic qualities. Contraindications for the use of hypnosis in depression that have been mentioned in the literature include the presence of suicidal ideation, severe endogenous depression, agitated melancholia, and the depressed phase of manic-depressive illness.

In our experience hypnosis is not a substitute for other appropriate clinical interventions. However, we have found that hypnotically facilitated ego-strengthening work is of unparalleled value with many suicidal patients. Brown and Fromm (1986) have recommended hypnosis and the accessing of an internal transitional space as an urgent intervention with the suicidal patient. The calming and soothing so provided could be life-saving in some cases.

Depression and Ego-Strengthening

When the underlying dynamics have been identified, and the therapeutic alliance is in place, both hypnotic and nonhypnotic ego-strengthening are strongly indicated. The emphasis is ego-strengthening, not symptom removal. The ego-strengthening can emphasize ways that the patient can learn to experience relaxation, calmness, inner peace, and inner strength. Many ego-strengthening scripts are also useful in dealing with low self-esteem, self-derogatory thoughts, and feelings of self-loathing. When suggestions are worded positively and combined with projective/evocative imagery, the patient is more likely to be receptive and able to find inner resources that exist apart from the feelings of depression. It is our experience that, when suggestions are presented in trance to the depressed patient, it is usually more effective. We routinely use hypnosis with depressed patients. Other aspects of ego-strengthening that are helpful to the depressed patient are mastery and affect release (e.g., the silent abreaction).

Each of the theorists presented earlier included ego-strengthening hypnotic techniques integrated with other hypnotic approaches in the treatment of depression. Ego-strengthening is helpful in each stage of treatment of depression. In the early stages of treatment, it is beneficial for accessing resources and providing relaxation and feelings of calmness. During the middle phase of treatment, ego-strengthening can provide a way to reframe a myriad of troublesome situations: Hypnotic ego-strengthening suggestions can help relabel or reformulate experiences. In the later stages of treatment, ego-strengthening can help fortify ego states, reinforce emerging new skills, increase self-confidence and self-esteem, and facilitate the establishment of integration and new identity. Chapters 13 and 14 address the use of ego-strengthening with another set of complex clinical situations, those that exist in posttraumatic and dissociative conditions.

Chapter 13

Ego-Strengthening With Posttraumatic and Dissociative Disorders I

Overview, Stabilization, and the Repair of Developmental Deficits

This chapter makes a brief tour into the land of dissociation and the contemporary treatment of dissociative disorders. The focus then shifts to selected issues in the use of ego-strengthening in the treatment of dissociative disorders. These disorders have become one of the most challenging contemporary problems encountered by both research scientists and psychotherapists. As history and cultural anthropology abundantly confirm (Ellenberger, 1970; Ross, 1989), they have always been present, and they can still be identified under their old names within primitive cultures.

In one form or another, pathological dissociation has always been a presence transculturally. It can manifest itself in many ways: in conversion disorders that manifest themselves with blindness, deafness, or paralyses, usually accompanied by *la belle indifference;* as somnambulism, and in posttraumatic symptoms; in fugue states and other amnesias; in a host of psychophysiologic disorders; and in various degrees of Dissociative Identity Disorder (DID; formerly known as Multiple Personality Disorder). Dissociative symptoms may be disguised (Frederick, 1990, 1993b; Phillips & Frederick, 1995) in the manifestations of problems not commonly thought of as dissociative (see chap. 11), such as depression (Frederick, 1993b), Obsessive Compulsive Disorder (Frederick, 1990, 1996c), eating disorders (Torem, 1987a), Posttraumatic Stress Disorder (PTSD; Phillips, 1993b), phobias (Malcolm, 1996), Panic Disorder (Frederick, 1993c), and a host of somatic difficulties (Phillips, 1993a) including excruciating pain (Gainer, 1992, 1997). The ability of dissociation to manifest itself in varieties of clinical symptoms appears to be limitless.

Ancient historical explanations for dissociative problems have included demon possession, loss of the soul, and wandering of the uterus inside the body. The healer-priest, shaman, and cleric were once considered the appropriate people to deal with such disturbances. However, by the turn of the last century, psychotherapy had come to replace the exorcisms, potions, and prayers used to treat them in earlier times (Ellenberger, 1970). Janet and many of his colleagues, as well as Freud and Jung, treated numerous patients with dissociative symptoms.

DOI:10.4324/9781003442585-13

Indeed, it was through the treatment of dissociation that psychoanalysis emerged (see chap. 1). In the face of the trends toward psychoanalysis and behaviorism, interest in dissociative difficulties waned and nearly vanished. Later, the conspicuous and demanding presence of posttraumatic symptoms in soldiers and other war victims made their reexamination necessary. The 1980s saw a vigorous revival of interest in dissociation, which has sparked numerous clinical and scientific studies as well as a great deal of debate as to the meaning and origins of dissociative disorders.

The causation of dissociative disorders appears to be quite complex (Lynn & Rhue, 1994). These disorders appear more frequently in individuals who have an innate (genetically determined) ability to dissociate (Braun, 1986; Frischholz, Lipman, Braun, & Sachs, 1992). A second factor thought by many to be crucial in their production is the presence of significant physical, sexual, or psychological trauma (Braun, 1986; Briere & Runtz, 1988; Chu & Dill, 1990; Kluft, 1985). A third assortment of factors, less frequently discussed, but equally important, involves the origins of such disorders within "the patient's construction of the event (internal efficient cause) and the socio-environmental context in which the event is embedded (external efficient cause)" (Tillman, Nash, & Lerner, 1994, p. 408). We believe that the concept of context is all too often overlooked in considerations of how dissociative disorders are formed. Khan (1963) has suggested that trauma need not be severe nor dramatic; it can have a strong impact when it occurs at certain developmental stages, and become cumulative. According to Khan (1963), *cumulative trauma* can seriously affect the intrapsychic structure of the individual.

The term *dissociation* is used by mental health professionals and behavioral scientists to mean a number of things (Cardeña, 1994). It has its origins in Janet's theory of desagregation. Janet was interested in what went on outside an individual's awareness. He used the term *subconscious* for the first time (Ellenberger, 1970; Janet, 1919/1976). This theory relied heavily on Janet's observations of patterns of feeling and cognitions in hypnotized patients. Janet concluded that when the mental apparatus became overwhelmed, certain mental processes and certain mental contents associated with the event did not become associated or integrated with the greater part of the mind.

In this century Hilgard's (1973) experimental work with hypnosis led him to create his theory of *neodissociation*. According to Hilgard, a number of "subordinate control systems" (p. 406) interact to produce cognitive functioning. Hilgard thought that there were two kinds of mental defense mechanisms that were available for dealing with unacceptable experiences and feelings. One was *repression*, which placed the undesirable material into the *unconscious*; the other was *dissociation*, which placed it into the *preconscious* where it was presumably more available.

Dissociation can be thought of as existing on a spectrum. Normal dissociation embraces the most normal of activities such as daydreaming, typing, or being absorbed in a good book. Also classified as normal are dissociations, at times severe, that occur in the presence of catastrophic events (Cardeña & Spiegel, 1993). When dissociation is at the pathological end of the spectrum, it can manifest itself in such clinical conditions as Posttraumatic Stress Disorder, amnesias, paralyses, blindness, deafness, fugue episodes, and Dissociative Identity Disorder (Multiple Personality Disorder (MPD). Some pathological dissociation is organically based (Phillips & Frederick, 1995; Ross, 1989).

Although dissociation is an adaptive response to what is perceived by the organism as overwhelming (Beahrs, 1982b; Kluft, 1984a, 1984b; Putnam, 1989; Spiegel, 1986), this adaptation carries a price with it. Dissociation has been shown to be damaging to ordinary functioning (Hilgard, 1973; Spiegel, 1986). As is seen later in this chapter, victims of the childhood trauma which is frequently connected with dissociation suffer from significant cognitive and emotional deficits.

The Treatment of Dissociative Disorders

The "cure" for the dissociative disorders, the way in which re-association takes place, has been held historically to come from the uncovering and abreaction of the dissociated material connected with the symptoms. Actually, the task is usually much more complex than that. The treatment of dissociation must be directed along several paths. Ego-strengthening is of the utmost importance with each of them. The first path is managing the patient's symptoms. No further work can be done until the patient is stable. The second path extends in the direction of dealing with the transference–countertransference manifestations of the attachment disorder (Holmes, 1996) that so frequently accompanies trauma and dissociation (Freyd, 1996; Marmer, 1980). Another path takes the therapist into the area of helping the patient repair the serious trauma-based neurobiological, cognitive, and emotional deficits that will probably be present. Yet another path leads to the uncovering and reassociating of the split-off or dissociated material with the rest of the mind. In each direction and at each step in the treatment process, ego-strengthening is a vital and essential element. Finally, integration of traumatic material and integration of ego states and of other structures must be facilitated.

In each area of the work with dissociative patients, memories reported in therapy with or without hypnosis can be problematic for both the patient and the therapist. Within today's climate there are political forces that appear to have a great stake in bringing therapeutic work designed to lift traumatic amnesia to a halt. Memory work can be complex and uncertain. Much of the uncertainty about memory has to do with its nature.

Memory

There are several kinds of memory. Memory can be short or long term. It can also embody a general fund of information and procedures a person possesses over the course of a lifetime. Such things as how to turn on the stove, how to drive a car, or what to do when one has both a stamp and an addressed envelope come from what is known as *procedural memory* (Tulving, 1985). Another kind of memory is the *semantic memory* (Tulving, 1972, 1985). This kind of memory represents a general sense of knowing about something without being aware, necessarily, of the source of that knowledge or the time of its acquisition. Much of the rules and regulations of a culture are held in semantic memory. For example, students in grammar school will probably know when the teacher is angry with the class even though the teacher may have not said a word. These two kinds of memory (procedural and semantic) do not even require the experience of recall or a sense of the past. They are often called implicit, or non-declarative, forms of memory. It is thought that these kinds of memory are developed early in life.

Episodic *memory* (which is also called *declarative* or *explicit memory*) is memory for the events that have occurred in one's life (Tulving, 1972). It is thought to develop later than semantic and procedural memory and is associated with the development of the hippocampus in the brain of the growing child. There may be little or no relationship between the individual's confidence about the accuracy of his memories and their reliability. Phenomena such as *confabulation*, in which one confidently invents a memory, and *cryptamnesia*, in which the individual with equal confidence recalls as his own what is actually someone else's material, are memory fabrications that can and do occur.

Memory has been the subject of many studies (Brown, Scheflin, & Hammond, 1997; Pettinati, 1988), and there seems to be some consensus for conceptualizing it as occurring in three stages. The first stage is the *stage of acquisition* in which memory becomes encoded into the mind. This encoding takes place in several ways. It may be either *superficial* or *deep*, and it may be either *holistic* or *detail-oriented* (Orne, Whitehouse, Dinges, & Orne, 1988). These factors always need to be kept in mind when one evaluates reports of memory experiments.

During the acquisition stage, what is actually acquired is subject to the influence of many external and internal factors. For example, the individual's expectation of what he will see may well influence what he does see. By the same token, one's state of health and mood, eyesight, and hearing, belief systems that include prejudices, as well as the physical conditions in which the event to be recalled occur are all relevant to what is taken in during the acquisition stage. Contingencies such as how far away the event or person is, how good the illumination is, and what else is happening at the time that could distort or distract are most significant. Further, there is evidence that deep processing of memory is more likely to yield memories that can be recalled and recognized at a later time than superficial processing (Craik & Lockhart, 1972).

Once memory has been acquired, it is held in a *retention phase*, where there are many ways in which it can be distorted. One possibility for memory distortion is that memories may fade or become less intense over a period of time. During the passage of time, the individual undergoes many experiences that can distort the memory. He may add, subtract, or distort the stored memory because of actual life experience he has had since the memory was acquired. Dreams and fantasies may become similarly linked with the memory. Thus, the memory may "be reworked, embellished, changed or transformed by the unconscious mind for a variety of reasons" (Phillips & Frederick, 1995, p. 8). There is some evidence that false information that is supplied after a *nontraumatic* event is recalled more easily than the event itself (Loftus, 1979; Loftus, Miller, & Burns, 1978).

Further opportunities for distortion exist during the *stage of memory retrieval*. Here the nature of the questioning and the relationship with the questioner can influence what is recalled. Leading questions are forms of information that may be false and are given after the fact. No matter how subtle the leading might be, it can have a strong influence on recall (Bowers & Hilgard, 1988; Loftus & Zanni, 1975).

The addition of hypnosis as an element in memory recall stirs the pot of confusion for many. This is because of evidence that suggests that hypnotic subjects relinquish their normal monitoring of reality and that they are more suggestible. More fantasy with which reality can become enmeshed exists in hypnosis, and confidence, even confidence that one's mistakes are correct, is also increased in hypnosis as may be critical judgment. The hypnotic subject is also fully capable of lying (Orne et al., 1988).

On the positive side, from the time of Janet and Freud hypnosis has been associated with *hypermnesia*, or heightened memory. Brown and Fromm (1986) have focused on the fact that, of all the altered states of conscious, hypnosis is the one most associated with cognitive activity. The use of hypnosis for memory retrieval is dramatically illustrated in Fromm's (1970) case of the man who was able to retrieve, hypnotically, the Japanese language he had not spoken since he was 3. Clinicians often encounter clear, albeit less dramatic, examples of the assistance hypnosis may give to memory retrieval.

Case Example: Phil

When Phil was a little boy, he had a dog. One day he was out with his dog, and he saw a car coming. Phil called his dog. But the very maneuver that had been intended to save the dog from the car backfired, and Phil's dog ran into the path of the car and was killed.

Phil had great difficulty recalling the events of his childhood as well as many details of significant events in his adult life. He also claimed to be out of touch with his feelings, incapable of feeling pain or grief, and unable to cry. One of Phil's goals for therapy was to be able to feel things and to be able to cry.

One day I (CF) was doing a hypnotic ego-strengthening exercise with Phil. I invited a shy and somewhat frightened child ego state to join Phil in the meadow that was his safe place. Suddenly, Phil exclaimed, "And the dog is there too! ... It's a collie!" Then Phil began to cry. I let him cry for some time. As his sobs subsided, I guided him back to the meadow and to the collie who was vibrantly alive in his imagination. When Phil came out of trance, he expressed doubt as to whether his dog had been a collie. I suggested that he check with family members who had been around at the time.

Phil began his next session by smiling and announcing, "It was a collie!" He had checked with his mother who recalled the dog quite well. During the hypnotic ego-strengthening in this session, it came to Phil that the dog's name had been Lassie. Again, he was encouraged to check it out.

Traumatic Memory

Although there is evidence that memory can be distorted and falsified, it is important to keep in mind that a great deal of memory research findings are not in agreement (Brown, Scheflin, & Hammond, 1997; Hammond, 1993). More importantly, there is much evidence that suggests that traumatic memory is encoded differently from nontraumatic memory (Brown, Scheflin, & Hammond, 1997; van der Kolk, 1996a, 1996b, 1997). There is now dramatic brain imaging evidence that traumatic flashbacks activate the amygdyla of the hypothalamus where memory for emotions and psychophysiological events is stored. The right hemisphere of the brain becomes activated as well, and left hemispheric activity is suppressed. This helps our understanding of why traumatic memory may not follow the same rules as nontraumatic memory as traumatic memory often features high affective and low cognitive components. Van der Kolk's (1997) brain imaging studies also demonstrate the positive changes that can occur with therapeutic reduction of trauma material. Daily perusal of the Internet will reveal that a great memory debate is still raging within the fields of psychotherapy and experimental psychology. There, van der Kolk's findings and his interpretation of them can become a focus of warm debate.

Memory Material or Memory Experiences

The clinician must assume a special position with regard to what is reported as memory. This holds true whether the material so labeled is retrieved hypnotically or nonhypnotically. The therapist must simultaneously be on the side of the patient, validate the patient's subjective experiences, and help the patient discover his own truth. At the same time, the therapist must safeguard the therapeutic process. In this position, he attempts to avoid the countertransference trap of taking a position that does not permit the patient to resolve his own uncertainties. This is a tall order, and it cannot be filled unless the therapist is willing and able to separate narrative truth from historical truth (Ganaway, 1989; Phillips & Frederick, 1995; Spence, 1982).

Phillips and Frederick (1995) have taken the position that what appears in therapy in or out of hypnosis should be called *memory material* or *memory experiences*. This material may have great validity for the patient, but it could be distorted or even completely false in the objective, historical realm. In the therapeutic situation the patient often appeals to the therapist to verify the memory material for him as objective fact. One overriding issue is that the therapist was not present at the time and cannot honestly validate the material for the patient.

The patient is encouraged to discover the meaning of the memory material for himself by exploring many other sources of information, such as independent corroboration, psychophysiological reactions, transference patterns, reenactments and repetitions, and family dynamics in order to make sense of what is going on within him (Frederick, 1994c; Phillips & Frederick, 1995). The therapist can and should assist the patient in these explorations.

Frederick (1994b) uses an informed consent for hypnosis in which she specifically addresses the issue of memory retrieval in hypnosis:

> She [Dr. Frederick] has also informed me that hypnosis is not a "truth serum." Some, many, or none of the memory material obtained under hypnosis may have a basis in objective reality. Such material could represent memories, distorted memories, fantasies symbolic of inner conflict, or combinations of memory and fantasy, or could have other bases. I acknowledge that decisions about whether memory material is "true" or not belong to me and not to Dr. Frederick.
>
> (p. 1)

When working with dissociative patients, it is vital that informed consent be obtained whenever hypnosis is used and that these issues be openly discussed in an ongoing fashion that extends and elaborates the informed consent over the course of treatment (Kluft, 1994).

The Sari Model

A number of models exist for treating dissociative patients (Braun, 1986; Kluft & Fine, 1993; Phillips & Frederick, 1995; Putnam, 1989; Ross, 1989). We use Phillips and Frederick's (1995) SARI model. It is a four-stage treatment model that was created for work with posttraumatic and dissociative patients (see chap. 1).

Stage 1: Safety and Stability

In this stage of treatment the symptomatic patient is stabilized and develops a sense of personal safety. It is essential that this take place before any uncovering work in Stage 2 occurs. Stabilization and safety can depend on both internal and external resources. Among the external resources that may be needed are such things as medication, hospitalization, 12-step work, and family therapy. Ego-strengthening is an integral part of this stage, and projective/evocative ego-strengthening that activates internal resources can be especially powerful here.

Stage 2: Accessing Trauma Material

In this stage of treatment, trauma material that has been separated from the rest of mental content is accessed. This can be done with formal hypnosis as well as with nonhypnotic therapy. In this stage, the therapist helps the patient access traumatic memory material. Usually only a small amount of memory material is accessed at a time. Although there are very sound and highly effective therapists who advocate full abreaction (Watkins & Watkins, 1997), it is our experience that most therapists are not able to carry out this kind of procedure without re-traumatizing their patients. Phillips and Frederick (1995) recommend safe remembering (Dolan, 1991) as well as accessing trauma material in a way that allows the patient to feel empowered. Uncovering sessions should be alternated with sessions in which ego-strengthening takes place. Material that is accessed in this way often needs to be dealt with, eventually, in Stage 3. Should the accessing destabilize the patient, a return to Stage 1 is in order.

Stage 3: Resolving Traumatic Experiences

Simply accessing trauma material is not enough. There needs to be some kind of re-processing of the traumatic material—a transmutation. This is the stage of working through. Here trauma can be renegotiated and processed, and the many components of trauma material (sensory, visual, behavioral, motoric, affective, and cognitive) can become connected with the mainstream of thought.

Certain corrective experiences can occur here as well. These would include desensitization and the re-working of trauma with the new ingredient of mastery. Should the patient destabilize at any time here, more Stage 1 work is done before moving on. When this stage is going well, the patient may return to Stage 2 to access more trauma material should this be necessary. Often Stage 2 and Stage 3 work are done together at the same time.

Stage 4: Integration and New Identity

In this stage integration of previously dissociated and reworked trauma material transpires. Ego states also integrate with one another, and other changing personality structures must integrate as well. At times this stage can be turbulent but can be an important locus for ego-strengthening—Stage 1 work.

The SARI model is a dynamic model. If at any time the patient destabilizes or feels unsafe, there is always a return to Stage 1 work. Should more uncovering need to precede integration (Stage 4), a return to Stage 2 work is indicated.

Ego-Strengthening for Dissociative Disorders

Ego-strengthening is vital in working with dissociative disorders. Dissociative and posttraumatic patients are like many other kinds of patients in that the therapist needs to begin to ego-strengthen the patient from the beginning of therapy. The SARI model requires that the Stage 1 issues of safety and stability must be attended before other work can be accomplished. Many dissociative patients are quite symptomatic when they enter treatment. Quite a few may be having flashbacks, a form of reliving or remembering traumatic events.

Stage 1: Ego-Strengthening Techniques for Stabilization

It is not uncommon for beginners to want to get into the real stuff (i.e., the trauma) by uncovering it. The truth is that many patients who present themselves to us are already having several kinds of flashbacks and their functioning is severely compromised by them. Horowitz (1979) has viewed flashbacks as a continuation of the information processing of traumatic material by individuals who have been overloaded with such material. The obvious illustrative patient is the Vietnam veteran who flings himself into the gutter at the sound of a car backfiring.

Other patients have less obvious kinds of flashbacks. Some of these are somatosensory, whereas others are affective. Such patients do not complain of intrusive memories. Rather, they are having intrusive experiences that may make no sense to them whatsoever. Often their anxiety levels become extremely high, for they do not know what is happening to them and they may often fear the disintegration of their personalities. These patients may confide that they believe they may be going crazy. Sensation and affect have become dissociated from cognition, imagery, and meaning in these patients. Thus, the nature of the complete underlying traumatic memory experience is not available to help these patients understand what is happening to them. When somatic components of flashbacks predominate, they may be misinterpreted and diagnosed as psychosomatic conditions (Herman, 1992).

It is the therapist's job to *teach the patient how to control and contain* flashbacks and other kinds of trauma material that may erupt in therapy. It takes considerable time and laborious work for this to occur. However, the therapist who fails to make this a central focus of his work with the posttraumatic patient has missed the boat. All of the techniques that patients learn to use for managing and eliminating traumatic symptoms are ego-strengthening and they can also be used during Stages 2, 3, and 4. Whenever the patient accesses traumatic material, there is always the possibility that it may become overwhelming. Should this occur, the therapy must be taken back to Stage 1, where further strengthening occurs.

Nonhypnotic techniques may assume prominence with patients who are having difficulties with identifiable flashbacks. What is being experienced with a flashback is a negative, or traumatic, trance (Gilligan, 1987), and it is the job of the therapist to teach the patient to dehypnotize himself and bring himself into the waking reality of the current calendar date and Greenwich time. Dolan (1991) has suggested that the patient be trained either to focus away from the intrusive memory material of the flashback into the material world about him or utilize the trance state for positive benefits. This can be accomplished in a number of ways. We find that the following ego-strengthening techniques may be essential to Stage 1 work with posttraumatic and dissociative patients. They can be used at any time that issues of safety and stabilization arise in therapy. Not every technique will have to be used with every patient.

Dehypnotize.   If the overwhelming symptoms such as flashbacks occur in a session, the therapist may decide that the best course of action is to firmly guide the patient away from them, to dehypnotize him. Like Dolan (1991), we strongly urge the patient to look about the office and name five things he can see. We also ask him to identify five sounds in the environment as well as five things that he feels. Then we ask him to name four things in each category, then three, then two, and then one. If there is still intrusion of traumatic material, we request that the patient repeat these maneuvers until there is improvement. In more severe cases, we also instruct the patient to do exercises such as jumping jacks or deep knee bends. There are many variations on this kind of technique.

Patients must be trained to transfer what they have learned in therapy to their life away from sessions and to take up other activities that will help dehypnotize them out of their traumatic trance experiences. As Dolan (1991) has suggested, such activities as deep breaths, performance of household chores, or a 5-minute walk may be sufficient to break intrusive experiences. It is crucial that the therapist not fall into the transference trap of taking care of all the patient's flashbacks or other intrusive symptoms. This only creates a dangerous dependency. The mastery that the patient experiences from learning to shut flashbacks off is beneficial and strongly ego-strengthening.

Case Example: Isabel

Isabel was in the process of beginning to uncover traumatic material in trance. Suddenly, she began to hyperventilate, and she exclaimed that she could see nothing but darkness around her. She said she was frightened of falling into a black hole. The therapist (SM) instructed her to "move your attention to the sensations you notice of your body in the chair and if you open your eyes you can see the familiar objects in the room ... and you may want to focus on the bookcase. There are some books inside the book case, and it will be interesting for us to see which one you select to focus upon ... now."

Utilize the Patient's Resources. However, some patients do not need to be dehypnotized because they are able to *utilize* their trance states and go to their inner worlds and safe places for calming and soothing. Thus, the spontaneous or the formal trance state in which the symptoms appear can be utilized by turning it into a positive trance experience. Patients can be trained to use symptoms as triggers for getting in touch with internal resources. This projective/evocative utilization can lead the patient to focus hypnotically on such things as positive age regressions; abilities and talents such as musical performance, athletic ability, or cooking skills; or interpersonal assets such as valuable friendships or close family relationships. Positive memories, relationships, achievements, and other positive resources can become symbolized in external objects that become emblems, souvenirs, or talismans of safety such as photographs, jewelry, or clothing.

Symptoms can be utilized as well. Phillips (1993c) uses the utilization technique very successfully with posttraumatic patients. In one of her reported cases, Phillips described a patient who was plagued by the recurrent frightening internal image of a horrible face. Phillips encouraged the patient to learn to make the face her best friend. Eventually the patient discovered that the appearance of the frightening face was a signal that she was emotionally overloaded and needed to use self-care maneuvers to relieve stress. It was only after the patient was comfortable with the face and stabilized that she and her therapist were able to uncover traumatic events that were symbolized by the face.

Utilize the Therapist's Resources. Flashbacks are traumatizing to the patient, as are many other posttraumatic and dissociative symptoms. During Stage 2 and Stage 3 work, there may be an exacerbation of symptoms as the "trauma material is being accessed and resolved. Frequently the therapist finds himself acting as a container for the patient's affect, experiencing projective identification, and displaying the signs and symptoms of vicarious traumatization" (Dolan, 1991; Pearlman & Saakvitne, 1995; Phillips & Frederick, 1995). Therapists are often called upon to enter fusional and transitional alliances and maintain strong boundaries (Frederick, 1997). A significant countertransference price the therapist may pay for this may be exhaustion (Geller, 1987; Kluft, 1984a; Pearlman & Saakvitne, 1995). It becomes important to the therapy that the therapist (a) use his own resources wisely, (b) avoid interminable transference–countertransference traps, and (c) constantly strive to move the patient into increasing autonomy. With extremely dependent patients it is necessary that the therapist place great emphasis on self-care and teach the patient self-care techniques. The challenge is to use the therapeutic alliance to facilitate this.

Utilize External Resources. Many external resources can be helpful. These include hospitalization and partial hospitalization, support, family, and 12-step groups (Phillips & Frederick, 1995; Spiegel, 1991). The value of such resources should not be ignored. They can be most helpful, and at times they are necessary to maintain a climate in which therapy can occur. Some of the external resources employed, like many interventions, may seem like "crutches" to the patient. They end up being ego-strengthening because they support the patient in a way that permits growth and healing. Other external resources include close relationships, friendships, social groups, spiritual groups, and associations that foster hobbies, and artistic, musical and other creative activities.

Train the Patient to Use and Master Imagery.   Patients who are learning to manage flashbacks are usually helped by trance work in which they learn how to control and master imagery. For example, the therapist will teach the patient how to mentally construct a lamp or a plant in the therapist's office bit by bit and then mentally cause it to disappear bit by bit. With certain patients this mastery over imagery can be applied to intrusive traumatic memory material.

Imagery training is also of great assistance to patients who can use imagery to construct and elaborate upon intrapsychic transitional space (Morton & Frederick, 1996, 1997a) and produce other kinds of transitional experiences (see chap. 7).

Identify Current Stressors.   The therapist can also assist the patient with the management of intrusive traumatic memory material by helping him understand what kinds of life events make the patient more vulnerable to such material. Fatigue, illness, and stress may bring on more troublesome symptoms (Phillips & Frederick, 1995) and patients need to be encouraged to take care of themselves. This and other self-caring activities ego-strengthen the patient further.

Interpret the Meaning of the Symptom.   Symptoms have meaning. They are about something that is momentous to the patient. The Stage 1 work that is necessary is only a step in the direction of accessing, resolving, and integrating the traumatic material that powers them. Symbolic communications of ego states may be confused with flashbacks at times (Frederick, 1994e; Frederick & Phillips, 1996; Phillips & Frederick, 1995). Such communications can usually be differentiated from flashbacks because they are not traumatizing.

Use Power Techniques to Remove Symptoms When Appropriate.   Techniques that reduce the psychological and physiological impact of traumatic memory material and remove or reduce symptoms can be most helpful. They are often referred to as the *power* techniques because they are often able to reduce or eliminate symptoms dramatically within a short period of time. Among these are Visual Kinesthetic Dissociation (VKD; Bandler & Grinder, 1979), Eye Movement Desensitization and Reprocessing (EMDR; Shapiro, 1995), Thought Field Therapy (Callahan, 1985), and Trauma Incident Reduction (French, 1993; Gerbode, 1989; R. Moore, 1993). EMDR has been studied empirically more than any of the other techniques, however. Some patients may need a certain amount of stabilization before they are able to utilize any of these techniques.

EMDR and Ego-Strengthening

Although Eye Movement Desensitization and Reprocessing (EMDR) is frequently grouped with the power therapies, its effects are distinctly different and extend beyond symptom removal; it often achieves comprehensive changes within personality.

EMDR is a treatment intervention that was developed by Francine Shapiro in 1989, stemming from her personal experiences during a walk in the park in May 1987. During that walk, Shapiro noticed that when disturbing thoughts spontaneously appeared within her mind, her eyes spontaneously began to move rapidly back and forth in an upward diagonal direction. When she then deliberately brought the thoughts back into consciousness, the negative affect seemed to be greatly reduced. She then began to experiment, using similar eye movements with other people; she noticed what happened when she moved her fingers rapidly back and forth and asked her subjects to follow the movement with their eyes. Because her orientation was behavioral and the initial focus of this work was on reducing anxiety, she called the procedure Eye Movement Desensitization (EMD; Shapiro, 1995).

Shapiro published a controlled study (Shapiro, 1989) in which she reported on the use of EMD with 22 trauma victims. Subjects in the treatment groups were asked to describe the disturbing images of their persistent traumatic memories along with their negative thoughts and beliefs, which she called the *negative cognition*. Then they were asked to rate their anxiety level on an 11-point Subjective Units of Disturbance Scale (SUDS), with 0 indicating the *least anxiety*, and 10, the *highest level*. She also asked subjects to verbalize a positive cognition that they would like to have about themselves (i.e., I did the best I could) and to rate how true they felt about the belief with a 7-point semantic differential scale, the Validity of Cognition Scale (VOC). A rating of 1 indicated *completely false* while a rating of 7 indicated *completely true*. EMD was performed with the treatment group. The control group received the same amount of interruptions and questions; however, they received no EMD and were only asked to describe their traumatic memory. The results showed decreased anxiety levels and increased perceptions of the truth of their positive cognitions. The EMD was administered to the control group, and the delayed treatment conditions also showed positive results. These results held up at 1-month and 3-month follow-ups, and were interpreted as demonstrating that substantial desensitization and cognitive restructuring had taken place.

Shapiro began to train licensed health care professionals in 1990, and the name of the procedure was changed to EMDR to emphasize the importance of the adaptive processing of disturbing memories. It became not only a technique to be used with Posttraumatic Stress Disorder (PTSD) patients, but also a methodology with far wider applications. The extension of the range of use of Eye Movement Desensitization and Reprocessing (EMDR) was an outgrowth of the feedback of trained clinicians who integrated EMDR into psychotherapy.

Shapiro (1995) has explained the theoretical basis of EMDR as follows:

there is a system inherent in all of us that is physiologically geared to process information to a state of mental health. This adaptive resolution means that negative emotions are relieved and that learning takes place, is appropriately integrated, and is available for future use. The system may become unbalanced due to a trauma or through stress engendered during a developmental period, but once it is appropriately activated and maintained in a dynamic state by means of EMDR, it transmutes information to a state of therapeutically appropriate resolution. Desensitization and cognitive restructuring are viewed as byproducts of the adaptive reprocessing taking place on a neurophysiological level.

(p. 13)

Shapiro's (1995) model now emphasizes accelerated information processing to explain how results are obtained so rapidly and consistently. As opposed to the earlier desensitization model, the information-processing model emphasizes the importance of early life experiences. These experiences produce a pattern of affect, behavior, and cognitions that are held in the nervous system in state-dependent form. Stimuli in present time elicit the negative affect and beliefs embodied in the memories, causing the patient to react in ways characteristic of the earlier event. EMDR seems to allow present affect and cognitions to become associated with the memories throughout the neurophysiological network. This leads, spontaneously, to new beliefs and behavior that are more appropriate to the present. Shapiro (1995) theorizes that pathology can be changed when the clinician targets the material that has been stored dysfunctionally in the nervous system, and intervenes with effective use of the (EMDR) method. Now the model is applied to many situations and disorders such as phobias, panic disorders, grief reactions, symptoms that follow assault or natural disaster, and accidents; it is also used with burn victims, patients with chemical dependency, as well as patients with dissociative disorders, Posttraumatic Stress Disorder, and even personality disorders.

It is interesting that what began as a behavioral model now includes theoretical principles that are cognitive and psychodynamic as well. It also includes ideas about the physiological aspects of memory such as those developed by van der Kolk (1996a) and Rossi (1993). There appears to be a link between EMDR and the rapid eye movement (REM) stage of sleep. Many sleep and dream researchers have interpreted their results as indicating that processing of emotional material may well occur during the REM stages of sleep, when subjects report that they were dreaming. The eye movements that occur during REM periods may be analogous to those that occur spontaneously when awake, such as the phenomena that led to Shapiro's initial discovery. However, it has also been shown that rhythmic tapping, lights, auditory stimuli, or other left-right stimulation can be utilized as part of the EMDR method. Thus, the eye movements themselves are not essential to stimulate the information processing that occurs.

Treatment With EMDR

EMDR treatment involves eight phases, and the number of sessions within each phase differs with the patient:

Phase 1:	History taking and treatment planning.
Phase 2:	Patient preparation including explaining EMDR procedures, theories, expectations about treatment effects and possible between-session experiences; establishing the therapeutic alliance and initiating relaxation and safety procedures.
Phase 3:	Determining the target, establishing positive and negative cognitions, and performing baseline assessment using the SUDS and VOC scales.
Phase 4:	Desensitization until the SUDS level is reduced to 1 or 0.
Phase 5:	Installation and cognitive restructuring, continuing until the rating of the positive cognition reaches 6 or 7 on the VOC scale, and then linking the positive cognition with the target memory.
Phase 6:	Body scan for evaluating residual body tension by holding the target memory and positive cognition in mind and mentally scanning the body.
Phase 7:	Debriefing and closure. The patient is told to keep a log of any disturbing thoughts, situations, dreams, or memories that might arise.
Phase 8:	Reevaluation to review whether treatment effects have been maintained.

Shapiro (1995) recognizes that EMDR is not for everyone. She cautions clinicians to evaluate carefully during Phase 1 whether the client is capable of withstanding high levels of emotional distress, and whether the patient is able and willing to use hypnosis, visualization, and relaxation techniques to restore emotional balance between sessions. Assessment of personal and environmental stability is especially important. Shapiro cautions clinicians not to use EMDR with DID patients unless they have been specially trained in the treatment of dissociative disorders.

EMDR-Assisted Ego-Strengthening

During Phases 2 and 3 ego-strengthening techniques can be introduced into standard EMDR treatment. Shapiro (1995) refers to what she calls *self-control techniques* which are used with the patient during Stage 1. Only if the patient responds favorably to these relaxation and visualization techniques should he be considered for EMDR. Shapiro emphasizes the importance of the safe place technique for patients who cannot relax because they have a need to remain vigilant. The eight-step EMDR procedure is modified and utilized to install an image of the calm safe place to which the patient can retreat. This is similar to the use of the safe place for calming, soothing, and affect regulation in hypnotic ego-strengthening as described in chapter 7.

Phillips (1997) has taught clinicians ego-strengthening techniques that can be utilized with EMDR to enhance patient safety and stability especially when treating patients with severe trauma and/or dissociative disorders. Phillips has used EMDR to install a positive image that the patient can evoke to promote consistency, stability, and object constancy. She suggests that the image to be selected should be a conflict-free image (an activity in the patient's present life in which all of him can participate, and that is associated with a feeling of unity and wholeness). This differs from the safe place, because it is an activity rather than a place and is something that is part of the patient's ongoing life rather than an imaginary place.

Both authors of this book have been trained in EMDR, and we feel comfortable using it in a variety of clinical situations. Like Phillips (1997), we use it to install and anchor positive memory material and the presence of conflict-free aspects of personality such as Inner Strength (McNeal & Frederick, 1993). We also use EMDR for other anchoring possibilities. Some of these may involve the conflict-laden sphere (see chap. 4). For example, we employ EMDR for the *anchoring of hope* with patients who may feel hopeless on the conscious level, but who produce positive unstructured age progressions. EMDR can anchor this ego-strengthening material in such a way that it is more available to the patient on a conscious level. Similarly, we use it to *anchor mastery*, especially with patients who have difficulty staying in touch with competent aspects of self, as well as to install and anchor internal commitments to practice certain self-care activities such as self-hypnosis (McNeal & Frederick, 1998).

We also utilize EMDR for dreamwork. Patients are asked to focus on dream images, as well as accompanying thoughts, affects, and bodily sensations (if present). During the eye movement sequences patients often become aware of associations that lead them to understand the underlying meaning of the dream. Like Phillips and Frederick (1995) we believe that EMDR can be a useful adjunct in treatment. It can be of special value when utilized with patients who, because of past trauma, want to remain fully conscious in an upright position while processing traumatic memories. However, as Shapiro (1995) has wisely observed, it is not for everyone, and many of the same considerations about patient selection for hypnosis are also relevant when deciding with whom to use EMDR.

Current research projects are attempting to determine the active ingredients of the power techniques (Figley & Carbonell, 1995). They are all generally considered helpful in the treatment of trauma. The main problem that can exist with some of the power techniques is that they are being used by certain technocrat practitioners as substitutes for therapy. For example, Thought Field Therapy has been presented as a way to successfully treat phobias and anxiety by telephone and radio (Callahan, 1987). There is no question that there are individuals with isolated symptom complexes who might need no more than that. However, many dissociative symptoms appear in disguise (see chaps. 11 and 12) and at times those seeking help for such symptoms may have much more extensive pathology and suffer from developmental problems as well.

It is often quite ego-strengthening to remove symptoms (as discussed later), and we do not believe that suffering is necessarily helpful to anyone. We recommend that the power therapies be used within well-planned therapy that is designed for the unique individual to whom it is addressed. We also recommend that these techniques be used by clinicians who have been properly trained to use them and always, like hypnosis, as an adjunct to therapy and not a substitute for it. Otani (personal communication, 1997) has reminded us of the old Zen proverb that says: "The right tool used for the wrong reason is the wrong tool." Some managed care organizations may not wish to hear that the posttraumatic or dissociative patient who has been ego-strengthened by and has benefited from symptom reduction from any of the power techniques has, in most cases, more Stage 2, Stage 3, and Stage 4 work to do in therapy.

Use Other Methods for Removing Symptoms. Symptom removal can be a significant milepost for certain patients. Posttraumatic and dissociative patients display a panoply of symptoms. These range from flashbacks to paralyses, from pseudoseizures to blindness and deafness. Although symptom removal has been viewed with great suspicion by many psychodynamic psychotherapists, there is much to suggest that it can be become ego-strengthening for many patients. Watkins (1987) has reviewed the pros and cons of symptom removal, which was considered impractical by Freud (1932/1964). He believed that symptoms could only be removed temporarily unless the underlying cause for the symptom had been resolved. There have been other psychoanalytic objections to symptom removal. One is that the symptom will be replaced by another in the absence of psychodynamic resolution. Another is that when hypnotic suggestions are used, hypnosis bypasses the ego. Consequently, the hypnotic suggestions that are made for symptom removal are not adequately egotized and integrated (Watkins, 1987).

Watkins (1987) believes that there are equally compelling psychodynamic reasons why symptom removal is desirable: (a) the underlying reason for the symptom may no longer be present, (a) the symptom may be maintained only for secondary gain, (c) the removal of a psychogenic symptom that is still based on a dynamic motivation could become permanent because the symptom removal may bring about changes in the individual's life that initiate a new motivational system that keeps the symptoms suppressed. The patient can and often does introject the therapist in the therapeutic process of symptom removal. This internalized "good therapist" may continue to suggest that a symptom not be present long after therapy has ended.

Frederick (1994f) has observed that, "Another useful way of looking at symptom removal is that it can be ego-strengthening in many patients for a variety of reasons" (p. 1). New motivational systems and introjected good therapists are certainly ego-strengthening as are the increased freedom provided by the loss of a symptom, a borrowed sense of mastery, and a less distracted, more open mind about the possibility of change.

All symptom removal should occur only after the patient has been thoroughly evaluated. Some questions that need to be asked by the therapist are:

- How would the patient function without the symptom? Are there other visible indications that the patient may require more uncovering psychotherapy instead?
- What are the patient's resources for uncovering therapy?
- What are his/her financial and ego resources?
- What are the patient's goals for therapy? Expectations about hypnotherapy?
- Can the patient be educated about a two-tiered approach that would involve trusting his unconscious mind to decide whether symptom removal might work in his case?
- What can be learned ideomotorically about the status of the symptom and the willingness of the unconscious mind to help the patient relinquish it?
- Could symptom removal be undesirable in a given patient, an offer of a magical cure that could work for a patient who really needs to pay attention to more significant symptoms for which he may be in denial?
- Is this the right time for symptom removal in the patient?

Watkins (1987) recommends several ways to remove symptoms suggestively. They can be employed with or without hypnosis:

- Indirect or nonspecific suggestions,
- Ego-strengthening,
- Linking suggestions together,
- Cumulative suggestions,
- Aligning suggestions with the patient's motives,
- Posthypnotic suggestion, and
- Symptom amelioration, substitution, or displacement.

"Symptom removal can often assist insight oriented therapy by changing the balance of energies, mobilizing resistances, and strengthening the ego" (Frederick, 1994f, p. 2).

The Management and Repair of Cognitive, Emotional, and Neurological Deficiencies

Trauma and dissociation have serious effects on the development of the individual. Ego deficits can be found within the realm of the neurobiological and the cognitive as well as that of the emotional. Certain defenses become exaggerated and overused, whereas others fail to develop or simply atrophy from lack of continued ongoing development. There is now evidence that trauma has an effect on the way the brain develops in children (Perry 1996, 1997).

The Nature of the Deficiencies

Severely physically abused children "often do suffer from deficits in intellectual and language development" (Zelikovsky & Lynn, 1995). They possess less ability to concentrate, have more learning problems, and measure with lower IQs than children who have not been abused (Toro, 1982). They also had delays in language development and degraded school achievement (Elmer, 1977; Elmer & Gregg, 1967). Traumatized children also develop attachment difficulties (Aber & Allen, 1987) and suffer from poor self-esteem (Oates, Forrest, & Peacock, 1985). Zelikovsky and Lynn (1995) have surveyed literature that indicates that they tend to be more depressed and display a panoply of affective symptoms, not infrequently have symptoms of Posttraumatic Stress Disorder, and "have a wide range of behavioral and interpersonal problems" (p. 200) as well as delinquency, substance abuse, criminality, and adult psychopathology. They also have higher levels of dissociative symptoms in adulthood (Chu & Dill, 1990).

Fine's (1990) investigation of the cognitive sequelae of incest reveals more of the nature of the cognitive problems. Core beliefs become shattered by the trauma, and the victim's world becomes reconstructed on a base of distorted beliefs and unreasoned and misguided assumptions. She has listed 10 common cognitive distortions that are commonly found in victims of childhood abuse. They include dichotomous thinking (which may reveal poor object constancy), selective abstraction, arbitrary inference, overgeneralization, catastrophizing, time distortion, distortions of self-perceptions, excessive responsibility, and misassuming causality (Fine, 1990). McCann and Pearlman (1990) have also discussed disrupted cognitive development with reference to frame of references for causality, hope for a better future, and locus of control as well those for "safety, trust-dependency, independence, power, esteem, and intimacy" (Phillips & Frederick, 1995, p. 133). Fish-Murray, Koby, and van der Kolk (1987) are also among those who have reported that there are measurable deficits present.

Use-Dependent Development of the Central Nervous System

There is a recurrent tendency in Western culture to see the violent and disturbed as different and perhaps genetically flawed (Ellenberger, 1970; Stone, 1997).

Explanations for this have invoked such determining factors as Satanic influence, phrenology, and genetics. There are those who still search for genetic markers or neurobiological traits to be found. Perry (1996, 1997) reminds us that millions of children in the United States are victims of and/or witnesses of many kinds of traumatic violence. This includes domestic violence, physical abuse, and violence in the community. Further, almost all of them, even the most disadvantaged, have inescapable and intimate relationships with television sets. As they watch TV, they are immersed with a great number of images of violence, usually in situations where violence has been overvalued as a solution to many kinds of conflicts.

Perry (1996, 1997) has presented a point of view that is interactional. It is the experience of children, usually with their primary caregivers, rather than genetic influences, that molds the core neurobiological organization of the brain. All traumatic behavior has an impact on children. It is interesting that the brain, like other organs, somehow creates its own adaptation to violence. It is able to do this because it is hierarchically structured (from lower to higher centers) and develops in sequence throughout life. Most of the critical structural organization of the brain takes place in childhood.

As the brain develops, higher functions assume more and more control over lower ones. When optimal developmental experiences from the environment are not available, cortical, subcortical, and limbic areas will not develop properly. Among environmental experiences that violence and other traumata can bring to children are a deprivation of normal and ordinary sensory experiences and a disruption or abnormal distribution of the necessary pattern of developmental cues. This leaves the lower and more primitive parts of the brain more on their own. Conspicuous symptoms of *emotional retardation*, such as a lack of empathy and refractory attachment difficulties, may appear. Activities such as literacy help develop higher levels of the brain, but our society is reading less now and watching more TV. There is accumulating evidence that *Sesame Street* and MTV may not be sufficiently stimulating for the adequate development of the cortex.

Trauma will cause stress responses to develop. If the stress continues, stress-response systems will work too much and behave too sensitively. This is exactly what has been observed in children with neurobiological trauma (Perry, 1996, 1997). These children are behaviorally impulsive and demonstrate cognitive distortions. They have chronic physiologic hyperarousal, increased muscle tone, heightened startle response, sleep disturbances that can be quite severe, generalized anxiety, and great difficulty regulating affect. They may also display chronic tachycardia and a chronic, slightly elevated body temperature. They frequently carry the labels of hyperactive or learning disabled (Perry, 1996, 1997).

Among children who are displaying these kinds of reaction patterns, there are differences based on sex. The females will often dissociate in the face of trauma, whereas the males tend to act out more, often violently. There is an impressive preponderance of clinical diagnoses, often of hyperactivity, in males during childhood. It is in the adult phase of life that women who have been traumatized develop depression, anxiety disorders, and dissociative disorders, and occupy the lioness' share of the patient population (Perry, 1996, 1997).

Revictimization and the Sitting Duck

Herman (1992) and Terr (1991) have reported their findings that trauma has serious effects on emotional development as well as upon the development of intrapsychic structure. Schetky (1992) has reviewed the literature concerning the tendency of trauma victims toward revictimization in later life. There are also other reenacts and repetitions of trauma. Kluft (1990a, 1990b) has noted that victims of incest are vulnerable to exploitation by therapists. He has termed such vulnerable individuals, *sitting ducks*. According to Kluft (1990b), the *sitting duck syndrome* occurs because of a conjunction of several factors: "1) severe symptoms and traits, 2) dysfunctional individual dynamics, 3) pathological object relations and family dynamics, and 4) deformation of the observing ego/ debased cognition" (p. 278).

The chain of revictimization can only be broken with the mitigation and repair of the neurobiological, cognitive, and emotional deficits. Their egos are characteristically in great need of strengthening. The primary ego-strengthening task for the therapist is to establish trust in the therapeutic alliance. Such a task can be accomplished only if the therapist is in touch with his own countertransference feelings because his work with posttraumatic patients may draw him into a *traumatic transference–countertransference matrix* (Chefetz, 1996). In this matrix the therapist and patient will experience the full range of expectations of abuser, victim, and protector in well-directed treatment. Each person involved must allow himself to be aware of the affect but not to act on it.

At times the task that the repair of neurobiological deficits occupies in therapy may seem overwhelming. The developmental work whose purpose is to facilitate their cognitive and emotional growth and development frequently needs to take place over a long period of time because altering the patient's internal environment that is characterized by use-dependent failure of the brain to develop normally takes time. The importance of the kind of developmental work provided by internal self-soothing and transitional experiences, establishing object permanence and constancy, and boundary development, strengthening, and management has been discussed in chapters 7, 8, and 9. The consistent use of these principles and techniques in such a way as to integrate them with the totality of therapy can help the patient move forward developmentally. It cannot be forgotten, however, that such work takes time.

We endorse using the full complement of projective/evocative ego-strengthening techniques with dissociative patients: positive age regressions including regressions to significant nurturing figures, age progressions, creative renurturing, boundary formation, and internal self-soothing as well as utilization techniques. We find that helping the patient access archetypal selfobjects such as

Inner Strength, Inner Love, and Inner Wisdom are of significant value in advancing development.

The value of uncovering and resolving trauma should not, however, under any circumstances, be underestimated. A tremendous amount of defensive energy is tied up in dissociated traumatic material. Further, the patient's ego is always strengthened immeasurably by mastery over trauma when it is eventually achieved.

Alienation From Inner Resources

It may be quite difficult for the clinician to evaluate the nature and availability of the dissociative patient's internal resources. Dissociation alienates patients from what is already there. Every time a resource is activated in therapy, another move in the direction of integration is made. For this reason, the projective/evocative ego-strengthening techniques may have greater potential in the treatment of these patients than techniques that are simply suggestive. The utilization of dissociation and posttraumatic symptoms (Phillips, 1993c; Phillips & Frederick, 1995) is another excellent way to strengthen the ego.

The Creation of Resources: Ego-Strengthening With the Severely Impoverished Patient

There are patients, however, who are severely impoverished (Phillips & Frederick, 1995). Their development has been so drastically compromised that the usual kinds of available resources are not present. With such patients, the therapeutic relationship may assume heightened significance. The patient can develop internal resources by internalizing the resources of the therapist in the identification process. Additionally, the severely impoverished patient can be helped by direct suggestive ego-strengthening. Transitional experiences in the therapeutic hour and mastery experiences based on everyday life are also recommended. This can be a time for the judicious use of metaphor, seeding, and embedding (see chap. 3). We have been pleased with the usefulness of creative renurturing (Murray-Jobsis, 1990a) exercises as well. The exercises of Baker (1981) for the development of object permanence and object constancy are also invaluable with severely impoverished patients (see chap. 9).

Chapter 14

Ego-Strengthening With Posttraumatic and Dissociative Disorders II

Uncovering and Integration

The therapist with a more or less *surgical* bend of mind likes to uncover and discover more than anything in the world. He only feels as if he is doing something when he is prying memory material out of the patient, often session by session. In most therapy this is definitely the way to keep dissociative patients symptomatic; in many cases, it worsens the clinical situation. The reason for this is that reliving traumatic experiences can be retraumatizing. Indeed, some patients can easily be turned into trauma junkies by well-intentioned therapists (Phillips & Frederick, 1995; van der Kolk, 1989). The trend in working with dissociative patients today is away from the affect-laden abreactions that were once in vogue (van der Hart & Brown, 1992). It must be said, however, that there are a few patients who respond only to complete abreaction and that there are some therapists (Watkins & Watkins, 1997) who are so inherently ego-strengthening in themselves that they are able to safely guide their patients through complete abreactions. We believe that most therapists should proceed cautiously in uncovering work, and we recommend that it be done in stages, a piece at a time.

Ego-strengthening is the secret to safely accessing trauma without retraumatizing the patient. Before any accessing can be done, the patient must be stable and feel safe. This means that the patient is involved in a good working alliance with the therapist and has learned to control symptoms such as flashbacks (with the help of medication, if indicated). She must also have been thoroughly evaluated and her hypnotic abilities and talents explored through a number of safe, ego-strengthening trance experiences. In trance she must have a safe place that is experienced as safe, peaceful, and nurturing. When the patient appears to be extremely fearful and has come to therapy with clear recollections of trauma, we also recommend the immediate additional reassuring presence of barrier imagery around the safe place.

We also believe that in most instances it is essential that the dissociative patient have a series of experiences with ego-strengthening, including varieties of projective/evocative ego-strengthening in formal trance, before any abreactive work be done. This not only strengthens the patient, but also gives her points of reference and internal boundaries for safety. Before the first uncovering

DOI:10.4324/9781003442585-14

experience takes place, the patient should first, in that session, have ideomotor signals established. This helps set up therapeutic alliances with deeper, more unconscious levels of mind, among which are the ego states. Like barrier imagery and positive ego-strengthening experiences, the ideomotor signals also help reinforce internal boundaries. This is of the utmost importance because the compelling question with dissociative patients at this point in treatment is: What will they do with the material they have uncovered? Will they be able to contain it? Disappear it? Put it into a far-away place?

Many patients do quite well with some kind of *control* apparatus in the safe place. This could feature a giant TV and VCR with controls for "On," "Off," "Freeze," "Fast Forward," and "Rewind." Like ideomotor signals, these are mechanisms for setting boundaries that establish more inner control. With the preliminary work out of the way, the therapist can now approach the "inner mind" or the ego states.

Ideomotor signals give a great deal of safety during the uncovering phase. We engage the deeper levels of mind in producing a positive age regression. Ideomotor signals are used to maintain continued communication with deeper levels of mind. If, at any time, a "no" reply occurs, we stop and work with that. Is it a "no" answer because the inner mind, or deeper levels of mind, does not understand the question? Because for some reason the inner mind does not want the patient to have a positive experience from the past? Because we, the therapists, are not trusted? Because something else is needed first?

The first kind of memory work to be done should be positive. Positive age regressions strengthen the patient and put her in touch with powerful internal resources. We may ask for even earlier and perhaps more helpful positive material after the first positive age regression has occurred. Once a climate of positive strengthening has been established in the session, we then request the ego state or the "inner mind" to allow the patient to access some of the painful internal material. If we get a "no" signal, we know that more strengthening has to occur. If there is a "yes" signal, we select one of many hypnoanalytic techniques for producing age regression.

Many patients, when strengthened this way, are able to retrieve significant and meaningful memory material. Others have difficulty with what they experience at this stage. They may feel overwhelmed, and they may require immediate ego-strengthening intervention in the session. The therapist may ask the patient to go to a safe place, put the material into a container, or enlist the help of inner allies such as Internal Self Helpers, guides, and members of the internal family of ego states. Some therapists interpolate themselves as inner protectors at these times (Watkins & Watkins, 1997). The patient may decide to hide, protect herself with stronger barrier imagery, or even leave formal trance. When the latter occurs, we help her complete her imagery work with her eyes open. We like to close every accessing or uncovering session with further ego-strengthening. This could be a return to the safe place, a transitional experience in trance, and/or an unstructured hypnotic age progression. It is wise to always move to unstructured hypnotic age progressions before ending the trance session because they are prognostic (Phillips & Frederick, 1992; see chap. 5) and can keep the therapist and the patient informed as to whether the treatment is on the right track.

Sufficient time must always be left in the session for processing the trance material. Although the temptation might be to return to uncovering trance work in the next session, this is truly a case where "Fools rush in where angels fear to tread." The patient might well need several sessions to adequately integrate what she has experienced in trance with the rest of her experiences. Many patients push at this, claiming that they "want to get it over." As therapists, we can understand this as a natural transference reaction springing from the trauma of the past. Our advice is to resist the push. The patient needs to understand how she feels about the material—whether she sees evidence of its influence in her interpersonal interactions, the transference, her family dynamics, and so forth. The therapist can help the patient with the additional task of examining how she feels about what she may discover next. The processing period should always include formal ego-strengthening, as it extends cooperation and mastery. If, for any reason, the patient has become destabilized after the uncovering work, a return to Stage 1 of the SARI model is essential. No further uncovering work should be contemplated until the patient is stable and safe once more.

Reprocessing Trauma: Corrective Emotional Experiences

Uncovering traumatic material is not necessarily enough to effect internal changes in dissociative patients, nor is it usually sufficient to allow them to gain the mastery that is essential to their recoveries over it. Indeed, without the patient's having acquired adequate mastery over traumatic material, she may discover that she has redissociated it.

Although the term *corrective emotional experience* has been historically attached to Franz Alexander (1930), it has acquired various meanings over time. Many therapists believe some kind of corrective experience to be essential to successful therapy (Watkins & Watkins, 1997), whereas others regard the concept as a meaningless trap. Stone (1997) has described Alpert's (1954) application of Alexander's concept in her work with children. Stone emphasized the importance of interacting with the child in more humane and adaptive ways than what the child has experienced at home. Another way of viewing the corrective emotional experience embraces that host of empathically driven interpretations (Geller, 1987) that arise from the therapist's understanding of the patient's experience. They are experienced as *real* by the patient, and they can be *transmutative* (Strachey, 1934) in the sense that they effect changes within the patient's intrapsychic life. The necessity for such kinds of healing experiences in psychotherapy should never be overlooked in favor of more dramatic approaches.

We believe that the corrective emotional experience should be interpreted in the broadest way. From our standpoint, the corrective emotional experience is any experience that results in internal changes in the patient's significant thoughts, beliefs, affects, expectations, internal structures, and ways of relating. For some patients, as with the woman who was the subject of the February Man study, the experience could center on some form of renurturing. For others, it might be a series of transitional experiences. Certain patients may need stronger boundaries as well and would benefit from Baker's (1981) exercises for increasing object relatedness. While still others might need experiences such as re-grieving or the silent abreaction.

We have found the silent abreaction (H. Watkins, 1980) to be an extremely valuable hypnotic imagery technique with dissociative patients. This technique facilitates the symbolic release of rage through an imaginary pounding and smashing rocks on a rock pile (H. Watkins, 1980) while the patient is in touch with feelings, thoughts, and bodily sensations associated with various degrees of anger and rage. Affect that has been previously pent up within the patient is released in a way that is manageable. The constructive management of the affect is as significant a part of this exercise as is its release. Many patients reprocess the trauma through internal interactions with the situation, with any abuser, or with persecutory or destructive ego states. Often ego states undergo profound identity changes in these interactions.

Stage 3 work emphasizes a number and variety of corrective experiences that allow the patient to renegotiate and reprocess traumatic memory material. To this end, the patient may discover that emerging creativity and socialization are also integral parts of the personality reorganization that is occurring. It is during this stage that the fragments of dissociated material begin to be reconnected. Both the BASK (Braun, 1988) and SIBAM (Levine, 1991) models help the patient have yet another kind of corrective emotional experience as the cognitive, affective, behavioral, and sensory components of the fragmented material become reassociated and are given meaning. This process continues to be prominent during Stage 4.

Ego-Strengthening in Stage 4: Integration

Patients are extremely vulnerable during the integration process. There are good reasons for this. The realignment of the ego states and the collapse of outworn defenses are often accompanied by oscillating shifts in identity and sense of the self. This is often a period characterized by outbursts of extensive anxiety, distress, and acting out, which may even jeopardize the therapy. Patients who are integrating are in a state of affairs that resembles the internal chaos of adolescence in many ways (Morton & Frederick, 1997a).

Morton and Frederick (1997a) have noted that the turbulence of integration rests on several factors. One is the collapse of the defenses that have previously helped the patient to survive. There is usually a host of defensive activities including repression, dissociation, massive numbing of affect, ubiquitous and penetrating denial, apathy, avoidance, and displacement into obsessive compulsive defenses such as addictive behavior. The collapse of the defenses can be seen as the result of trauma resolution and personality growth and maturation. The emergence of a more intact and adult personality brings with it many new threats. The more adult personality is tempted by the growth it is experiencing to venture into new ways of relating to others. The patient now has the possibility of engaging in the appropriate expression and management of sexuality. She can begin to tolerate intimacy. Pleasure and success are, for the first time, within her reach: "all of these indicate to the patient that he/she has entered a terra incognita that can be as confusing and frightening as it may be enticing" (Morton & Frederick, 1997a, p. 4).

Furthermore, the energy that abounds from the fall of the defenses is new and strange. Patients in the integration stage of therapy may often misinterpret this energy as anxiety. Because integration is a process that takes place over days and weeks and months, the released energy may not have had time to attach itself to the ego functions it will best serve. Hence, the ego has not "filled out" and can even be considered to be impoverished because the energy has not become sufficiently *egotized* (J. G. Watkins, 1992; Watkins & Watkins, 1997).

The psychodynamic viewpoint emphasizes the advent of a healthier system of defenses. Internal objects are also undergoing changes as new structures are formed (McNeal, 1993) and adequate nurturing selfobjects are developed. Cognitive-behaviorists would identify cognitive consonance, better reality testing, and interpretation, and more adaptive behavior. All of this is accompanied by the integration of ego states into a cooperative and harmonious internal family with shared consciousness (Phillips & Frederick, 1995; Watkins & Watkins, 1997) and many other changes in identity that have come about as the result of the interpersonal interaction with the therapist (Frederick, 1996b).

Morton and Frederick (1997a) have identified one of the primary problems in the process of integration as a "rigidity or opacity of the boundaries between conscious and unconscious processes" (Gilligan, 1987). They have noted that Jung was aware of this problem, which he called a "dysfunction of conscious and unconscious mental processes" (Jung, 1956, p. 235). Finally, the Stage 3 work of connecting the fragments must be extended into Stage 4. The dissociated material must also be integrated into the personality (Phillips & Frederick, 1995). This fragmented material, like fragmented aspects of the self, needs to be reconnected multimodally (into behavior, affect, sensation, cognition, and meaning) as represented by the BASK (Braun, 1988) or the SIBAM (Levine, 1991) models.

With the formation of a new identity,

the experiences of the self, even in painful events or self reflections, in unacceptable wishes, and in tormenting memories, are observed and acknowledged by the self. The price of this new maturity is pain. The counterbalances for the patient in this process are a new sense of self, greatly increased problem solving energy and repertoire, and an expanded ego that can negotiate and coordinate both conscious and unconscious material to its benefit.

(Morton & Frederick, 1997a, pp. 7–8)

The stage of integration (SARI Stage 4) is characteristically accompanied by a recrudescence of symptoms, reemergence of conflicts at every level of the psyche (Glover, 1955; Nunberg, 1955), acting out, and, at times, severe anxiety. There may be sleep disturbances and nightmares as well as psychophysiological manifestations such as diarrhea, vomiting, abdominal pain, and headache (Phillips & Frederick, 1995). Although integration is frequently troubled, its manifestations are often misinterpreted by therapists.

The Hypnotic Facilitation of Integration

Morton and Frederick (1997a) believe that there is much that can be done to "help the patient negotiate the often alien and troubled psychic countryside" (p. 9). They recommend that the entire process be discussed with the patient so that the patient's understanding and cooperation can be enlisted on the conscious level. However, it is their observation that what can help most in the integration stage is the facilitation of conscious–unconscious complementarity. They cite Gilligan's (1987) metaphorical description of the boundaries between the conscious and the unconscious mind as softer or translucent and harder or opaque. According to Gilligan, softer, more translucent boundaries allow the two aspects of mental functioning to communicate and to interact with one another so that they can complement rather than oppose one another. This is in keeping with Erickson's (1948/1980) thoughts on the matter: "There is a tremendous need of enabling the patient to integrate the unconscious with the conscious or of making the new understandings of the unconscious fully accessible, upon need, to the conscious mind. Comparable to this failure would be an appendectomy with failure to close the incision" (p. 40).

Morton and Frederick (1997a) have offered suggestions as to how the therapist can facilitate conscious–unconscious complementarity in the integrating patient. As this complementarity is increased, the patient gets more in touch with the nature of the process in whose grips he is. At this point, he can also begin to take measures that increase his mastery and are ego-strengthening. Many of Morton and Frederick's suggestions employ hypnosis. Hypnosis is already a step in the direction of increasing complementarity. However, therapists and patients who are not employing direct hypnosis in treatment can work indirectly with the material suggested by Morton and Frederick, who have made recommendations concerning approaches and attitudes that can be helpful to the integrating patient.

Education. Educating the patient about the nature of the integration process should always be done initially with the patient in a conscious, awake, nonhypnotized state. However, the use of trance as a vehicle for the message may bring it to the attention of the unconscious mind more effectively. Morton and Frederick (1997a) recommend that both nonhypnotic and hypnotic education occur as a model for conscious–unconscious complementarity:

> As we just take an opportunity now to review what has been going on with you, to review what improvement can do to someone. You know you are now improving as the parts are getting closer together, as you are reaching out into new worlds for yourself. You know that at times you experience a lot of anxiety, and sometimes you even find that you're getting angry.... You can accept that it isn't bad for you.
>
> (Morton & Frederick, 1997a, pp. 11–12)

The use of metaphor to explain this process to the patient is also recommended. Metaphor has the ability to touch deep unconscious associations:

> I don't know if you have ever really thought about what happens to the caterpillar when it forms a cocoon. These days people use that word, cocoon, to represent safety and protection. But, you know, the caterpillar in the cocoon risks all that he has.... He loses all of his familiar shape and structure and becomes an amorphous mass of tissue. He really gives his all so that one day he will have a different form of locomotion, so that he will be able to fly instead of crawl. It's only through the drastic, reorganizing, transforming activities of the cocoon that he develops new and better sense organs, and a new body, and wonderful wings ... and when we see the butterfly we always think, "How beautiful!"
>
> (Morton & Frederick, 1997a, p. 12)

Respect for the Sacredness of the Process. As we discuss the process with patients, we should never overlook the fact that we are witnessing a unique and sacred event: The birth of a new identity or self. This is the result of the therapy the patient has been working at; this is the new, strengthened ego. Although we can explain a lot about this process, there is a certain aspect that is ineffable. It has to do with the individual becoming more of his potential.

We find it important to remind our patients of the sacredness of the process with statements such as: (a) "You are becoming the person you were always meant to be" (Morton & Frederick, 1997a, p. 14), or (b) "You have waited a long time to discover who you really are." Such comments, described by Morton and Frederick (1997a) as "'wise and profound' declarations" (p. 13), speak to both conscious and unconscious processes. They have a mythic ring to them, and they seed hope (Dolan, 1991) about the outcome of the painful process of integration.

Reframing Anxiety as Energy. There are many ways to help the patient re-channel his newly emerging energy. He needs to change his concept about the anxiety he may be feeling. He must come to understand that, although he may have many reasons to be anxious, some of what he is identifying as anxiety is really new energy. This should be presented in the general education of the patient about integration. However, it should be repeated in trance. The use of metaphor and symbolism is most helpful.

> Take a little time to reflect on the anxiety you have been experiencing lately in your body.... Search your memory in recent days for just where and how you have felt it ... you may discover that as you do, you are beginning to re-experience some of it.... Now let yourself picture in your mind those feelings you have called "anxiety" as pulsing rays of energy, golden energy.... You can see it circulating throughout your mindbody ... filling you with strength, with new ideas, new appreciations.... You might want to picture it entering your body through the top of your head ... and circulating ... and leaving through the soles of your feet ... there seems to be an endless supply ... and isn't it interesting that you can have all that energy and still be able to relax yourself profoundly whenever you want to ...
>
> (Morton & Frederick, 1997a, p. 14)

Encouragement to Utilize Transitional Phenomena. As patients integrate, they become more independent in terms of their activities and feeling states. The purpose of transitional phenomena in the growth process is to allow the individual to move into more emotional independence (see chap. 7).

Patients can be encouraged to use self-hypnosis for transitional experiences. They can also be helped to discover and create appropriate transitional situations for them in their everyday life. "For some patients the actual use of a talisman or object (Dolan, 1991; Watkins & Watkins, 1997) in the external world to represent and trigger this kind of transitional affective state is often of great assistance in keeping the conscious and the unconscious in close contact with one another" (Morton & Frederick, 1997a, p. 15).

Permission to Experience Regression as Part of the Process.   Because regression into symptomatology is a common feature of integration, it can be helpful for the therapist to *normalize* this phenomenon and remind the patient that it is only temporary:

> With these perspectives that you can have in trance, you know that it's all right for you to have symptoms. It's okay if frightened parts need to express whatever fears they might have ... fears of change ... fears of becoming anni-hilated just by losing some of their more independent functions as they move into more cooperative positions. It's all right for you to have the symptoms

again. When you have symptoms, you can accept that this is just part of the process. You can accept that it isn't bad for you, and you can use the symptoms as an occasion to stabilize and soothe yourself, an occasion to take some time for you and every part of you ...

(Morton & Frederick, 1997a, p. 15)

This approach utilizes the symptoms as it directs the patient to the future—to a time when the integration process has been completed.

Permission to Wish to Have the Therapist Closer as Part of the Process. An aspect of the regression often seen in integration is a return of the patient's more childlike transferences to the therapist. This can produce wishes to cling to the therapist and often carries with it, at this stage of therapy, a sense of shame on the patient's part. He may find himself needing the therapist more but feeling that he shouldn't or that, if he does, it really means he is getting worse, not better. For some patients, regressive feelings about the therapist may only exist on an unconscious level and may manifest themselves in other ways: "... you can even recall that I am with your recovery. I am with you. [There can be times] when it's okay to recall that. Okay to see me there" (Morton & Frederick, 1997a, p. 16). Again, the temporary nature of these regressive wishes should be stressed.

Self-Hypnosis. Self-hypnosis (see chap. 7) offers ways for the patient to (a) calm and soothe himself, (b) create transitional spaces and experiences, (c) enter into objective thinking, (d) reframe anxiety as energy, and (e) mentally draw close to the therapist. It increases conscious–unconscious complementarity through these activities. Additionally, the patient is able to become more receptive to his internal processes and their unconscious component. He also learns to trust them more. Morton and Frederick (1997a) have noted that Fromm and Kahn (1990) found that, in self-hypnosis, there is a greater ease in the alternation of ego activity and ego receptivity.

Posthypnotic Suggestions. Posthypnotic suggestions can be thought of as ways of locking into place gains that have been made in heterohypnosis. The patient can be given cues that can automatically activate healing responses:

And should you notice that memories of that event you have just dealt with so well here in trance should come to you in a troublesome way when you are in a waking state, you will discover that you will be able, at the first opportunity, to enter a self-hypnotic state and effectively deal with any remnants you may discover ...

(Morton & Frederick, 1997a, p. 17)

Age Progressions.   Age progressions have been discussed in detail in chapter 5. Unstructured age progressions provide the patient with anchors into the future—a view of the future self that comes from within the patient's unconscious mind. The phenomena of experiencing integration and a new identity take on more reality for the patient and seem more believable. This vision of the future reinforces conscious–unconscious complementarity and offers soothing, positive feelings of hope.

Unconscious Learning.   The therapist can help reinforce the patient's confidence in the unconscious mind's ability to learn, understand, and problem solve. The patient is encouraged to turn his doubts, pain, and concerns over to his unconscious with the confidence that there are abundant resources. It is usually helpful to give the patient examples of his having functioned well in this respect on previous occasions.

Awake-Alert Trance.   Patients in awake-alert trance (see chap. 11), also called *eyes-open trance* by some clinicians, experience "increased alertness, enhancement of positive emotional tone, and perceptions of more active participation on active-alert hypnosis as compared with traditional hypnosis" (Banyai, Zseni, & Tury, 1993, p. 292). Awake-alert trance is a practical way to facilitate conscious–unconscious complementarity. Sometimes we like to tell our patients that such a trance state allows them to live in two worlds at the same time. A patient facing both external and internal stress could elect to spend some time in awake-alert trance as a way of getting through the day.

Walking the Tightrope.   Most patients engage in many automatic behaviors in which they function quite competently. Morton and Frederick (1997a) have termed such activity as *walking the tightrope*. They use the image of the tightrope walker as a paradigm for the successfulness of certain automatic activities that would certainly go amiss if the individual performing them brought conscious control into the picture. The tightrope artist does not think about walking the tightrope. She just does it. Everyone has innate abilities to perform well on automatic pilot. Most patients relate well to examples of touch typing, riding a bike, driving a car, or dancing. We like to remind patients in and out of trance that they are on automatic pilot, and can go on automatic pilot. We encourage them to walk the tightrope. This means that we guide our patients in the integration stage to greater trust in conscious–unconscious complementarity. The ensuing script was used with one of the authors' (CF) patients and is cited by Morton and Frederick (1997a). The patient had actually walked a tightrope unsuccessfully while she was in a wilderness rope course. She had failed because she was focusing on a perfect performance. This caused her to conduct her actions too much under the control of her conscious attention. She recognized what she had done, and then walked the tightrope again, this time properly. In order to do it successfully she had to throw the switch and allow conscious–unconscious complementarity to prevail.

Case Vignette

Most importantly, when symptoms return, as they often do during integration, or when you feel anxious or brimming with something that is so confusing to you, it's going to be important for you to do that thing we talked about. To go with the flow. And since you told me about the rope course that you took 5 or 6 years ago, I'll just remind you of what you told me. How you were climbing in the rope course, and you found yourself confronted with the job of walking across a high wire. Even though you were secured to safety ropes, as you began to cross on the wire, you noticed fear. Fear that caused you to begin to think about where you would put your foot so that you could do it perfectly ... and then the other foot. And then you discovered you just couldn't manage that. You were starting to fall. And isn't it wonderful that when you were finally holding onto the support ropes and made your way to the other side ... that you turned around and walked back, turning all of that over to your inner mind and the parts. Remember, you told me you didn't think about it. You just did it. And you know it's like the waves and the wind. The waves that carry and the wind that propels a boat. They don't think about it. They just do it.

Morton and Frederick's (1997a) techniques for increasing conscious–unconscious complementarity are ego-strengthening. They encourage the patient to use his whole mind. Although they have scrutinized the usefulness of the techniques in the integration process, they have hypothesized that increasing the permeability of the boundaries between conscious and unconscious minds could also bring about an "increase in creativity and healthy play, more frequent use of self hypnosis, access to deeper levels of mind, enhanced therapeutic alliance, and in some patients, increased spirituality, are promoted by this focus on increased flow between conscious and unconscious process" (Morton & Frederick, 1997a, p. 23).

The posttraumatic and dissociative patient who has moved into integration has come a long way, into a process that continues for the rest of a lifetime (Erikson, 1964; Young-Eisendrath & Hall, 1991). The next chapter addresses how a strengthened ego might become replaced by a transpersonal self in the process of successful living, as well as how much integration may be necessary for certain individuals to die well.

Chapter 15

The Strengthened Ego and the Transpersonal Self in Living and Dying

Discovery and change do not cease to be vital life forces simply because formal integration has occurred. Identity tends to undergo changes over a life span. Jung (1935/1971) attributed this ongoing process to the amazing power of the unconscious mind. It is rich in undreamed-of resources; as a person ages, more of his potential, hitherto stored in the unconscious, is allowed to come out. For many, therapy accelerates this process, catches them up, or, at the very least, puts them farther along the road than they would otherwise be. Patients who have integrated the developmental progress that has been the fruit of their therapy often experience themselves as changed. They have new identities, and they are no longer so narcissistically involved with themselves.

Stages of Psychological Development

Hartley (1993) has reviewed a number of models for assessing psychological development. The earliest ones were the psychosexual model, the ego-psychological model, and the psychosocial model of Erik Erikson (1959). Erikson's psychosocial model has been most helpful for understanding how ego states mature and integrate (Phillips & Frederick, 1995; see chap. 13). Later models that were based on both clinical and normative observations of infants and children emerged. Subsequent models were not restricted to childhood observations, but rather were based on the observation of psychic development over a life span (Hartley, 1993). A number of empirical scales have been created to measure the level of psychological development. One of the best known models for assessing the level of ego development is that of Loevinger (1976).

Loevinger (1976) conceptualized development as occurring in stages. Chronological age is not a consideration in her measurements. Loevinger's stages of ego development are:

- Presocial
- Symbiotic

DOI:10.4324/9781003442585-15

- Impulsive: This stage is characterized by intense affect. Relationships sought are immediate and need-gratifying.
- Self-Protective: This stage is pleasure-oriented, and characterized by opportunism, short-term rewards, and avoidance of responsibility.
- Conformist: In this stage the norm of the group rules. Thinking tends to be stereotypical and conventional.
- Conscientious: The individual who has progressed to this stage is capable of complex thinking and has internalized rules. He has a sense of responsibility, possesses values, and has long-term goals. He experiences fine shades of emotion.
- Autonomous: In this stage there is an awareness of conflict and a capacity for ambiguity. Individual differences are highly valued, and emotional interdependence rather than emotional dependence prevails.
- Integrated: The individual who has reached this level of development has transcended conflict and is involved in self-actualization.

The Development of the Transpersonal

As the patient with the strengthened ego progresses through the stages of ego development, he may discover that he is beginning to develop perceptions and concerns that are more universal and less particular, may experience deeper connections with the rest of the human race, with nature, and with the cosmos. He also has been able to shift his energies from maintaining repression and other defenses, he has a better intrapsychic structure, and within his mind conscious–unconscious complementarity will be greatly increased. Expanded contact with his unconscious mind may lead him to become much more aware of what Jung (1939) called the collective unconscious.

Jung (see chap. 6) has received much less attention than Freud in the United States. Nevertheless, Jung had influenced the development of modern thought so pervasively that the man or woman on the street frequently expresses Jungian ideas without having any idea of their origin. For example, the terms *introvert*, *extrovert*, and *inferiority complex* are ones that no one would find alien. Jung has had marked influence outside his own fields of psychiatry and psychoanalysis. "Contemporary studies of cultural history and mythology are profoundly indebted to Jung" (Munroe, 1955, p. 539). Jung viewed humankind as living in a world of symbols. The function of the symbol was to express mystery, the unknown. Jung observed that symbols occur everywhere: in arts and crafts, folklore, fantasy, and dreams. He observed that the unconscious mind seems to form the same symbols all over the world. The recurrent appearance of certain symbols led Jung to create his theory of the *collective unconscious*.

> This psychic life is the mind of our ancient ancestors, the way in which they thought and felt, the way in which they conceived of life and the world, of gods and human beings. The existence of these historical layers is presumably

the source of the belief in reincarnation and in memories of past lives. As the body is a sort of a museum in its phylogenetic history, so is the mind. There is no reason for believing that the psyche, with its peculiar structure, is the only thing in the world that has no history beyond its individual manifestation. Even the conscious mind cannot be denied a history extending over at least five thousand years. It is only individual ego-consciousness that has forever a new beginning and an early end. But the unconscious psyche is not only immensely old, it is also able to grow increasingly into an equally remote future. It forms, and is part of, the human species just as much as the body, which is also individually ephemeral, yet collectively of immeasurable duration.

(Jung, 1939, p. 24f)

The individual becomes acquainted with his collective unconscious through universal symbols known as the archetypes. The archetypal symbols, or images, are not commonly experienced; when they are, the encounter is distinct and vivid. Many individuals who have archetypal experiences realize that such experiences expand their sense of the transpersonal. The transpersonal can be defined as that which transcends or reaches beyond the personal or individual. We have observed many times that as the ego is strengthened, the sense of the *transpersonal* increases. It is not unusual for one to experience the transpersonal as part of a spiritual dimension that expands and changes our patients' sense of identity in a positive way.

There can be no doubt that the individual who functions from a transpersonal base has developed an expanded sense of self. The popular or cliché ego, or narcissistic self-concern, begins to vanish and reveal in its place an emerging transcendent self. It is our belief that this transcendent self is better able to negotiate the waters of living and dying than is the self-involved ego. However, patients who have progressed in their intrapsychic development and are becoming interested in spirituality may bring these inclinations to a halt because they may fear losing what they have so laboriously gained. Most commonly, patients who stand on this brink of spiritual development may feel that they have to turn back to avoid having to lose their hard-won personhood or to escape engulfment by God. Such are the effects of old and erroneous belief systems. One of the authors (Phillips & Frederick, 1995) previously has explored spiritual issues from the standpoint of the guidelines for happiness offered by the French philosopher Pierre Teilhard de Chardin (1957/1960, 1964, 1966/1973, 1969). Another, somewhat different look at Teilhard de Chardin is now offered as a different kind of perspective that encourages us to become more of ourselves as we become more spiritual. This is followed by a discussion of an Eastern approach to spirituality, that of Tibetan Buddhist practice which also promotes adventure, curiosity, humor, and living very much in the present.

Teilhard de Chardin was a paleontologist who was on the Peking Man digs; he was also a Jesuit priest. Just as his biological and paleontological orientations were developmental, so also was his original and creative spiritual philosophy. His church silenced his writings. However, Teilhard de Chardin willed them to Thomas Huxley because he knew this was a certain way to get them published. De Chardin suggested several parallel lines of developmental progression. He called one of them "The Theoretical Axes of Happiness" (Teilhard de Chardin, 1966/1973, p. 13), and he categorized happiness into three types:

- The Happiness of Tranquility: "No worry, no risk, no effort. Let us cut down our contacts, let us restrict our needs, let us dim our lights, toughen our protective skin, withdraw into our shell. The happy man ... attains a minimum of thought, feeling and desire" (Teilhard de Chardin, 1966/1973, p. 21).
- The Happiness of Pleasure: This kind of happiness is opportunistic and totally oriented to the individual's obtaining as much and as many kinds of pleasure as she can obtain in the present.
- The Happiness of Growth: "The happy man is therefore the man who, without any direct search for happiness, inevitably finds joy as an added bonus in the act of forging ahead and attaining the fullness and finality of his own life" (Teilhard de Chardin, 1966/1973, p. 23). This is the kind of happiness that corresponds to self-actualization.

As to *how* one achieves that happiness, de Chardin is succinct: "first, *be*. Secondly, *love*. Finally, *worship*" (Teilhard de Chardin, 1966/1973, p. 42). Teilhard de Chardin was well aware of internal fragmentation, and he viewed the installation of internal harmony as his *first stage of happiness*. The individual who had achieved this much internal integration could now presumably turn from the isolation of self-love to the love of another human being in the *second stage of happiness*. In the *third stage of happiness*, termed *worship* by Teilhard de Chardin, the individual actualizes herself and becomes a partner of the divine by fulfilling her evolutionary destiny. For Teilhard de Chardin, worship is what the astronauts did when they took off for the moon; Lewis and Clarke were worshipping when they explored an unknown part of a great continent. Scientist worship when they work for new breakthroughs, artists when they paint, and writers when they write. Worship is no longer relegated to a few specific ritualistic activities. Worship is becoming one's best self. When self-actualization is pursued, human life becomes divinised.

Teilhard de Chardin believed that the rhythm of spiritual growth began with "first develop yourself" (Teilhard de Chardin, 1957/1960, p. 70). He was concerned with the call to renunciation of the world and of one's talents that some experience; he was also concerned with the tensions in each consciousness between development and renunciation and attachment and detachment. He did not believe that these opposites were mutually exclusive. He pictured self-actualizing humans as "... continually passing from attachment to detachment as they faithfully mount the ladder of human endeavor" (Teilhard de Chardin, 1957/1960, p. 72).

Another way of developing one's spiritual or transpersonal self in the project of living comes from the somewhat similar, yet somewhat different, perspective of Tibetan Buddhism as provided by Pema Chodron (Chodron, 1991), a Tibetan Buddhist renunciate. Like Teilhard de Chardin, Chodron invites us to an interesting and adventurous life, one in which our curiosity and humor are prominent features. "To lead a life that goes beyond pettiness and prejudice and always wanting to make sure that everything turns out on our own terms, to lead a more passionate, full and delightful life than that, we must realize that we can endure a lot of pain and pleasure for the sake of finding out who we are ..." (Chodron, 1991, p. 3). At the very heart of the Buddhist principle of loving-kindness is self-acceptance—a commonly agreed upon desirable outcome of therapy. *Loving-kindness* means that the patient does not have to become perfect and lose all of his symptoms. As he has moved into a more transpersonal perspective, he sees that he must treat himself with loving-kindness and complete acceptance. He is not expected to become selfless or egoless, but rather to learn more of who he really is. In order to do this he must learn to live in the present. There is what may seem to be surprising similarity between Tibetan Buddhist practice and the Christian philosophy of Pierre Teilhard de Chardin. We believe that, on the main, many of the truly great spiritual traditions tend to strive toward many of the same goals.

Living in the present accentuates the sense of being alive. One way of learning to live in the present is to use meditation with mindfulness techniques. These, interestingly enough, can be used productively with ego states as well as with the greater personality (Dickey, Nungary, & Frederick, 1998). "While we are sitting in meditation, we are simply exploring humanity and all of creation in the form of ourselves" (Chodron, 1991, p. 7). In the Tibetan Buddhist tradition the individual is led to accept the self, to know that it is impossible to separate wisdom, for example, from our own flaws, crazinesses, neuroses, and hang-ups. Everything in us that is good and desirable is jumbled up with all that is wrong with us. The goal is to discover, not judge ourselves. This kind of self-discovery is not solely self-centered, for as we do this, we realize that we are also engaged in a search for understanding everyone else as well. We are in a strange way plunging into the collective unconscious.

Also important in the Tibetan Buddhist tradition is the acceptance of our feelings—the understanding that even our negative emotions are exactly what we need at the time. At times these feelings lead us to wish that we could be better than we really are, that we should be more adept at spiritual practices, and that we should learn faster to see into the heart of things. Chodron (1991) reminds us that there is a tradition in Tibetan Buddhist called the *mishap lineage*. This lineage of venerable and wise teachers is known for its history, from generation to generation, of "blowing it." One was a madman, another almost paralyzed by his obsessionalism, another was bad-tempered, stubborn, and a drunk, yet another was a murderer. Like Augustine in the Christian tradition, they were flawed vessels. Unlike Augustine, their behaviors underwent no sudden, dramatic changes.

Their tradition did not feature sudden conversion to model behavior as a necessity. What did these teachers do in order to learn to live with loving-kindness?

They used mindfulness techniques. These meditative techniques induce a trance state whose purpose is only to focus on the present time. For example, the meditator concentrates on the ordinary exhaled breath—that is all. When the mind wanders in to thinking about anything, the meditator mentally says, "thinking," and then returns his attention to his exhaling breath. This gentle technique is used to bring the meditator into the present fully, just as he is. It is not about change or perfection. In the present, he is encouraged to take the time to appreciate the things that he encounters that give him joy: the beauty of some flowers, the smell of freshly baked bread, or the strains of a wonderful piece of music. Joy is a version of loving another. It is an emotion that springs from an encounter with that which is outside of us.

Eventually the practice of meditation leads to changes. "Meditation begins to open up your life, so that you're not caught in self-concern, just wanting life to go your way" (Chodron, 1991, p. 29). The meditative process is a path to waking up to a more intense, more vivid now into which greater awareness has crept. We learn that it is our emotions that often stand between us and a larger perspective of the world. "The more sensitive we become to this, the more we realize that when we start getting angry or denigrating ourselves or craving things in a way that makes us feel miserable, we begin to shut down, shut out, as if we were sitting on the edge of the Grand Canyon but we had put a big black bag over our heads" (Chodron, 1991, pp. 30–31).

Within the Tibetan Buddhist tradition, it is recognized that doctrinaire attitudes are soul killing and often lead us to harm others who do not share our beliefs. No matter how important our beliefs are to us, there is always the possibility that they may be blinding us and lulling us into dead existences. Living in the present, we are able to see our beliefs as simply our interpretations of reality. The Tibetan Buddhist tradition is based on their interpretation of Buddha's *Four Noble Truths*.

- The *First Noble Truth* tells us that there is discomfort in every human life. This discomfort can be regarded as part of the dynamism of life that simply comes with the human condition. It does not have to anchor or deter us from exploration or adventure.
- The *Second Noble Truth* tells us that our egos cause suffering by resisting life through our attachments.
- The *Third Noble Truth* is that the cessation of suffering comes from our letting go of our attachments. "By 'cessation' we mean the cessation of hell as opposed to just weather …" (Chodron, 1991, p. 41). Meditation brings the practitioner back from the brink of fear and despair over this into an elemental appreciation of the breath in the present moment, and "that original fluttering feeling that might be very edgy but is basically the wind, the fire, the earth, the water" (Chodron, 1991, pp. 41–42).

- The *Fourth Noble Truth* is the eightfold path. It tells us that all of our medi-
  tations, our careers and livelihoods, our discipline, our work can be used by
  us to help us realize our unity with all things—and that the same "… energy
  that causes us to live and be whole and awake and alive is just the energy that
  creates everything, and we're part of that"

  (Chodron, 1991, p. 42).

The similarity of this orientation with Teilhard de Chardin (1973) is striking.
Both tell us that, to be truly spiritual, we only need to accept who we are and
become as much of that as we can—to become deeply and excitingly involved
with the richness of life, a richness we could not comprehend before our enlightenment. The *enlightenment* is a multimodal realization that we are connected
with all the energies and manifestations of existence. It is our transpersonal self
that we then begin to experience.

The Question of Spirituality

The transpersonal self leads the individual into pathways of spiritual development that bring great joy to life; it can greatly assist in development and divini-
sation, or sensing oneself as a cocreator of the universe. The transpersonal self
leads a different life. It is a life that is truly alive and energized, even though
there may be *weather*. It is a life in which love and acceptance are prominent
features, and in which self-acceptance frees the individual to deep and appropriate self-love and self-regard, as well as deep acceptance for others—even those
who are alien and different. These issues frequently emerge as therapy becomes
increasingly successful and the ego becomes stronger. How should therapists
deal with them when they arise in therapy? We find that a few simple rules are
helpful. It is essential that the therapist not impose any religious orientation or
views upon any patient. Although many of the goals embodied in what follows
can be espoused by individuals of no religious beliefs at all, they can also be
utilized to enhance spirituality.

1. The path belongs to the patient, not the therapist. Validate what the patient is
   experiencing.
2. It is appropriate to teach the patient about psychological development and let
   him know that often people who are involved in self-actualization have many
   of the same kinds of thoughts and feelings he has.
3. If necessary, indicate to the patient that some kind of spiritual direction—
   instruction that he may wish to have in his life—is all right with you. Strict
   and fearful fundamentalism of any kind is a symptom of failure to develop
   psychologically. The ego is stuck at Loevinger's (1976) conformist stage, and
   the patient has a long way to go in treatment. It is important not to directly
   disagree with the patient who is so involved.

4. Allow yourself to get in touch with your own transpersonal self. We believe that the more you develop this aspect of your self, the more sensitive you will be to all of your patients' needs.
5. Be prepared that not every patient is able to travel as far as he needs to go. Some patients will terminate therapy, some will move to other geographies, and others may simply not improve as much as we have wished them to. There is a special category of patient who has not arrived at a discovery of his transpersonal self before he is told that he is going to die. Death can be the occasion for great psychological as well as spiritual development.

From Strengthened Ego to Transpersonal Self in the Terminally Ill Patient

Death, a natural part of the life cycle, comes to each of us in time. Although a few prophets and some children foresee the season and manner of their deaths, this kind of knowledge is not usually given to us in advance in our adult lives. According to Kubler-Ross (1969) the patient who receives the verdict that she is terminally ill classically undergoes a complex series of reactions that culminates in the acceptance of approaching death.

However, there is another tradition in medicine that has the terminally ill patient reject the death sentence, undergo certain processes that effect internal changes, and regain her health. Among these are the psychotherapeutic understanding of the meaning of her illness and lifestyle changes (Fawzy et al., 1993; Fawzy, Fawzy, Arndt, & Pasnau, 1995; McDaniel, Musselman, Porter, Reed, & Nemeroff, 1995; Spiegel, 1991), and the utilization of hypnotherapeutic techniques such as imagery (LeShan, 1989; Siegel; 1969, 1989; Simonton, Matthews-Simonton, & Creighton, 1978), ideodynamic healing (Rossi & Cheek, 1988), and the development of high-level awareness (Brigham, 1994) to turn the course of the illness and escape from the sentence of terminal illness. Outside of the Western medical tradition, patients so motivated may seek recovery with spiritual practices, shamans, psychic surgeons, macrobiotic diets, and a host of other interventions.

A variation of acceptance of death that is important for the therapist to recognize is one in which the patient utilizes techniques for recovery in the interests of prolonging life and improving its quality to accomplish significant developmental, interpersonal, and/or spiritual tasks before leaving the planet.

It is often quite perplexing for the clinician to decide whether he should be helping the patient work from a *life perspective* or from a *death perspective* (H. Watkins, personal communication, 1994). For this reason, many clinicians eschew life perspective, or getting well strategies, because they fear that they might build false hopes in their patients, fill them with cruel and undeserved guilt for causing their own illnesses, and increase the sense of helplessness of their caregivers (Peter, 1994).

The power of personal beliefs to kill or cure in a primitive culture has been described dramatically by Cannon (1957). He related this to the effects of mind on the human autonomic nervous system. Currently, acceptance of the relevance of belief systems to physical health and the possibility that recovery techniques will work for patients is widely held (Alexander, 1950; Cousins, 1983; Rossi, 1993). Yet the job of discovering what the patient's deepest beliefs might be can often seem impossible in as much as they are usually unconscious, and the evidence for their existence may be absent or confusing (Frederick, 1995b; Frederick & Phillips, 1992). For example, a patient may speak in the language of hope and determination about recovery, while unconsciously he is truly fatalistic and thinks his number is up.

It can be most helpful to utilize the therapeutic relationship to help patients discover which path they have chosen and assist them in reaching the levels of maturation and integration necessary for a successful journey into life or into death. The following clinical examples show how variations of the life perspective and the death perspective may appear in clinical practice.

Case Example: Mattie

Mattie had been diagnosed with breast cancer when she was only 27 years old. When I (CF) first saw her several years later, she had bone metastases in several sites and had been through several remissions and exacerbations. Mattie, an Asian American, told me that she had developed cancer during her marriage to a very attractive young Anglo man who had won her heart and that of her family. Although he had wooed her intensely, Mattie became aware that he was volatile. At one point she broke off their engagement because he had been seeing another woman. He became disconsolate, and Mattie reinstated the engagement and went through with the marriage despite considerable doubts that she kept from her protective family.

After the marriage, Mattie discovered that her new husband was severely controlling and was also a batterer. She concealed this from her family and friends because she did not wish any blemish to appear on the surface of what they had come to perceive as the dream marriage. The husband she described to me may well have had a dissociative disorder, as she reported that he switched a great deal from Dr. Jekyll to Mr. Hyde, and then to a sobbing child.

When Mattie discovered the cancer had metastasized into her skeletal system, she informed Jim that she was going to get well and that he would have to change his behavior toward her. That failing, she would leave him. For a magical year, Jim's behavior was exemplary; he was a loving, considerate, attentive husband. All of Mattie's skeletal lesions swiftly and miraculously vanished within this period of time. However, when she finally informed Jim of her dramatic improvement, he reverted to his earlier sadistic and controlling behavior. Within a short period of time, the skeletal metastases reappeared. After this kind of interaction and its consequent effect on the appearance of metastases had occurred several times, Mattie was convinced that she could not live if she stayed with Jim.

I saw her after she had left him, filed for divorce, and moved to another geographic location. She was seeking help for her clinical depression and control of the spread of the cancer. She was concomitantly in treatment with an oncologist who told me that she was in the terminal phase of her illness and would live for only a matter of a few months.

Mattie's initial hypnotic experiences were frightening to her, and I wondered if she had experienced trauma in her early life. She had visualizations of a furious witch who threatened her. Out of trance she explained, "I can't visualize!" By this she meant that she could not voluntarily produce helpful visualizations and felt at the mercy of the witch. Her first hypnotic task was to learn how to use hypnosis to produce simple, familiar, and stabilizing visualizations such as those of lemons, oranges, basketballs, and Mickey Mouse. When I saw her smile at the Mickey Mouse visualization, I added the rest of the Mouse family as well as Dorothy, Toto, and all the friendly characters from the land of Oz. The patient was able to incorporate them as ego-strengthening companions. More visualization training and formal ego-strengthening work was done. When the patient was considerably less depressed and not at all frightened about what might transpire in a hypnotic experience, formal direct suggestive and projective/evocative ego-strengthening was done. Mattie began to display pride and confidence at her ability to take charge of her hypnotic experiences. It was within this climate of stability that ego-state exploration was begun.

The witch represented an ego state that felt Mattie should be punished. She had, in her grammar school years, been sexually molested by an older, frightening, developmentally challenged male student. Mattie felt she had brought disgrace on her family through her victimhood. The witch also felt Mattie should be punished because she wasn't a boy like her brother, not as pretty as her sister, and because she hadn't been a good wife to Jim.

Another ego state, Cancer, said she produced both the cancer and the depression in attempts to force nurturing attention on Mattie from Jim, as well as from her family.

Indeed, although she had recently lost Jim, her family was more involved with her than it had ever been before in her entire life. As these ego states were worked with therapeutically, Mattie's X-rays changed in a positive direction again. There was a noticeable waxing and waning of metastatic activity as she uncovered and then worked through both internal and family issues.

Eventually, Mattie got both a roommate and a dog. She became stronger, healthier, and more assertive, and began to attend support groups. After she had been in treatment with me for approximately 2 years, she was aware of the progression of her consciousness from that of a child-victim to that of an adult who was intimately involved with her own destiny and who felt very much in charge of her own life. She understood many of her family's dynamics and the role of her illness in those changing dynamics. Mattie felt that her death sentence had become a call to life.

Mattie's internal progress continued as she became involved with spiritual awareness and development for the first time in her life. She began to work with other cancer patients and read books on spirituality. In trance, Mattie had beautiful hypnotic age progressions: pastoral scenes permeated with golden light. She viewed them as transpersonal experiences. She radiated happiness. As her third year of treatment was nearly ended, it was time for me to make a long anticipated geographical move. A transition was made to another therapist with whom Mattie felt comfortable. As we worked on the termination process and the grief it involved for both of us, Mattie told me that, whether she lived or died, her therapy had been a success because she had been able to become an adult and reach her own spiritual experiences. "I'm not sure that I would ever have had to grow this much if I hadn't had to face the possibility of my dying. It doesn't matter how long your life is, if you are really living it."

Case Example: Jonas

When I (CF) first saw Jonas he was in an agitated depression because he believed that he had cancer although his physicians had not been able to locate it. The basis for his belief was a PSA laboratory test for antibodies to prostatic cancer he'd insisted he be given. His physician had referred him to me for help with his depression as well as his obsession with an illness no one could locate and most of his physicians suspected did not exist.

Jonas was 80 years old, and terrified of dying. He had multiple physical complaints, anxiety attacks, and insomnia. When he frequently complained of a variety of somatic preoccupations, he appeared to be extremely frightened. A talented and gregarious man, Jonas was a retired radio/TV producer and artist who had, until recently, worked on a multitude of artistic and performance projects.

The immediate therapeutic goal was to allay the anxiety and depression Jonas was feeling, because they constituted barriers to his psychotherapeutic work. Medications were used to help with this. The next project was to work with Jonas about his fear of death. I had a sense that this morbid fear was not a symptom of depression. Instead, it seemed to be an underlying issue that was an important cause of the anxious depression. I wondered what his fear was about. My own idea was that, on some unconscious level, he probably was aware of a life-threatening situation somewhere within his body. If this were the case, then the threat of approaching death had precipitated earlier unfinished business. I had no hard medical evidence for my intuition whatsoever, but I experienced countertransference wishes never to see him again, and I erroneously scheduled him on one occasion.

I suspected that the therapeutic relationship had become a hologram for Jonas' internal situation (feeling thrown away and not being able to look at it) and that, with careful work, it could be turned around and made holographic for information that would lead to the resolution of his situation. In time the story of a man with many intrapsychic difficulties and a lifelong history of a succession of symptoms emerged. When Jonas was a young man, his favorite brother, a Jesuit priest, had died at an early age of a cerebral aneurysm. This experience was pivotal in his life because this brother had represented stability to him in a severely dysfunctional family. Jonas' father had been alcoholic, and his mother had been quite disturbed and unavailable.

I introduced Jonas to self-hypnosis and encouraged him to fight his depressive symptoms and resocialize. I made audiotapes of hypnotic sessions for him to use at home for self-hypnosis. Ego-strengthening techniques including Inner Strength (McNeal & Frederick, 1992) and internal self-soothing (McNeal & Frederick, 1994) were used. The tapes of these inductions served double duty as transitional objects and experiences (Baker, 1994; McNeal & Frederick, 1994). Jonas' fear of death diminished dramatically. He began to feel and act better, and he eagerly looked forward to our talks. I had given him an adequate holding environment. He still seemed to be walking on eggs, however, and we discussed how one part of a personality could have one point of view and a certain set of feelings, while another part might have another. It came as no real surprise to either of us when Jonas was finally diagnosed with advanced bronchogenic carcinoma.

Although Jonas spoke of the Simonton method and visualization techniques, and of friends who had achieved cures in this way, his heart was not in any of it. His language and the nature of my countertransference responses within the hypnotherapeutic relationship led me to believe that he felt overwhelmed by his physical illness and was already looking spontaneously at an earthly future that existed for others but not for Jonas, as he would be dead and gone. We talked openly about this, and I conducted a life review with him. He was a man who had brought joy and laughter to millions of people. We focused on this and the many other contributions he had made to the world during the course of his life. It became as clear to Jonas as it was to me that he had been an extremely generative man in Erik Erikson's sense (Erikson, 1959). I decided to continue to use indirect approaches with ego states. Jonas and I talked about how stronger parts of his personality could help more childlike parts with their fears and how more spiritual parts could also help the entire inner family. I seeded our conversations with brief anecdotes, sometimes only a sentence or two long, that had transpersonal implications. For example, one day I simply said, "When I look out at the lake and the mountains, I know I am part of it all." Jonas nodded his head.

We also discussed practical ways in which some of his concerns for his wife could be managed after he had died. We were now able to use the words death and dying. Throughout this phase of his treatment, we continued to use ego-strengthening techniques including the powerful Inner Strength technique (McNeal & Frederick, 1993).

Within the therapeutic relationship, Jonas was given a combination of ego-strengthening, direct interpretations, indirect Ego State Therapy, and education for letting go. As he turned to me to experience the kind of close and unconditional relationship he had been unable to have with his mother I provided him with a number of transitional experiences. His interests began to turn to the spiritual dimension. I noticed that I had not felt reluctant to see Jonas for some time. My comfort with him increased dramatically. As he was able to mature and integrate personality parts, we grew quite close. Finally, I gave Jonas a tape I had once been asked to make for a cancer hospital in London. The tape contained many ego-strengthening suggestions and metaphors for transformation and letting go. Jonas listened to this tape at home, and several hours later died quietly and peacefully in his sleep, much sooner than his family or physicians had expected. His death had occurred within an atmosphere of integrity rather than despair (Erikson, 1959).

The Importance of an Open Mind

A description of stages through which cancer patients progress can be applied with modification to many patients with terminal illnesses. In general, cancer patients can be divided into those who show no remission and do not survive at all and those who survive for varying periods of time. Within this latter group are those who have acute remissions, those who have extended remissions, and those who have enduring remissions also known as cures (Fleishman, 1994).

Many terminally ill patients come to the attention of a therapist because of depression, delirium, and other psychological manifestations associated with their illnesses. Current psychiatric practice does not offer much to the terminally ill patient beyond support and compassion. Breitbart (1994) admonished the medical profession that the priorities in the care of patients with advanced cancer should be symptom control and supportive care. This point of view is laudable as far as it goes; there is no doubt that far too many patients are left to die in humiliation and pain. What is ignored in this pure medical model is the active and dynamic work that many terminally ill patients need—may require—before they can die peacefully. It is fortunate that, within the therapeutic relationship, the patient and the therapist have the opportunity to discover together what it is that the patient truly needs. The therapist who works with the terminally ill in this fashion must be free of prejudice that either life or death is necessarily a desirable outcome. Both aspects of the life cycle must be seen as having equal importance. This freedom will allow the therapist to utilize the therapeutic relationship to help the patient discover the nature of her framework.

Within the therapeutic relationship, there are many sources of information about the direction the patient wishes to take. Among them are ideodynamic signaling (used in a tactful manner and not with direct questions about living and dying, initially), the programming of dreams (Peter, 1994), the use of the active imagination, ego-state exploration, and careful examination of the transference and countertransference.

The Role of Ego-Strengthening

Ego-strengthening is of the utmost importance with terminally ill patients. These patients require every bit of available strength, and then more, to confront their momentous life and death decisions and issues. In the case of Jonas, the role of ego-strengthening was particularly important because it was necessary for the therapist to function as a transitional object and supplier of transitional experiences (Baker, 1983b, 1994; McNeal & Frederick, 1997) as well as a container to hold many of Jonas' affects and impulses for him until he was strong enough to deal with them (Baker & McColley, 1982). I (CF) believe that at times our alliance was *fusional* (Diamond, 1983, 1984) so that growth could occur at the earliest developmental level for Jonas. The patient who has been sufficiently strengthened is able to tune in to unconscious information about where she needs to go; that is, which perspective she shall embrace.

Hypnotic Age Progressions

The anxious therapist, like the anxious patient, would like to have a crystal ball. Everyone could feel more comfortable knowing what was ahead. However, the use of formal hypnotic age progressions is usually contraindicated for determining life versus "death" framework orientations with patients formally diagnosed as terminally ill. This is true for several reasons. Severe anxiety about dying can, at times, activate needs to overcontrol, thus allowing the conscious mind to enter the process and produce inaccurate or confusing material. Even accurate perceptions at this stage, if negative, could be quite disruptive to the therapeutic process when they are premature. However, the therapist must be vigilant for spontaneous age progressions as they can supply information that may be quite helpful in understanding the patient. For example, a patient who says: "What will happen to Cathy after I'm gone?" is producing a spontaneous age progression whose future orientation is toward her death. The inauspicious use of hypnotic age progressions, once a medical sentence has been given to the patient, can be extremely dangerous. A patient not ready to die and in denial might not be able to cope with the sight of herself in a coffin early in treatment.

With regard to the *sentence*, however, ideomotor signals may be quite helpful when used with patients who have a good potential for recovery, but whose early life and/or trauma issues may make them extremely susceptible to suggestions made by a medical authority. In this kind of situation, the medical authority becomes the witch doctor, and the diagnosis-prognosis becomes the witch doctor's curse. Ideomotor work can help identify any connections between the condemning medical expert and analogous (in the mind of the patient) childhood experiences.

Frederick and Phillips (1992) have used unstructured hypnotic age progressions as urgent interventions with patients with acute psychosomatic disorders. The terminally ill patient is a good candidate for age progressions once the life or death framework has been clearly established. We suggest caution in the extreme for using them too early in treatment. Direct ideomotor questioning about commitment to life and healing must also be avoided early in treatment. Such approaches only reflect the anxiety of the therapist. They unnecessarily and inhumanely pressure the patient, and can be devastating to her.

Later in treatment, formal hypnotic age progressions become valuable therapeutic tools. For patients aimed toward life as well as those aimed toward death, they can be ego-strengthening, integrating, and prognostic for how the treatment is going (Phillips & Frederick, 1992). Like Inner Strength (McNeal & Frederick, 1993; Frederick & McNeal, 1993), they frequently provide patients, and at times ego states, with experiences they identify as transpersonal. Such experiences infuse extraordinary energy into the therapeutic process. Levitan (1985) has reported utilizing formal, structured hypnotic age progressions known as *hypnotic death rehearsal* with the terminally ill. This is a desensitizing procedure that has been reported to be useful with certain patients, but it is a technique with which neither of us has personal experience. We recommend that it be considered only with patients who have been carefully selected and then with great caution. We believe that it can be of great benefit to patients to discuss openly with them what they think death will be like for them.

At this point, patients may wish to discuss their transpersonal thoughts and feelings. Because the dying patient is moving into a new identity, the therapist should be aware that there may be evidences of the transcendent function at work. As with the development of new identity and the transpersonal self, the transcendent function "… mediates opposites—real and imaginary, rational and irrational, and conscious and unconscious" (Cwick, 1991, p. 106). "It facilitates a transition from one psychological attitude or condition to another" (Samuels, Shorter, & Plaut, 1986, p. 150). Thus, it helps bridge the gap between the personal and the transpersonal, between life and death.

Other Ego-Strengthening Uses of the Hypnotic Relationship

Ego State Therapy. We frequently use the ego-state approach (Watkins & Watkins, 1997) with terminally ill patients. Because the goal of Ego State Therapy, integration, is a state of harmony and co-consciousness among the parts, ego-state interventions can effect crucial differences in the patient's being able to achieve necessary developmental tasks before dying, or continuing to live, whichever the case may be. The patient who is more integrated can often mobilize herself into making important and necessary decisions.

Ego-state work can be critical with a patient who really wants to fight for life but has one or several frightened and paralyzed child ego states or a demonic state that thinks she should be punished with death. By the same token, it can be invaluable with a patient who is ready to die but is unable to prepare herself for that great transition because the loss of self is so terrifying to some child ego states. The utilization of Internal Self Helpers (Allison, 1974; Comstock, 1991) as well as observer states (Watkins & Watkins, 1997) can facilitate both decision making as well as the maturational and other work that must follow it.

With some patients Ego State Therapy is of great assistance with transpersonal or spiritual issues (Phillips & Frederick, 1995). We believe that therapists should speak with dying patients about their views concerning an afterlife. Ego-state conflict can exist on this level, and it is important to the dying patient to have such conflicts resolved.

Holographic Transference and Countertransference. Another valuable way of utilizing the hypnotherapeutic relationship was described in the case of Jonas. Smith (1990) has given us a model of what transpires within the hypnotherapeutic relationship as a holographic paradigm for what is going on within the patient. Frederick (1995a, 1995c) has extended this concept so that what is experienced as having to do with the patient or in the countertransference may also be holographic in some way for what is present in family processes or among the patient's healthcare givers who, like ego states, may or may not be in conflict with one another. Observations about the patient's family and its interactions, about what is going on within the immediate health care team, and about the nature of transferences and countertransferences may be intensely relevant to understanding what is going on with the patient.

For the patient who is moving toward life, the therapeutic relationship can be the matrix for beginning lifestyle changes, stress management, or hypnoanalytic work; it can be a school for visualization and ego-strengthening as well as for transpersonal experiences that cast living into a new and transformed light. For many seriously ill patients, the therapeutic relationship may be used to introduce techniques that can afford the patient help with pain management and with treatment side effects such as those of radiation therapy and chemotherapy. It can help patients adjust to dismaying consequences of surgery that may mutilate, such as amputations and colostomies, and it can assist in the restoration of self-esteem that has been damaged by the ravages of devastating illness. It can be a vehicle for the use of active imagination in the resolution of family and other dynamic problems and as a conveyance for prayer and spiritual experiences.

For some terminally ill patients confronting death the therapeutic relationship may be the container for many affects and impulses. The fusional alliance (Diamond, 1983) and transitional experiences (McNeal & Frederick, 1997; Smith, 1990) may accelerate growth spurts that allow the patient to progress into the realm of the transpersonal. Within the therapeutic relationship, the patient can examine those forces that may propel him in the direction of choosing to end his life voluntarily or choosing not to. It can be a locus where these choices can be affirmed, and it can be a safe place for the patient to feel and work through anticipatory grief over losing himself as it is now, as well as losing current relationships. Within the therapeutic relationship, the patient has an opportunity to discover who he truly is, and to find what is of importance for living and dying. In interactive trance (Gilligan, 1987) the therapist can share all of this with the patient: as a facilitator, container, nourisher, helper, and witness.

Case Example: Nora

I (CF) had known Nora since she came to me for stress management after she had had surgery for a particularly aggressive type of breast cancer. When she returned, she was terminally ill and desperately seeking a radical procedure—stem cell rescue. Unfortunately, Nora was unable to have this procedure as she had developed brain metastases. Together we worked on the issues she needed to solve before she died: Her sorrow at leaving her husband, her troubled relationship with her daughters, and her rage for her glamorous, talented, famous, and rejecting narcissistic mother.

One day she was assisted to my office by her husband. The three of us discussed some practical matters briefly, as I had made a commitment to Nora to be with her as she negotiated the new passage she faced, and a few home visits might be necessary. Then Al retired to the waiting room.

"I'm ready for it," Nora told me. She was calmly smiling. "It came to me while I was watching Maya Angelou on television. She said you should make a space, a great big space so wide" (She held her arms as far apart as she could) "to let the spirit, or whatever you want to call it, God, in! And I have! I'm ready. Look at my fingernails. For the first time in my life they're not bitten off."

Nora's nails were long and lovely. "All of my affairs are in order. I even have my memorial service planned ... I want to ask you something. You don't have to answer if you don't want to ... How old are you? ... You know if we had met under different circumstances we would have been ... "

I answered, "... the best of friends."

"Yes," said Nora, "that's it. As it is, I really need to thank you for all of this instead, and I really thank you."

When Nora left that day I knew that I had been speaking with someone new. Her ego had been strengthened, and her transpersonal self stood firmly in its place.

Appendix

The plethora of offerings for training in the field of hypnosis could be confusing to therapists who would like to acquire or to amplify a knowledge of hypnosis. One reason for this is that in the United States many organizations and individuals have the legal right to train in hypnosis. In the state of California, for example, a high school graduate who takes certain courses in hypnosis and passes an examination given by the state can become certified as a hypnotherapist under the Department of Secondary Education. We believe this term to be extremely misleading, as hypnosis training alone does not turn anyone into a therapist.

The psychotherapist who seeks hypnosis training will have no difficulty, however. There are several professional organizations whose membership consists only of trained psychotherapists, physicians, nurses, and dentists who utilize hypnosis in clinical practice and/or research. A term frequently associated with the hypnosis training that is received in such groups is "medical hypnosis." Its use serves to separate this kind of training and use from those of lay hypnosis.

It is possible to obtain a basic knowledge of hypnosis and the tools to begin to use it in clinical practice with 20 to 40 hours of workshop training. After an intermediate workshop of the same length has been taken, the professional is able to move into a wide array of advanced material. The rate at which training is acquired is a function of the individual. It is possible to move into advanced training within a six-month period. Most professionals proceed at a slower pace. We recommend the following organizations for the training of psychotherapists and other professionals:

The American Society of Clinical Hypnosis
East Devon Avenue, Suite 291
Des Plaines, IL 60018
(847) 297–3317

The American Society of Clinical Hypnosis (ASCH) was founded by Milton Erickson and his associates because they felt there was a need for a society that was more clinically oriented than The Society for Clinical and Experimental

Hypnosis whose membership was more geared to academia and research. Both the authors are American Society of Clinical Hypnosis Approved Consultants in Clinical Hypnosis. One of us is on their Regional Workshop Faculty. The Regional Workshops are taught by the American Society of Clinical Hypnosis a number of times a year in various cities in the U.S., Canada, and Mexico. The American Society of Clinical Hypnosis trains at basic, intermediate, and advanced levels. It also certifies licensed professionals in hypnosis and qualifies consultants in clinical hypnosis. These consultants participate in a mentoring consultant program. At its annual meeting workshops are taught at all levels, and there is a scientific program as well. The society publishes *The American Journal of Clinical Hypnosis*.

***

The Society for Clinical and Experimental Hypnosis
3905 Vincennes Road, Suite 304
Indianapolis, IN 46268
(800) 214–1738

The Society for Clinical and Experimental Hypnosis (SCEH) was the first national society for professionals (doctors, dentists, and research scientists). It has a heavy emphasis on the scientific and research aspects of hypnosis. However it does offer clinical training in hypnosis at several levels. This society also has an annual meeting that features both workshops and scientific presentations. It publishes the *International Journal of Clinical and Experimental Hypnosis*.

***

Local Societies

There are many local professional hypnosis societies in existence at this time. They are usually affiliated with the American Society of Clinical Hypnosis, and a number of them have Society for Clinical and Experimental Hypnosis affiliations as well. Training at the local level can be quite good. These societies also offer a collegiate atmosphere for the sharing and development of ideas and case discussion. The American Society of Clinical Hypnosis can tell the reader the location of the closest component society.

***

The European Society of Hypnosis

If you like to travel, you might wish to consider the European Society of Hypnosis. It has meetings every three years. We have participated in several of these meetings. Again, there is a great deal of workshop training, and there are abundant scientific offerings. Recent meetings have been in Konstanz (Germany), Vienna, and Budapest. The next meeting (1999) will be held in Amsterdam.

***

The International Society of Hypnosis
Level I, South Wing, A & RMC, Repat Campus
Locked Bag I, West Heidelberg VIC 3081

AUSTRALIAThe International Society of Hypnosis (ISH) offers opportunities for travel and contact with professionals who use hypnosis around the globe. Their annual meetings can be quite exciting. We have both presented at ISH meetings in Jerusalem, Melbourne, and San Diego.

***

The Milton H. Erickson Foundation
3606 N. 24th St.
Phoenix, AZ 85016–6500
(602) 956–6196

Therapists with particular interests in the thinking and techniques of Milton H. Erickson find the Erickson Foundation an excellent place to get training in Ericksonian hypnosis as well as to hear clinical presentations. The annual meeting is in Erickson's home town, Phoenix, Arizona. The Foundation puts on other meetings during the year. The Erickson Foundation publishes the Milton H. Erickson Foundation Newsletter.

***

Local Erickson Foundations

Just as there are American Society of Clinical Hypnosis component societies on the local level, so also are there local Erickson societies. The parent organization in Phoenix can supply information about their locations.

References

Aber, J. L., & Allen, J. P. (1987). Effects of maltreatment on young children's socioemotional development: An attachment theory perspective. *Developmental Psychology, 23*, 406–414.

Achterberg, J. (1985). *Imagery and healing*. Boston: New Science.

Alexander, F. (1930). The psychoanalysis of the total personality. *Nervous and Mental Disease Monographs, 32.*

Alexander, F. (1950). *Psychosomatic medicine*. New York: Norton.

Allison, R. B. (1974). A new treatment approach for multiple personalities. *American Journal of Clinical Hypnosis, 17*, 15–32.

Allison, R. B., & Schwarz, T. (1980). *Minds in many pieces*. New York: Rawson, Wade.

Alman, B., & Carney, R. E. (1980). Consequences of direct and indirect suggestion on success of posthypnotic behavior. *American Journal of Clinical Hypnosis, 23*, 112–118.

Alman, B. M., & Lambrou, P. (1992). *Self-hypnosis: The complete manual for health and self change* (2nd ed.). New York: Brunner/Mazel.

Alpert, A. (1954). Observations on the treatment of emotionally disturbed children in a therapeutic center. *Psychoanalytic Study of the Child, 9*, 334–343.

American Psychiatric Association. (1987). *Diagnostic and statistical manual of mental disorders* (3rd rev. ed.). Washington, DC: American Psychiatric Press.

American Psychiatric Association. (1994). *Diagnostic and statistical manual of mental disorders* (4th ed.). Washington, DC: American Psychiatric Press.

Angel, K. (1967). On symbiosis and pseudosymbiosis. *Journal of the American Psychoanalytic Association, 15*, 294–316.

Ansbacher, H. L., & Ansbacher, R. R. (Eds.). (1985). *The individual psychology of Alfred Adler*. New York: Basic Books.

Aroaz, D. L. (1981). Negative self-hypnosis. *Journal of Contemporary Psychotherapy, 12*, 45–52.

Assagioli, R. (1965). *Psychosynthesis: A manual of principles and techniques*. New York: Penguin.

Atwood, G., & Stolerow, R. (1992). *Contexts of being: The intersubjective foundations of psychological life*. Hillsdale, NJ: The Analytic Press.

Azima, H., & Wittkower, E. D. (1956). Gratifications of basic needs in schizophrenia. *Psychiatry, 19*, 121–129.

Baer, L. (1993). Behavior therapy for obsessive compulsive disorder in the office-based practice. *The Journal of Clinical Psychiatry, 54*, 10–14.

Baker, E. L. (1981). An hypnotherapeutic approach to enhance object relatedness in psychotic patients. *International Journal of Clinical and Experimental Hypnosis, 124,* 136–147.

Baker, E. L. (1983a). Resistance in hypnotherapy of primitive states: Its meaning and management. *International Journal of Clinical and Experimental Hypnosis, 31,* 82–89.

Baker, E. L. (1983b). The use of hypnotic dreaming in the treatment of the borderline patient: Some thoughts on resistance and transitional phenomena. *The International Journal of Clinical and Experimental Hypnosis, 31,* 19–27.

Baker, E. L. (1985). Ego psychology and hypnosis: Contemporary theory and practice. In *Psychotherapy in private practice* (*Vol. 3,* pp. 115–122). New York: Haworth.

Baker, E. L. (1994, March). *The therapist as transitional object in intensive hypnotherapy.* Paper presented at the annual meeting of the American Society of Clinical Hypnosis, Philadelphia, PA.

Baker, E. L., & McColley, S. (1982). Therapeutic strategies for the aftercare of the schizophrenic: An object relations perspective. *International Journal of Partial Hospitalization, 1,* 119–129.

Ballenger, J. C., Burrows, G. D., & Dupont, R. L. (1988). Alprazolam in panic disorder and agoraphobia: Results from a multicenter trial: I. Efficacy in short-term treatment. *Archives of General Psychiatry, 43,* 413–442.

Bandler, R., & Grinder, J. (1975). *Patterns of the hypnotic techniques of Milton H. Erickson, M.D.* (*Vol. 1*). Cupertino, CA: Meta Publications.

Bandler, R., & Grinder, J. (1979). *Frogs into princes: Neuro-linguistic programming.* Moab, UT: Real People Press.

Bandura, A. (1977). Self-efficacy: Toward a unifying theory of behavior change. *Psychological Review, 84,* 191–215.

Banyai, E. I. (1980). *A new way to induce a hypnotic-like altered state of conscious: Active alert induction.* Paper presented at the fourth meeting of Psychologists from the Danubian Countries, Budapest.

Banyai, E. I. (1985). A social psychophysiological approach to the understanding of hypnosis: The interaction between the hypnotist and the subject. *Hypnos, 12,* 186–210.

Banyai, E. I. (1991). Toward a social psychobiological model of hypnosis. In S. J. Lynn & J. W. Rhue (Eds.), *Theories of hypnosis: Current modes and perspectives* (pp. 564–598). New York: Guilford Press.

Banyai, E. I., & Hilgard, E. (1976). A comparison of active-alert hypnotic induction with traditional relaxation induction. *Journal of Abnormal Psychology, 85,* 218–224.

Banyai, E. I., Zseni, A., & Tury, F. (1993). "Active–alert" hypnosis in psychotherapy. In J. Rhue, S. Lynn, & I. Kirsh (Eds.), *Handbook of clinical hypnosis* (pp. 271–290). Washington, DC: American Psychological Association.

Barber, J. (1980). Hypnosis and the unhypnotizable. *American Journal of Clinical Hypnosis, 23,* 4–9.

Barlow, D. H. (1997). Cognitive-behavioral therapy for panic disorder: Current Status. *The Journal of Clinical Psychiatry, 58* [suppl. 2], 32–36.

Barlow, D. H., & Cerny, J. A. (1988). *Psychological treatment of panic.* New York: Guilford.

Beahrs, J. O. (1982a). Understanding Erickson's approach. In J. K. Zeig (Ed.), *Ericksonian approaches to hypnosis and psychotherapy* (pp. 58–84). New York: Brunner/Mazel.

Beahrs, J. O. (1982b). *Unity and multiplicity*. New York: Brunner/Mazel.

Beahrs, J. O. (1986). *Limits of scientific psychiatry: The role of uncertainty in mental health*. New York: Brunner/Mazel.

Beck, A. G., & Emery, G. (1985). *Anxiety disorders and phobias: A cognitive perspective*. New York: Basic Books.

Benedek, T. (1949). The psychosomatic implications of the primary-unit: mother–child. *American Journal of Orthopsychiatry, 19,* 642–654.

Berne, E. (1961). *Transactional analysis in psychotherapy*. New York: Grove.

Bibring, E. (1937). On the theory of the results of psychoanalysis. *International Journal of Psychoanalysis, 18,* 170–189.

Binet, A. (1977). *On double consciousness*. Washington, DC: University Publications of America. (Original work published 1890)

Binet, A. (1977). *Alterations of personality*. Washington, DC: University Publications of America. (Original work published 1896)

Blatt, S. J., & Wild, C. M. (1976). *Schizophrenia: A developmental analysis*. New York: Academic Press.

Bliss, E. L. (1984). A symptom profile of patients with multiple personalities, including MMPI results. *Journal of Nervous and Mental Disease, 172,* 197–202.

Borges, J. L. (1964). A new refutation of time. In E. Editores (Trans.), *Labyrinths: Selected stories and other writings* (pp. 217–334). New York: New Directions. (Original work published 1941)

Bowen, M. (1960). A family concept of schizophrenia. In D. D. Jackson (Ed.), *The etiology of schizophrenia* (pp. 346–372). New York: Basic Books.

Bowen, M. (1978). *Family therapy in clinical practice*. New York: Jacob Aronson.

Bower, G. H. (1981). Mood and memory. *American Psychologist, 36,* 129–148.

Bower, G. H., & Gilligan, S. G. (1979). Remembering information related to one's self. *Journal of Research in Personality 13,* 420–432.

Bowers, K. S., & Hilgard, E. R. (1988). Some complexities in understanding memory. In H. M. Pettinati (Ed.), *Hypnosis and memory* (pp. 3–18). New York: Guilford.

Bowlby, J. (1988). *A secure base: Clinical applications of attachment theory*. London: Routledge.

Boyer, B. L., & Giovacchini, P. L. (1967). *Psychoanalytic treatment of characterological and schizophrenic disorders*. New York: Science House.

Braun, B. G. (Ed.). (1986). *Treatment of multiple personality disorder*. Washington, DC: American Psychiatric Press.

Braun, B. G. (1988). The BASK model of dissociation: II. Treatment. *Dissociation, 1,* 16–84.

Breitbart, W. (1994, May). *Symposium on psychiatric oncology*. Paper presented at the annual meeting of the American Psychiatric Association, Philadelphia, PA.

Bresler, D. E. (1990). Meeting an inner advisor. In D. C. Hammond (Ed.), *Handbook of therapeutic suggestions and metaphors* (pp. 318–320). New York: Norton.

Breuer, J., & Freud, S. (1964). Studies on hysteria. In J. Strachey (Ed. & Trans.), *The standard edition of the complete psychological works of Sigmund Freud* (*Vol. 2,* pp. 1–181). London: Hogarth. (Original work published 1893–1895)

Briere, J. D., & Runtz, M. (1988). Multivariate correlates of childhood psychological and physical maltreatment among university women. *Child Abuse and Neglect, 12,* 331–341.

Brigham, D. D. (1994). *Imagery for getting well*. New York: Norton.

Brown, D. P., & Fromm, E. (1986). *Hypnotherapy and hypnoanalysis*. Hillsdale, NJ: Lawrence Erlbaum Associates.

Brown, D. P., Scheflin, A. W., & Hammond, D. C. (1997) *Memory, trauma, treatment, and the law*. New York: Norton

Callahan, R. (1985). *Five minute phobia cure*. Wilmington, DE: Enterprise.

Callahan, R. (1987). Successful treatment of phobias and anxiety by telephone and radio. *Collected papers of the International College of Applied Kinesiology*, Winter.

Calnan, R. B. (1977). Hypnotherapeutic ego-strengthening. *Australian Journal of Clinical Hypnosis, 5*, 105–118.

Campbell, J. (Ed.). (1971). *The portable Jung*. New York: Viking Press.

Cannon, W. (1953). *Bodily changes in pain, hunger, fear, and rage* (2nd ed.). Boston: Charles T. Branford.

Cannon, W. (1957). "Voodoo" death. *Psychosomatic Medicine, 19*, 182–190.

Cardeña, E. (1994). The domain of dissociation. In S. J. Lynn & J. W. Rhue (Eds.), *Dissociation: clinical and theoretical perspectives* (pp. 15–31). New York: Guilford.

Cardeña, E., & Spiegel, D. (1993). Dissociative reactions to the San Francisco bay area earthquake of 1989. *American Journal of Psychiatry, 150*, 474–478.

Caul, D., Sachs, R. G., & Braun, B. G. (1986). Group therapy in treatment of multiple personality disorder. In B. G. Braun (Ed.), *The treatment of multiple personality disorder* (pp. 145–156). Washington, DC: American Psychiatric Press.

Cheek, D. (1959). Unconscious perception of meaningful sounds during surgical anesthesia as revealed under hypnosis. *American Journal of Clinical Hypnosis, 1*, 101–113.

Chefetz, R. A. (1996, November). *The erotic transference and countertransference: The view through the sado-masochistic matrix*. Paper presented at the 13th International Fall Conference of the International Society for the Study of Dissociation, San Francisco, CA.

Chevreul, M. (1854). *De la baguette divinatoire, du pendule explorateur, de tables tournant, au point de vue de l'histoire, de la critique et de la méthode expérimentale*. Paris: Mallet-Bachelier.

Chodron, P. (1991). *The wisdom of no escape*. Boston: Shambala.

Chu, J. A., & Dill, D. L. (1990). Dissociative symptoms in relation to childhood physical and sexual abuse. *American Journal of Psychiatry, 147*, 887–892.

Clarke, J. C., & Jackson, A. (1983). *Hypnosis and behavior therapy: The treatment of anxiety and phobias*. New York: Springer.

Clements, F. E. (1932). Primitive concepts of disease. *University of California Publications in American Archaeology and Ethnology, 32*, 185–252.

Coe, W. C., & Sarbin, T. R. (1966). An experimental demonstration of hypnosis as role enactment. *Journal of Abnormal Psychology, 71*, 400–416.

Coe, W. C., & Sarbin, T. R. (1991). Role theory: Hypnosis from a dramaturgical and narrational perspective. In S. J. Lynn & J. W. Rhue (Eds.), *Theories of hypnosis: Current modes and perspectives* (pp. 303–323). New York: Guilford.

Comstock, C. (1987). Internal self helpers or centers. *Integration, 3(1)*, 3–12.

Comstock, C. (1991). The inner self helper and concepts of inner guidance: Historical antecedents, its role within dissociation, and clinical utilization. *Dissociation, 4*, 165–177.

Comstock, C., & Vickery, D. (1993). The therapist as victim: A preliminary discussion. *Dissociation, 5*, 155–158.

Cooper, L. (1948). Time distortion in hypnosis: I. *Bulletin of the Georgetown University Medical Center, 1*, 214–221.

Cooper, L., & Erickson, M. H. (1950). Time distortion in hypnosis: II. *Bulletin of the Georgetown University Medical Center, 41*, 50–68.

Cooper, L., & Erickson, M. H. (1959). *Time distortion in hypnosis.* Baltimore: Williams & Wilkins.

Coué, E. (1922). *Self-mastery through conscious autosuggestion.* New York: American Library Service.

Courtois, C. A. (1988). *Healing the incest wound: Adult survivors in therapy.* New York: Norton.

Cousins, N. (1983). *The healing heart.* New York: Norton.

Cowley, D. S. (1992). Alcohol abuse, substance abuse, and panic disorder. *American Journal of Medicine, 92 [suppl. A]*, 415–485.

Craik, F. I. M., & Lockhart, R. S. (1972). Levels of processing: A framework for memory research. *Journal of Verbal Learning and Verbal Behavior, 11*, 671–684.

Crasilneck, H. B., & Hall, J. A. (1975). *Clinical hypnosis: Principles and applications.* New York: Grune & Stratton.

Crits-Christoph, P., Barber, J. P., Miller, N. E., & Beebe, K. (1993). Evaluating insight. In N. E. Miller, L. Luborsky, J. P. Barber, & J. P. Docherty (Eds.), *Psychodynamic treatment research: A handbook for clinical practice* (pp. 407–466). New York: Basic Books.

Curtis, J. (1996, November). *Table talk: Metaphors for internal healing of ego states.* Paper presented at the annual meeting of the International Society for the Study of Dissociation, San Francisco, CA.

Cwick, A. J. (1989). *Jung, active imagination and hypnosis.* Unpublished manuscript.

Cwick, A. J. (1991). Active imagination as imaginal play-space. In N. Schwartz-Salant & M. Stein (Eds.), *Liminality and transitional phenomena* (pp. 99–114). Wilmette, IL: Chiron.

D'Eslon, C. (1780). *Observations sur le magnétisme animal.* London & Paris: Didot.

De Shazer, S. (1978). Brief hypnotherapy of two sexual dysfunctions: The crystal ball technique. *American Journal of Clinical Hypnosis, 20*, 203–208.

De Shazer, S. (1985). *Keys to solution in brief therapy.* New York: Norton.

De Shazer, S. (1988). *Clues: Investigating solutions in brief therapy.* New York: Norton.

Diamond, M. J. (1983, August). *Reflections on the interactive nature of the hypnotic experience: On the relational dimensions of hypnosis.* Presented at the 91st annual convention of the American Psychological Association, Anaheim, CA.

Diamond, M. J. (1984). It takes two to tango: Some thoughts on the neglected importance of the hypnotist in an interactive hypnotherapeutic relationship. *American Journal of Clinical Hypnosis, 27*, 3–13.

Diamond, M. J. (1986). Hypnotically augmented psychotherapy: The unique contributions of the hypnotically trained clinician. *American Journal of Clinical Hypnosis, 28*, 238–247.

Dickey, T., Nungary, V., & Frederick, C. (1998, March). *You must be present to win: Attentional training for the management of serious ego-state problems.* Paper presented at the annual meeting of the American Society of Clinical Hypnosis, Ft. Worth, TX.

Dimond, R. E. (1981). Hypnotic treatment of a kidney dialysis patient. *American Journal of Clinical Hypnosis, 23*, 284–288.

Dolan, Y. M. (1991). *Resolving sexual abuse*. New York: Norton.

Dossey, L. (1982). *Space, time, and medicine*. Boston: Shambala.

Edelstien, M. G. (1981). *Trauma, trance, and transformation: A clinical guide to hypnotherapy*. New York: Brunner/Mazel.

Edgette, J. H., & Edgette, J. S. (1995). *The handbook of hypnotic phenomena in psychotherapy*. New York: Brunner/Mazel.

Edmonston, W. E., Jr. (1991). Anesis. In S. J. Lynn & J. W. Rhue (Eds.), *Theories of hypnosis: Current modes and perspectives* (pp. 197–237). New York: Guilford.

Einstein, A. (1905). Zur Elektrodynamik bewegter Körper. *Annalen der Physik, 18(ser. 4)*, 549–560.

Einstein, A. (1916). Die Grundlage der allgemeinen Relativitätstheorie. *Annalen der Physik, 49(4)*, 769–822., pt. 2, 831–839.

Eisen, M. R., & Fromm, E. (1983). The clinical use of self-hypnosis in hypnotherapy: Tapping the functions of imagery and adaptive regression. *International Journal of Clinical and Experimental Hypnosis, 31*, 243–254.

Ellenberger, H. F. (1970). *The discovery of the unconscious*. New York: Basic Books.

Elmer, E. (1977). A follow-up study of traumatized children. *Pediatrics, 59*, 273–279.

Elmer, E., & Gregg, G. S. (1967). Developmental characteristics of abused children. *Pediatrics, 40*, 596–602.

Emmelkamp, P. M. G. (1979). The behavioral study of clinical phobias. *Progress in Behavior Modification, 8*, 55–125.

Erickson, M. H. (1954). Pseudo-orientation in time as a hypnotherapeutic procedure. *Journal of Clinical and Experimental Hypnosis, 2*, 261–283.

Erickson, M. H. (1959). Further techniques of hypnosis. Utilization techniques. *American Journal of Clinical Hypnosis 2*, 3–21.

Erickson, M. H. (1961). Historical note on the hand levitation and other ideomotor techniques. *American Journal of Clinical Hypnosis, 3*, 196–199.

Erickson, M. H. (1965a). Hypnosis and examination panics. *American Journal of Clinical Hypnosis, 7*, 356–358.

Erickson, M. H. (1965b). The hypnotic corrective emotional experience. *American Journal of Clinical Hypnosis, 7*, 242–248.

Erickson, M. H. (1966). The interspersal hypnotic technique for symptom correction and pain control. *American Journal of Clinical Hypnosis, 8*, 198–209.

Erickson, M. H. (1979). *International congress on Ericksonian approaches to hypnosis and psychotherapy* [Brochure]. Phoenix, AZ: Milton H. Erickson Foundation.

Erickson, M. H. (1980). Hypnotic psychotherapy. In E. L. Rossi (Ed.), *The collected papers of Milton H. Erickson on hypnosis* (*Vol. 4*, pp. 35–48). New York: Irvington. (Original work published 1948)

Erickson, M. H. (1980a). Age regression: Two unpublished fragments of a student's study. In E. L. Rossi (Ed.), *The collected papers of Milton H. Erickson on hypnosis* (*Vol. 3*, pp. 104–111). New York: Irvington. (Original work published 1924–1931)

Erickson, M. H. (1980b). Hypnotic psychotherapy. In E. L. Rossi (Ed.), *The collected papers of Milton H. Erickson on hypnosis* (*Vol. 4*, pp. 35–48). New York: Irvington.

Erickson, M. H. (1980c). The clinical discovery of a dual personality. In E. L. Rossi (Ed.), *The collected papers of Milton H. Erickson on hypnosis* (*Vol. 3*, pp. 261–270). New York: Irvington. (Original work unpublished manuscript, circa 1940s)

Erickson, M. H. (1980d). The interspersal hypnotic technique for symptom correction and pain control. In E. L. Rossi (Ed.), *The collected papers of Milton H. Erickson on hypnosis* (*Vol. 4*, pp. 282–1279). New York: Irvington. (Original work published 1966)

Erickson, M. H., & Kubie, L. S. (1940). The translation of the cryptic automatic writing of one hypnotic subject by another in a trancelike dissociated state. *The Psychoanalytic Quarterly*, *9*, 51–63.

Erickson, M. H., & Kubie, L. S. (1980). The permanent relief of obsessional phobia by means of communications with an unsuspected dual personality. In E. L. Rossi (Ed.), *The collected papers of Milton H. Erickson on hypnosis* (*Vol. 3*, pp. 231–260). New York: Irvington. (Original work published 1939)

Erickson, M. H., & Rossi, E. L. (1976). Two level communication and the microdynamics of trance and suggestion. *American Journal of Clinical Hypnosis*, *18*, 153–171.

Erickson, M. H., & Rossi, E. L. (1977). Autohypnotic experiences of Milton H. Erickson. *American Journal of Clinical Hypnosis*, *20*, 36–54.

Erickson, M. H., & Rossi, E. L. (1979). *Hypnotherapy: An exploratory case book.* New York: Irvington.

Erickson, M. H., & Rossi, E. L. (1989). *The February Man: Evolving consciousness and identity in hypnotherapy.* New York: Brunner/Mazel.

Erickson, M. H., Rossi, E. L., & Rossi, S. I. (1976). *Hypnotic realities: The induction of clinical hypnosis and forms of indirect suggestion.* New York: Irvington.

Erikson, E. (1959). Identity and the life cycle, selected papers. In G. S. Klein (Ed.), *Psychological issues* (*Vol. 1*). New York: International Universities Press.

Erikson, E. (1964). *Insight and responsibility.* New York: Norton.

Escalona, S. K. (1962). The study of individual differences and the problem of state. *Journal of the American Academy of Child Psychiatry*, *1*, 11–37.

Ewin, D. M. (1983). Emergency room hypnosis for the burned patient. *American Journal of Clinical Hypnosis*, *26*, 5–8.

Fairbairn, W. R. D. (1952). Endopsychic structure considered in terms of object-relationships. In W. R. D. Fairbairn (Ed.), *Psychoanalytic studies of the personality* (pp. 82–136). London: Tavistock. (Original work published 1944)

Fairbairn, W. R. D. (1954). *An object relations theory of the personality.* New York: Basic Books.

Fairbairn, W. R. D. (1958). On the nature and aims of psychoanalytic treatment. *International Journal of Psychoanalysis*, *39*, 374–385.

Fawzy, F. I., Fawzy, N. W., Arndt, L. A., & Pasnau, R. O. (1995). Critical review of psychosocial interventions in cancer care. *Archives of General Psychiatry*, *52*, 100–113.

Fawzy, F. I., Fawzy, N. W., Hyun, C. S., Elashoff, R., Guthrie, D., Fahey, J. L., & Morton, D. L. (1993). Malignant melanoma: Effects of an early structured psychiatric intervention, coping, and affective state on recurrence and survival 6 years later. *Archives of General Psychiatry*, *50*, 681–689.

Federn, P. (1952). *Ego psychology and the psychoses.* New York: Basic Books.

Fenichel, O. (1941). *Problems of psychoanalytic technique.* Albany, NY: The Psychoanalytic Quarterly, Inc.

Ferenczi, S. (1949). Ten letters to Freud (J. Riviere, Trans.). *International Journal of Psychoanalysis*, *30*, 243–245.

Ferenczi, S. (1950). Introjection and transference. *Sex in Psychoanalysis*. New York: Basic Books. (Original work published 1909)

Figley, C. R. (Ed.). (1995). *Compassion fatigue: Coping with secondary traumatic stress disorder in those who treat the traumatized*. New York: Brunner/Mazel.

Figley, C. R., & Carbonell, J. (1995). *The "Active Ingredient" Project: The systematic demonstration of the most efficient treatments of PTSD, A research plan*. Tallahassee: Florida State University Psychosocial Stress Research Program and Clinical Laboratory.

Fine, C. (1993). A tactical integrationist perspective on the treatment of multiple personality disorder. In R. P. Kluft & C. G. Fine (Eds.), *Clinical perspectives on multiple personality disorder*. Washington, DC: American Psychiatric Press.

Fine, C. G. (1990). The cognitive sequelae of incest. In R. P. Kluft (Ed.), *Incest related syndromes of adult psychopathology*. Washington, DC: American Psychiatric Press.

Fink, D. (1993). Observations on the role of transitional objects and transitional phenomena in patients with multiple personality disorder. In R. P. Kluft & C. G. Fine (Eds.), *Clinical perspectives on multiple personality disorder* (pp. 241–251). Washington, DC: American Psychiatric Press.

Fish-Murray, C. C., Koby, E. V., & Van der Kolk, B. A. (1987). Evolving ideas: the effect of abuse on children's thought. In B. A. Van der Kolk (Ed.), *Psychological trauma* (pp. 89–110). Washington, DC: American Psychiatric Press.

Fleishman, S. (1994, May). *Symposium on psychiatric oncology*. Paper presented at the annual meeting of the American Psychiatric Association, Philadelphia, PA.

Fowler, W. L. (1961). Hypnosis and learning. *International Journal of Clinical and Experimental Hypnosis*, 9, 223–232.

Frank, A. (1990). Metapsychology. In B. Moore & B. Fine (Eds.), *Psycho-analysis: The major concepts* (pp. 508–520). New Haven, CT: Yale University Press.

Fraser, G. (1991). The dissociative table technique: A strategy of working with ego states in dissociative disorders and ego state therapy. *Dissociation*, 4, 205–213.

Fraser, G. A. (1993). Special treatment techniques to access the inner personality system of multiple personality disorder patients. *Dissociation*, 6, 193–198.

Frederick, C. (1990, March). *The rapid treatment of obsessive compulsive disorder with ego state therapy: A case study*. Paper presented at the annual meeting of the American Society of Clinical Hypnosis, Orlando, FL.

Frederick, C. (1992, April). *Bringing up baby: A developmental approach to the management and maturation of child ego states*. Paper presented at the annual meeting of the American Society of Clinical Hypnosis, Las Vegas, NV.

Frederick, C. (1993a). *Ego-strengthening techniques*. Unpublished workshop handout.

Frederick, C. (1993b). Pools and wellings: The resolution of refractory intermittent depression with ego-state therapy. *Hypnos*, 20, 221–228.

Frederick, C. (1993c, March). *Who's afraid of the big bad wolf: Ego-state therapy for panic disorder with and without agoraphobia*. Paper presented at the annual meeting of the American Society of Clinical Hypnosis, New Orleans, LA.

Frederick, C. (1994a). *Ego state therapy*. Unpublished workshop handout.

Frederick, C. (1994b). *Informed consent for hypnosis*. Unpublished document.

Frederick, C. (1994c). *Reconstructing the patient's history in psychodynamic hypnotherapy: Tradition and practice*. Unpublished workshop handout.

Frederick, C. (1994d, March). *The safety of the therapist: Aspects of the hypnotherapeutic relationship*. Paper presented at the annual meeting of the American Society of Clinical Hypnosis, Philadelphia, PA.

Frederick, C. (1994e). Silent partners: The hypnotherapeutic relationship with non-verbal ego states. *Hypnos, 21,* 141–149.

Frederick, C. (1994f). *Symptom removal.* Unpublished workshop handout.

Frederick, C. (1994g, March). *When weight means wait: The hypnotherapeutic treatment of eating disorders induced by ptsd.* Paper presented at the annual meeting of the American Society of Clinical Hypnosis, Philadelphia, PA.

Frederick, C. (1995a). A holographic approach to holism. *Journal of Interprofessional Care, 9,* 9–13.

Frederick, C. (1995b). *Ideodynamic healing and the mind-molecule-gene connection.* Unpublished workshop handout.

Frederick, C. (1995c). *Ideomotor signals: Getting started.* Unpublished workshop handout.

Frederick, C. (1995d, March). *Summoning the healing messenger of time: Hypnotic age progressions for psychosomatic and psychiatric emergencies.* Paper presented at the annual meeting of the American Society of Clinical Hypnosis. San Diego, CA.

Frederick, C. (1995e, March). *The internal family and the external family: Perspectives on family systems aspects of ego state therapy.* Paper presented at the annual meeting of the American Society of Clinical Hypnosis, San Diego, CA.

Frederick, C. (1996a). Functionaries, janissaries, and daemons: A differential approach to the management of malevolent ego states. *Hypnos, 23,* 37–47.

Frederick, C. (1996b). *Hypnotic facilitation of new identity formation.* Unpublished workshop handout.

Frederick, C. (1996c, March). *Liberating Sisyphus: Ego state therapy in the treatment of obsessive-compulsive disorder revisited.* Paper presented at the annual meeting of the American Society of Clinical Hypnosis, Orlando, FL.

Frederick, C. (1996d). *Memory, trauma, and dissociation.* Unpublished workshop handout.

Frederick, C. (1996e). *Stress diathesis model.* Unpublished workshop handout.

Frederick, C. (1996f, March). *Resolving overwhelming positive transferences in the therapeutic relationship with dissociative disorder patients.* Paper presented at the annual meeting of the American Society of Clinical Hypnosis, Orlando, FL.

Frederick, C. (1996g). *The activation of positive or helpful ego states.* Unpublished workshop handout.

Frederick, C. (1996h). *The facilitation of ideomotorically activated positive age regression.* Unpublished workshop handout.

Frederick, C. (1996i, March). *With a little help from our friends: Ego states as resources for ego-strengthening.* Paper presented at the annual meeting of the American Society of Clinical Hypnosis, Orlando, FL.

Frederick, C. (1997). Resolving overwhelming positive transferences in the hypnotherapeutic relationship with post-traumatic patients. *Hypnos, 24,* 82–93.

Frederick, C., & Kim, S. (1993). Heidi and the little girl: The creation of helpful ego states for the management of performance anxiety. *Hypnos: 20,* 49–58.

Frederick, C., & McNeal, S. (1993). From strength to strength: Inner strength with immature ego states. *American Journal of Clinical Hypnosis 35,* 250–256.

Frederick, C., & Morton, P. (1998, March). *Welcome to Oz: Ideodynamic healing and ego states.* Paper presented at the annual meeting of the American Society of Clinical Hypnosis, Ft. Worth, TX.

Frederick, C., & Phillips, M. (1992). The use of hypnotic age progressions as interventions with acute psychosomatic conditions. *American Journal of Clinical Hypnosis, 35,* 89–98.

Frederick, C., & Phillips, M. (1994). *Hypnosis and memory*. Unpublished workshop handout.

Frederick, C., & Phillips, M. (1996). Decoding mystifying signals: Translating symbolic communications of elusive ego-states. *American Journal of Clinical Hypnosis, 38*, 187–196.

French, G. D. (1993). *Traumatic incident reduction workshop manual*. Menlo Park, CA: IRM.

Freud, A. (1936). *The ego and the mechanisms of defense*. New York: International Universities Press. (Original work published 1936)

Freud, S. (1961). The dynamics of transference. In J. Strachey (Ed. & Trans.), *The standard edition of the complete works of Sigmund Freud* (*Vol. 12*, pp. 97–108). London: Hogarth. (Original work published 1912)

Freud, S. (1961). Beyond the pleasure principle. In J. Strachey (Ed. & Trans.), *The standard edition of the complete psychological works of Sigmund Freud* (*Vol. 18*, pp. 3–64). London: Hogarth. (Original work published 1920)

Freud, S. (1961). The ego and the id. In J. Strachey (Ed. & Trans.), *The standard edition of the complete psychological works of Sigmund Freud* (*Vol. 18*, pp. 67–143). London: Hogarth. (Original work published 1923)

Freud, S. (1964). Recommendations to physicians practicing psychoanalysis. In J. Strachey (Ed. & Trans.), *The standard edition of the complete psychological works of Sigmund Freud* (pp. 235–254). London: Hogarth. (Original work published 1912)

Freud, S. (1964). On narcissism: An introduction. In J. Strachey (Ed. & Trans.), *The standard edition of the complete psychological works of Sigmund Freud* (*Vol. 14*, pp. 73–102). London: Hogarth. (Original work published 1914)

Freud, S. (1964). A metapsychological supplement to the theory of dreams. In J. Strachey (Ed. & Trans.), *The standard edition of the complete psychological works of Sigmund Freud* (*Vol. 14*, pp. 222–235). London: Hogarth. (Original work published 1917)

Freud, S. (1964). Group psychology and the analysis of the ego. In J. Strachey (Ed. & Trans.), *The standard edition of the complete psychological works of Sigmund Freud* (*Vol. 18*, pp. 111–116). London: Hogarth. (Original work published 1921)

Freud, S. (1964). Two encyclopedia articles. In J. Strachey (Ed. & Trans.), *The standard edition of the complete psychological works of Sigmund Freud* (*Vol. 23*, pp. 209–253). London: Hogarth. (Original work published 1923)

Freud, S. (1964). Inhibitions, symptoms, and anxiety. In J. Strachey (Ed. & Trans.), *The standard edition of the complete psychological works of Sigmund Freud* (*Vol. 20*, pp. 77–175). London: Hogarth. (Original work published 1926)

Freud, S. (1964). New introductory lectures on psychoanalysis. In J. Strachey (Ed. & Trans.), *The standard edition of the complete psychological works of Sigmund Freud* (*Vol. 22*, pp. 3–182). London: Hogarth. (Original work published 1932)

Freud, S. (1964a). An outline of psychoanalysis. In J. Strachey (Ed. & Trans.), *The standard edition of the complete psychological works of Sigmund Freud* (*Vol. 23*, pp. 141–207). London: Hogarth. (Original work published in 1940)

Freud, S. (1964b). The technique of psychoanalysis. In J. Strachey (Ed. & Trans.), *The standard edition of the complete psychological works of Sigmund Freud* (*Vol. 23*, pp. 172–182). London: Hogarth. (Original work published 1940)

Freyd, J. J. (1996). *Betrayal trauma: The logic of forgetting childhood abuse*. Cambridge, MA: Harvard University Press.

Friesen, J. G. (1991). *Uncovering the mystery of mpd*. San Bernadino, CA: Here's Life Publishers.

Frischholz, E. J. (1996, March). *Hypnotizability and psychopathology*. Paper presented at the annual meeting of the American Society of Clinical Hypnosis, Orlando, FL.

Frischholz, E. J., Lipman, L. S., Braun, B. G., & Sachs, R. G. (1992). Psychopathology, hypnotizability, and dissociation. *American Journal of Psychiatry, 149*(11), 1521–1525.

Fromm, E. (1970). Age regression with unexpected reappearance of a repressed childhood language. *Journal of Clinical and Experimental Hypnosis, 18*, 79–88.

Fromm, E. (1984). Hypnoanalysis—with particular emphasis on the borderline personality. *Psychoanalytic Psychology 1*, 61–76.

Fromm, E., & Kahn, S. (1990). *Self-hypnosis: The Chicago paradigm*. New York: Guilford Press.

Fromm, E., & Nash, M. (1997). *Psychoanalysis and hypnosis*. New York: International Universities Press.

Gainer, M. J. (1992). Hypnotherapy for reflex sympathetic dystrophy. *American Journal of Clinical Hypnosis, 34*, 227–232.

Gainer, M. J. (1997, June). *Ego state therapy for pain control*. Paper presented at the 14th International Congress of Hypnosis. San Diego, CA.

Gainer, M. J., & Torem, M. S. (1993). Ego state therapy for self-injurious behavior. *American Journal of Clinical Hypnosis, 35*, 257–266.

Ganaway, G. K. (1989). Historical versus narrative truth: Clarifying the role of exogenous trauma in the etiology of mpd and its variants. *Dissociation, 2*, 205–220.

Gardner, G. G. (1976). Hypnosis and mastery: Clinical contributions and directions for research. *International Journal of Clinical and Experimental Hypnosis, 24*, 202–214.

Gazzaniga, M. S. (1989). Organization of the human brain. *Science, 245*, 947–952.

Gazzaniga, M. S. (1995, March). *Consciousness is an instinct*. Plenary address presented at the annual meeting of the American Society of Clinical Hypnosis, San Diego, CA.

Gelder, M. G. (1990). Psychological treatment of panic anxiety. *Psychiatric Annals, 20*, 529–532.

Geller, J. D. (1987). The process of psychotherapy: Separation and complex interplay among empathy, insight, and internalization. In J. Bloom-Feshbach & S. Bloom-Feshbach (Eds.), *The psychology of separation and loss: Perspectives on development, life transitions, and clinical practice* (pp. 459–514). San Francisco: Jossey-Bass.

Gerbode, F. A. (1989). *Beyond psychology: An introduction to metapsychology*. Menlo Park, CA: IRM.

Gil, E. (1988). *Treatment of adult survivors of childhood abuse*. Walnut Creek, CA: Launch Press.

Gill, M. M., & Brenman, M. M. (1959). *Hypnosis and related states: Psychoanalytic studies in regression*. New York: International Universities Press.

Gilligan, S. G. (1987). *Therapeutic trances: The cooperation principle in Ericksonian hypnotherapy*. New York: Brunner/Mazel.

Gilligan, S. G. (1997). *The courage to love*. New York: Norton.

Giovacchini, P. L. (1996). *The transitional space in mental breakdown and creative integration.* Northvale, NJ: Jason Aronson.

Gitelson, M. (1962). The curative functions in psychotherapy. *International Journal of Psychoanalysis, 43,* 194–205.

Glover, E. (1955). *The technique of psychoanalysis.* New York: International Universities Press.

Goldstein, A. J., & Chambless, D. I. (1978). A reanalysis of agoraphobia. *Behavior Therapy, 9,* 47–59.

Goodman, W. K., McDougle, C. J., Barr, L. C., Aronson, S. C., & Price, L. H. (1993). Biological approaches to treatment-resistant obsessive compulsive disorder. *The Journal of Clinical Psychiatry, 53,* 16–26.

Goodman, W. K., McDougle, C. J., & Price, L. H. (1992). Pharmacotherapy of obsessive compulsive disorder. *The Journal of Clinical Psychiatry, 53,* 29–37.

Goodnick, P. J. (1997). Medical illness and depression. *Psychiatric Annals, 27,* 339–340.

Goodwin, D. W. (1986). *Anxiety.* New York: Oxford University Press.

Gorman, J. M., & Coplan, J. D. (1996). Comorbidity of depression and panic disorder. *Journal of Clinical Psychiatry, 57* [suppl. 10], 34–41.

Gorman, J. M., Liebowitz, M. R., Fryer, A. J., & Stein, B. A. (1989). A neuroanatomical hypothesis for panic disorder. *The American Journal of Psychiatry, 146,* 148–161.

Goulding, R. A., & Schwartz, R. C. (1995). *The mosaic mind: Empowering the tormented selves of child abuse survivors.* New York: Norton.

Gravitz, M. A. (1991). Early theories of hypnosis: A clinical perspective. In S. J. Lynn & J. W. Rhue (Eds.), *Theories of hypnosis: Current modes and perspectives* (pp. 19–42). New York: Guilford.

Gravitz, M. A. (1994). The first use of self-hypnosis: Mesmer mesmerizes Mesmer. *American Journal of Clinical Hypnosis 37,* 49–52.

Greenacre, P. (1969). The fetish and the transitional object. *Psychoanalytic Study of the Child, 24,* 144–164.

Greenacre, P. (1971). The fetish and the transitional object, the transitional object and the fetish: With special reference to the role of illusion. *Emotional Growth 1,* 1315–1334.

Greenbaum, T. (1978). The "analysing instrument" and the transitional object. In S. Grolnick, L. Barkin, & W. Muensterberger (Eds.), *Between reality and fantasy: Transitional objects and phenomena.* Northvale, NJ: Jason Aronson.

Greenberg, J. R., & Mitchell, S. A. (1983). *Object relations and psychoanalytic theory.* Cambridge, MA: Harvard University Press.

Greenleaf, E. (1969). Developmental-stage regression through hypnosis. *American Journal of Clinical Hypnosis, 12,* 20–36.

Greenson, R. R. (1965). The working alliance and the transference neurosis. *Psychoanalytic Quarterly, 34,* 155–181.

Greenson, R. R. (1967). *The technique and practice of psychoanalysis (Vol. 1).* New York: International Universities Press.

Gregory, J. (1997). *Revivifying archetypal selfobject functioning in hypnotic trance: An integrative approach for early intervention in a brief therapy mode.* Unpublished doctoral dissertation, Pacifica Institute of Graduate Studies, Carpenteria, CA.

Greist, W. K. (1992). Obsessive compulsive disorder: Integrating theory and practice. *The Journal of Clinical Psychiatry, 53,* 3–10.

Grinker, R. R., & Spiegel, J. P. (1945). *War neuroses.* Philadelphia: Blakiston.

Groddek, G. (1950). *The book of the it*. London: Vision Press. (Original work published 1923)

Grotjahn, M. (1966). George Groddek: The untamed analyst. In F. Alexander, S. Eisenstein, & M. Grotjahn (Eds.), *Psychoanalytic pioneers* (pp. 308–320). New York: Basic Books.

Gruenewald, D. (1971). Agoraphobia: A case study in hypnotherapy. *International Journal of Clinical and Experimental Hypnosis, 19*, 10–20.

Grunhaus, L. (1988). Clinical and psychobiological characteristics of simultaneous panic disorder and major depression. *American Journal of Psychiatry, 145*, 1214–1221.

Guntrip, H. (1969). *Schizoid phenomena, object relations, and the self*. New York: International Universities Press.

Gurgevich, S. (1990). Hypnotic suggestion/metaphor to begin reframing. In D. C. Hammond (Ed.), *Handbook of therapeutic suggestions and metaphors* (p. 167). New York: Norton.

Hall, J. A. (1989). *Hypnosis: A Jungian perspective*. New York: Guilford Press.

Hamilton, N. G. (1988). *Self and others: Object relations theory and practice*. London: Aronson.

Hammond, D. C. (1984). Myths about Erickson and Ericksonian hypnosis. *American Journal of Clinical Hypnosis, 26*, 236–245.

Hammond, D. C. (1986). Evidence of Erickson's effectiveness. In B. Zilbergeld, M. G. Edelstien, & D. L. Aroaz (Eds.), *Hypnosis: Questions and answers* (pp. 232–236). New York: Norton.

Hammond, D. C. (Ed.). (1990). *Handbook of therapeutic suggestions and metaphors*. New York: Norton.

Hammond, D. C. (1990a). Anxiety, phobias, and dental disorders. In D. C. Hammond (Ed.), *Handbook of therapeutic suggestions and metaphors* (pp. 153–197). New York: Norton.

Hammond, D. C. (1990b). Ego-strengthening: Enhancing esteem, self-efficacy, and confidence. In D. C. Hammond (Ed.), *Handbook of therapeutic suggestions and metaphors* (pp. 109–151). New York: Norton.

Hammond, D. C. (1990c). Formulating hypnotic and posthypnotic suggestions. In D. C. Hammond (Ed.), *Handbook of therapeutic suggestions and metaphors* (pp. 11–44). New York: Norton.

Hammond, D. C. (1990d). Time reorientation: Age regression, age progression, and time distortion. In D. C. Hammond (Ed.), *Handbook of therapeutic suggestions and metaphors* (pp. 509–558). New York: Norton.

Hammond, D. C. (1993). False memories, misrepresentations, & ritual abuse. *The American Society of Clinical Hypnosis Newsletter, 34*, 3.

Hammond, D. C., & Cheek, D. B. (1988). Ideomotor signaling: A method for rapid unconscious exploration. In D. C. Hammond (Ed.), *Hypnotic inductions & suggestion: An introductory manual* (pp. 90–97). Des Plaines, IL: American Society of Clinical Hypnosis.

Hammond, D. C., Haskins-Bartsch, C., Grant, C. W., & McGhee, M. (1988). Comparison of self-directed and tape-assisted self-hypnosis. *American Journal of Clinical Hypnosis, 1*, 129–137.

Harlow, H. F. (1960). Primary affectional patterns in primates. *American Journal of Orthopsychiatry, 30*.

Harriman, P. L. (1942a). The experimental induction of a multiple personality. *Psychiatry, 5,* 179–186.

Harriman, P. L. (1942b). The experimental production of some phenomena related to multiple personality. *Journal of Abnormal Psychology, 37,* 244–255.

Harriman, P. L. (1943). A new approach to multiple personalities. *American Journal of Orthopsychiatry, 13,* 638–643.

Hartland, J. (1965). The value of "ego strengthening" procedures prior to direct symptom removal under hypnosis. *American Journal of Clinical Hypnosis, 8,* 89–93.

Hartland, J. (1971). Further observations on the use of ego-strengthening techniques. *American Journal of Clinical Hypnosis 14,* 1–8.

Hartley, D. (1993). Assessing psychological development level. In N. E. Miller, L. Luborsky, J. P. Barber, & J. P. Docherty (Eds.), *Psychodynamic treatment research* (pp. 152–176). New York: Basic Books.

Hartmann, H. (1961). *Ego psychology and the problems of adaptation.* New York: International Universities Press.

Hartmann, H. (1965). *Essays on ego psychology.* New York: International Universities Press.

Hartmann, H., Kris, E., & Lowenstein, R. M. (1946). Comments on the formation of psychic structure. In *The psychoanalytic study of the child* (*Vol. 2,* pp. 11–338). New York: International Universities Press.

Havens, R. (1986). Posthypnotic predetermination of therapeutic progress. *American Journal of Clinical Hypnosis, 26*(2), 78–83.

Hegeman, E. (1995). Transferential issues in the psychoanalytic treatment of incest survivors. In J. L. Alpert (Ed.), *Sexual abuse recall: Treating trauma in the era of the recovered memory debate* (pp. 185–212). Northvale, NJ: Jason Aronson.

Herman, J. L. (1992). *Trauma and recovery.* New York: Basic Books.

Hilgard, E. R. (1973). A neodissociation interpretation of pain reduction in hypnosis. *Psychological Review, 80,* 396–411.

Hilgard, E. R. (1977). *Divided consciousness: Multiple controls in human thought and action.* New York: Wiley.

Hilgard, E. R. (1984). The hidden observer and multiple personality. *The International Journal of Clinical and Experimental Hypnosis, 32,* 248–253.

Hilgard, E. R. (1991). A neodissociation interpretation of hypnosis. In S. J. Lynn & J. W. Rhue (Eds.), *Theories of hypnosis: Current modes and perspectives* (pp. 83–104). New York: Guilford.

Hilgard, E. R., & Hilgard, J. R. (1994). *Hypnosis in the relief of pain* (rev. ed.). New York: Brunner/Mazel. (Reprinted from 1983 edition, published by William Kaufmann, Inc., Los Altos, CA)

Hillman, J. (1976). *Revisioning psychology.* New York: Harper & Row.

Hillman, J. (1996). *The soul's code: In search of character and calling.* New York: Random House.

Holmes, J. (1996). *Attachment, intimacy, autonomy.* Northvale, NJ: Jason Aronson.

Horner, A. J. (1995). *Object relations and the developing ego in therapy* (2nd ed.). New York: Jason Aronson.

Horowitz, M. J. (1979). Psychological response to serious life events. In V. Hamilton & D. M. Warburton (Eds.), *Human stress and cognition* (pp. 235–263). New York: Wiley.

Horwitz, L. (1974). *Clinical prediction in psychotherapy.* New York: Jason Aronson.

Hovarth, A., Gaston, L., & Luborsky, L. (1993). The therapeutic alliance and its measures. In N. E. Miller, L. Luborsky, J. P. Barber, & J. P. Docherty (Eds.), *Psychodynamic treatment research* (pp. 247–273). New York: Basic Books.

Hunter, M. E. (1994). *Creative scripts for hypnotherapy*. New York: Brunner/Mazel.

Husserl, E. D. (1964). *The phenomenology of internal time consciousness* (M. Heidigger, Ed., & J. S. Churchill, Trans.; Part 1, pp. 21–124). Bloomington, IN: Indiana University Press. (Original work published 1906)

Jacobson, E. (1973). *The self and the object world*. New York: International Universities Press.

James, W. (1961). *The varieties of religious experience*. New York: Macmillan. (Original work published 1902)

James, W. (1983). *The principles of psychology*. Cambridge: Harvard University Press. (Original work published 1890)

Janet, P. (1897). L'Influence somnambulique et la besoin de direction. *Revue Philosophique, XLIII(1)*, 113–114.

Janet, P. (1976). *Psychological healing: A historical and clinical study* (2 vols.; E. Paul & C. Paul, Trans.). New York: Arne. (Original work published 1919)

Jenkins, J. (1974). Remember that old theory of memory? Well, forget it! *American Psychologist, 29*, 785–795.

Johnson, G. M., & Hallenbeck, C. E. (1985). A case of obsessional fears treated by brief hypno-imagery intervention. *American Journal of Clinical Hypnosis, 27*, 232–236.

Johnson, L. S., Dawson, S. L., Clark, J. L., & Sikorsky, C. (1983). Self-hypnosis versus hetero-hypnosis: Order effects and sex differences in behavioral and experiential impact. *International Journal of Clinical and Experimental Hypnosis, 31*, 139–154.

Johnson, L. S., & Weight, D. G. (1976). Self-hypnosis versus hetero-hypnosis: Experimental and behavioral comparisons. *Journal of Abnormal Psychology, 85*, 523–526.

Jones, E. (1953). *The life and work of Sigmund Freud*. New York: Basic Books.

Jung, C. G. (1939). *The integration of the personality*. New York: Farrar & Rinehart.

Jung, C. G. (1956). *Active imagination: Two essays on analytical psychology*. New York: The World Publishing Co.

Jung, C. G. (1957). *Psychiatric studies* (R. F. C. Hull, Trans.). New York: Pantheon.

Jung, C. G. (1960). *The psychogenesis of mental disease* (R. F. C. Hull, Trans.). New York: Pantheon.

Jung, C. G. (1964). *Man and his symbols*. New York: Doubleday.

Jung, C. G. (1965). *Memories, dreams, reflections*. New York: Vintage Books.

Jung, C. G. (1966). Two essays on analytic psychology. In R. F. C. Hull (Ed. & Trans.), *The collected works of C. G. Jung (Vol. 7)*. Princeton, NJ: Princeton University Press. (Original work published 1926)

Jung, C. G. (1967). The structure and dynamics of the psyche. In R. F. C. Hull (Ed. & Trans.), *The collected works of C. G. Jung (Vol. 8)*. Princeton, NJ: Princeton University Press. (Original work published 1958)

Jung, C. G. (1969). A review of the complex theory. In R. F. C. Hull (Ed. & Trans.), *The collected works of C. G. Jung (Vol. 8, pp. 92–104)*. Princeton, NJ: Princeton University Press.

Jung, C. G. (1971). The transcendent function. In J. Campbell (Ed.), *The portable Jung* (pp. 273–300). New York: Viking Press. (Original work published 1916)

Jung, C. G. (1971). The Tavistock lectures. In *The collected works of C. G. Jung* (*Vol. 18,* pp. 5–182). Princeton, NJ: Princeton University Press. (Original work published 1935)

Jung, C. G. (1971). Answer to Job. In J. Campbell (Ed.), *The portable Jung* (pp. 519–650). New York: Viking Press. (Original work published 1954)

Jung, C. G. (1990). *The collected works of C. G. Jung* (H. Read, M. Fordham, & G. Adler, Eds.). Princeton, NJ: Princeton University Press.

Kahn, S., & Fromm, E. (1992). Self-hypnosis, personality, and the experiential method. In E. Fromme & M. Nash (Eds.), *Contemporary hypnosis research* (pp. 390–404). New York: Guilford.

Kampman, R. (1976). Hypnotically induced multiple personality: An experimental study. *International Journal of Clinical and Experimental Hypnosis, 24,* 215–227.

Kant, I. (1929). *Critique of Pure Reason* (abridged ed.; N. K. Smith, Trans.). New York: Random House. (Original work published 1781)

à Kempis, T. (1987–1997). The imitation of Christ. In *Columbia Dictionary of Quotations. Microsoft Bookshelf 98.* Bellevue, WA: Microsoft Corp. (Original work published 1471)

Kernberg, O. F. (1975). *Borderline conditions and pathological narcissism.* Northvale, NJ: Jason Aronson.

Kernberg, O. F. (1976). *Object relations: Theory and clinical psychoanalysis.* Northvale, NJ: Jason Aronson.

Kernberg, O. F. (1982). Self, ego, affects, and drives. *Journal of the American Psychoanalytic Association, 30,* 893–917.

Kerr, M. E., & Bowen, M. (1988) *Family evaluation: An approach based on Bowen theory.* New York: Norton.

Kessler, R. S., & Miller, S. D. (1995). The use of a future time frame in psychotherapy with and without hypnosis. *American Journal of Clinical Hypnosis, 38,* 39–46.

Khan, M. M. R. (1963). The concept of cumulative trauma. *The psychoanalytic study of the child* (*Vol. 18,* pp. 286–306). New York: International Universities Press.

Kirsch, I., Montgomery, G., & Sapirstein, G. (1995). Hypnosis as an adjunct to cognitive-behavioral psychotherapy: A meta analysis. *Journal of Counseling and Clinical Psychology, 63,* 214–220.

Klein, D. F. (1980). Anxiety reconceptualized. *Comprehensive Psychiatry, 6,* 411–427.

Klein, M. (1948). *The psychoanalysis of children.* London: Hogarth.

Kluft, R. P. (1983). Hypnotherapeutic crisis intervention in multiple personality. *American Journal of Clinical Hypnosis, 26,* 73–83.

Kluft, R. P. (1984a). Multiple personality disorder in childhood. *Psychiatric Clinics of North America, 7,* 135–148.

Kluft, R. P. (1984b). Treatment of multiple personality disorder: A study of 33 cases. *Psychiatric Clinics of North America, 7,* 9–29.

Kluft, R. P. (1985). Development of multiple personality disorder: Predisposing, precipitating, and perpetuating factors. In R. P. Kluft (Ed.), *Childhood antecedents of multiple personality disorder* (pp. 37–64). Washington, DC: American Psychiatric Press.

Kluft, R. P. (1989). Playing for time: Temporizing techniques in the treatment of multiple personality disorder. *American Journal of Clinical Hypnosis, 32,* 90–98.

Kluft, R. P. (1990a). Dissociation and subsequent vulnerability: A preliminary study. *Dissociation, 3,* 167–173.

Kluft, R. P. (1990b). Incest and subsequent revictimization: The case of therapist–patient sexual exploitation, with description of the sitting duck syndrome. In R. P. Kluft (Ed.), *Incest-related syndromes of adult psychopathology* (pp. 263–293). Washington, DC: American Psychiatric Press.

Kluft, R. P. (1993). Clinical approaches to the integration of multiple personalities. In R. P. Kluft & C. Fine (Eds.), *Clinical perspectives on multiple personality disorder* (pp. 101–133). Washington, DC: American Psychiatric Press.

Kluft, R. P. (1994, March). *Preparing the patient for uncertainty: Informed consent as an ongoing process in the use of hypnosis with trauma patients.* Paper presented at the annual meeting of the American Society of Clinical Hypnosis, Philadelphia, PA.

Kluft, R. P., & Fine, C. (Eds.). (1993). *Clinical perspectives on multiple personality disorder.* Washington, DC: American Psychiatric Press.

Kohut, H. (1971). *The analysis of the self.* New York: International Universities Press.

Kohut, H. (1977). *The restoration of the self.* New York: International Universities Press.

Kripke, D. (1982). Ultradian rhythms in behavior and physiology. In F. Brown & R. Graeber (Eds.), *Rhythmic aspects of behavior* (pp. 313–344). Hillsdale, NJ: Lawrence Erlbaum Associates.

Krippner, S. (1963). Hypnosis and reading improvement among university students. *American Journal of Clinical Hypnosis, 5,* 189–193.

Kris, E. (1951). Ego psychology and interpretation in psychoanalytic therapy. *Psychoanalytic Quarterly, 20,* 15–30.

Kris, E. (1972). *Psychoanalytic explorations in art.* New York: International Universities Press. (Original work published 1936)

Kroger, W. (1977). *Clinical and experimental hypnosis* (2nd ed.). Philadelphia: Lippincott.

Kroger, W., & Fezler, W. D. (1976). *Hypnosis and behavior modification: Imagery and conditioning.* Philadelphia: J. B. Lippincott.

Krystal, J. H., Deutsch, D. N., & Charney, D. S. (1996). The biological basis of panic disorder. *Journal of Clinical Psychiatry, 57* [suppl. 10], 23–31.

Kubler-Ross, E. (1969). *On death and dying.* New York: Macmillan.

Lankton, S. (1980). *Practical magic.* Cupertino, CA: Meta Publications.

Lankton, S. R. (1986). Choosing the right metaphors for particular clients. In B. Zilbergeld, G. Edelstien, & D. Aroaz (Eds.), *Hypnosis: Questions and answers* (pp. 261–267). New York: Norton.

Lazarus, A. (1989). *The practice of multi-modal therapy* (rev. ed.). Baltimore: Johns Hopkins University Press.

Leavitt, H. D. (1947). A case of hypnotically produced secondary and tertiary personalities. *Psychoanalytic Review, 34,* 274–295.

LeCron, L. (1954). A hypnotic technique for uncovering unconscious material. *International Journal of Clinical and Experimental Hypnosis, 2,* 76–79.

LeCron, L. (1963). The uncovering of early memories by ideomotor responses. *International Journal of Clinical and Experimental Hypnosis, 11,* 137–142.

LeShan, L. (1989). *Cancer as a turning point.* New York: Dutton.

Levine, P. (1991). The body as healer: A revisioning of trauma and anxiety. In M. Sheets-Johnson (Ed.), *Giving the body its due* (pp. 85–108). Stonybrook: State University of New York Press.

Levitan, A. A. (1985). Hypnotic death rehearsal. *American Journal of Clinical Hypnosis, 27,* 211–215.

Lindner, R. (1954). The jet-propelled couch: The story of Kirk. In *The fifty minute hour* (pp. 163–216). New York: Dell.

Loevinger, J. (1976). *Ego development*. San Francisco: Jossey-Bass.

Loftus, E. F. (1979). The reality of repressed memories. *American Psychologist, 48,* 518–537.

Loftus, E. F., Miller, D. G., & Burns, H. J. (1978). Semantic integration of verbal integration into a visual memory. *Journal of Experimental Psychology: Human Learning and Memory, 4,* 19–31.

Loftus, E. R., & Zanni, G. (1975). Eyewitness testimony: The influence of the wording of a question. *Bulletin of the Psychonomic Society, 5,* 86–88.

Lorand, S. (1966). Sandor Ferenczi: Pioneer of pioneers. In F. Alexander, S. Eisenstein, & M. Grotjahn (Eds.), *Psychoanalytic pioneers* (pp. 14–35). New York: Basic Books.

Luborsky, L. (1990, June). *Therapeutic alliance measures as predictors of future benefits of psychotherapy*. Paper presented at the annual meeting of the Society for Psychotherapy Research, Wintergreen, VA.

Ludwig, A. M. (1966). Altered states of consciousness. *Archives of General Psychiatry, 15,* 225–234.

Lynn, S. J., Mare, C., Kvaal, S., Segal, D., & Sivec, H. (1994). The hidden observer, hypnotic dreams, and age regression: Clinical implications. *American Journal of Clinical Hypnosis, 37,* 130–142.

Lynn, S. J., & Rhue, J. W. (Eds.). (1991). *Theories of hypnosis: Current modes and perspectives*. New York: Guilford.

Lynn, S. J., & Rhue, J. W. (1994). *Dissociation*. New York: Guilford.

Mahler, M. S. (1968). *On human symbiosis and the vicissitudes of individuation* (*Vol. 1*). New York: Norton.

Mahler, M. S., Pine, F., & Bergman, A. (1975). *The psychological birth of the human infant*. New York: Basic Books.

Malcolm, N. (1996). Fear of flying—The use of ego state therapy—Two case studies. *Hypnos, 23,* 202–205.

Mar, S. (1997, May–June). Stress and the string player. *Practical Musician,* 28–32.

Markowitz, J. S., Weissman, J. M., Oulette, R., Lish, J. D., & Klerman, G. L. (1989). Quality of life in panic disorder. *Archives of General Psychiatry, 46,* 984–991.

Marks, I. M. (1981). Review of behavioral psychotherapy: I. Obsessive compulsive disorders. *American Journal of Psychiatry, 5,* 548–592.

Marlatt, G. A., & Gordon, J. R. (Eds.). (1985). *Relapse prevention*. New York: Guilford.

Marmer, S. S. (1980). Psychoanalysis of multiple personality disorder. *International Journal of Psychoanalysis, 61,* 439–459.

Marshall, J. R., Pollack, M. H., & Otto, M. W. (1997). Panic disorder: A treatment update. *The Journal of Clinical Psychiatry, 58,* 36–37.

Matthews, W. J. (1998). Ericksonian hypnosis: A review of the empirical data. In W. J. Matthews & J. Edgette (Eds.), *Current thinking and research in brief therapy: Solutions, strategies, and narrative* (*Vol. 2*). New York: Brunner/Mazel.

Matthews, W. J., & Mosher, D. L. (1988). Direct and indirect hypnotic suggestion in a laboratory setting. *British Journal of Clinical and Experimental Hypnosis, 5,* 63–71.

McCann, I. L., & Pearlman, L. A. (1990). *Psychological trauma and the adult survivor. Theory, therapy, and transformation*. New York: Brunner/Mazel.

McConkey, K. (1984). The impact of an indirect suggestion. *International Journal of Clinical and Experimental Hypnosis, 32*, 307–314.

McDaniel, J. S., Musselman, D. L., Porter, M. R., Reed, D. A., & Nemeroff, C. B. (1995). Depression in patients with cancer: Diagnosis, biology, and treatment. *Archives of General Psychiatry, 52*, 89–99.

McFarlane, A. C., & Van der Kolk, B.A. (1996). Conclusions and future directions. In B. A. Van der Kolk, A. C. McFarlane, & L. Weiseath (Eds.), *Traumatic stress: The effects of overwhelming experience on mind, body, and society* (pp. 559–575). New York: Guilford.

McMahon, E. (1986). Creative self-mothering. In B. Zilbergeld, G. Edelstien, & D. Aroaz (Eds.), *Hypnosis: Questions and answers* (pp. 150–155). New York: Norton.

McNeal, S. (1986, April). *How I do it; how I view it: Hypnosis for ego-strengthening.* Lecture to the San Francisco Academy of Hypnosis Academic Assembly, San Francisco, CA.

McNeal, S. (1989, March). *Ego-strengthening.* Lecture to the annual workshop, San Francisco Academy of Hypnosis, San Francisco, CA.

McNeal, S. (1993, March). *Coming together: Facilitating the integration process in psychotherapy.* Paper presented at the annual meeting of the American Society of Clinical Hypnosis, New Orleans, LA.

McNeal, S., & Frederick, C. (1993). Inner strength and other techniques for ego-strengthening. *American Journal of Clinical Hypnosis, 35*, 170–178.

McNeal, S., & Frederick, C. (1994, March). *Internal self-soothing: Other implications of ego-strengthening with ego states.* Paper presented at the annual meeting of the American Society of Clinical Hypnosis, Philadelphia, PA.

McNeal, S., & Frederick, C. (1995, March). *Good fences make good neighbors: Boundary formation in ego states as precursors to integration.* Paper presented at the annual meeting of the American Society of Clinical Hypnosis, San Diego, CA.

McNeal, S., & Frederick, C. (1996, March). *Inner love: Projective/evocative ego-strengthening of ego states with inner resources of unconditional love.* Paper presented at the annual meeting of the American Society of Clinical Hypnosis, Orlando, FL.

McNeal, S., & Frederick, C. (1997, June). *New vintages in old vessels: Activating and utilizing transitional phenomena with ego states.* Paper presented at the 14th International Congress of Hypnosis, San Diego, CA.

McNeal, S., & Frederick, C. (1998, March). *The land of milk and honey: Self-hypnosis and ego state therapy.* Paper presented at the annual meeting of the American Society of Clinical Hypnosis, Ft. Worth, TX.

Miles, J. (1995). *God: A biography.* New York: Alfred A. Knopf.

Moore, B. E. (1995). Narcissism. In B. E. Moore & B. D. Fine (Eds.), *Psychoanalysis: The major concepts* (pp. 229–251). New Haven, CT: Yale University Press.

Moore, R. H. (1993). Traumatic incident reduction: A cognitive-emotional treatment of post-traumatic stress disorder. In W. Dryden & L. Hill (Eds.), *Innovations in rational-emotive therapy.* Newbury Park, CA: Sage.

Moore, T. (1992). Self-love and its myth. *Care of the soul: A guide for cultivating depth and sacredness in everyday life.* New York: Harper Collins.

Morton, P., & Frederick, C. (1996, March). *Transitional space in the integration process in hypnotherapy: A preliminary report.* Paper presented at the annual meeting of the American Society of Clinical Hypnosis, Orlando, FL.

Morton, P., & Frederick, C. (1997a). Intrapsychic transitional space: A resource for integration in hypnotherapy. *Hypnos, 24*, 32–41.

Morton, P., & Frederick, C. (1997b, June). *Re-alerting in the middle of a tightrope: Promoting conscious/unconscious complementarity during the integration process in ego state therapy.* Paper pesented at the 14th International Congress of Hypnosis, San Diego, CA.

Munroe, R. L. (1955). *Schools of psychoanalytic thought.* New York: Dryden.

Murray-Jobsis, J. (1984). Hypnosis with severely disturbed patients. In W. C. Wester, II, & A. H. Smith, Jr. (Eds.), *Clinical hypnosis: A multidisciplinary approach* (pp. 368–404). Philadelphia: J, B. Lippincott.

Murray-Jobsis, J. (1985). Exploring the schizophrenic experience with the use of hypnosis. *American Journal of Clinical Hypnosis, 29*, 34–42.

Murray-Jobsis, J. (1990a). Renurturing: Forming positive sense of identity and bonding. In D. C. Hammond (Ed.), *Handbook of hypnotic suggestions and metaphors* (pp. 326–328). New York: Norton.

Murray-Jobsis, J. (1990b). Suggestions for creative self-mothering. In D. C. Hammond (Ed.), *Handbook of hypnotic suggestions and metaphors* (p. 328). New York: Norton.

Murray-Jobsis, J. (1990c). Ego building. In D. C. Hammond (Ed.), *Handbook of hypnotic suggestions and metaphors* (pp. 136–139). New York: Norton.

Murray-Jobsis, J. (1991). An exploratory study of hypnotic capacity of schizophrenic and borderline patients in a clinical setting. *American Journal of Clinical Hypnosis, 33*, 150–160.

Mussen, P. H. (1963). *The psychological development of the child.* Englewood Cliffs, NJ: Prentice-Hall.

Napier, N. J. (1990). *Recreating yourself: Help for adult children of dysfunctional families.* New York: Norton.

Nash, M. R. (1991). Hypnosis as a special case of psychological regression. In S. J. Lynn & J. W. Rhue (Eds.), *Theories of hypnosis: Current modes and perspectives* (pp. 171–194). New York: Guilford.

Nash, M. R. (1992). Hypnosis, psychopathology, and psychological regression. In E. Fromm & M. R. Nash (Eds.), *Contemporary hypnosis research* (pp. 149–169). New York: Guilford.

Nash, M. R., Drake, S. D., Wiley, S., Khalsa, S., & Lynn, S. J. (1986). Accuracy of recall by hypnotically age-regressed subjects. *Journal of Abnormal Psychology, 95*, 298–300.

Nash, M. R., Johnson, L. S., & Tipton, R. D. (1979). Hypnotic age regression and the occurrence of transitional object relationships. *Journal of Abnormal Psychology, 88*, 547–555.

Nash, M. R., Lynn, S. J., Stanley, S., Frauman, D., & Rhue, J. (1985). Hypnotic age regression and the importance of assessing interpersonally relevant affect. *International Journal of Clinical and Experimental Hypnosis, 33*, 224–235.

National Institutes of Health. (1991). *Consensus development conference: statement: Treatment of panic disorder.* Bethesda, MD: U. S. Government Printing Office.

Nemiah, J. (1981). A psychoanalytic view of phobias. *American Journal of Psychoanalysis, 41*, 115–120.

Newey, A. B. (1986). Ego state therapy with depression. In B. Zilbergeld, M. G. Edelstien, & D. L. Aroaz (Eds.), *Hypnosis: Questions and answers.* New York: Norton.

Noyes, R., Crowe, R. R., Harris, E. L., Hamra, B. J., McChesney, C. M., & Chaudry, B. R. (1986). Relationship between panic disorder and agoraphobia. *Archives of General Psychiatry, 43,* 227–232.

Nunberg, H. (1955). *Principles of psychoanalysis.* New York: International Universities Press.

Oates, R. K., Forrest, D., & Peacock, A. (1985). Self esteem of abused children. *Child Abuse and Neglect, 9,* 159–163.

Oetting, E. R. (1964). Hypnosis and concentration in study. *American Journal of Clinical Hypnosis, 7,* 148–151.

Oetting, E. R. (1990). Alert trance suggestions for concentration and reading. In D. C. Hammond (Ed.), *Handbook of therapeutic suggestions and metaphors* (pp. 446–448). New York: Norton.

O'Hanlon, W., & Weiner-Davis, M. (1989). *In search of solutions.* New York: Norton.

Orne, M. T., Whitehouse, W. G., Dinges, D. F., & Orne, E. C. (1988). Reconstructing memory through hypnosis: Forensic and clinical implications. In H. M. Pettinati (Ed.), *Hypnosis and memory* (pp. 21–63). New York: Guilford.

Ornstein, R. (1987). *Multimind: A new way to look at human behavior.* New York: Houghton Mifflin.

Overton, D. (1978). Major theories of state dependent learning. In B. Ho, D. Richards, & D. Chute (Eds.). *Drug discriminatory and state dependent learning* (pp. 283–318). New York: Academic Press.

Oyle, I. (1975). *The healing mind.* Milbrae, CA: Celestial Arts.

Palan, B. M., & Chandwani, S. (1989). Coping with examination stress through hypnosis: An experimental study. *American Journal of Clinical Hypnosis, 31,* 173–180.

Pavlov, I. P. (1923). The identity of inhibition with sleep and hypnosis. *Scientific Monthly, 17,* 603–608.

Pearlman, L. A., & Saakvitne, K. W. (1995). *Trauma and the therapist: Countertransference and vicarious traumatization in psychotherapy with incest survivors.* New York: Norton.

Perry, B. D. (1996). *Maltreated children: Experience, brain development, and the next generation.* New York & London: Norton.

Perry, B. D. (1997). Incubated in terror: Neurodevelopmental factors in the cycle of violence. In J. D. Osofsky (Ed.), *Children in a violent society* (pp. 124–149). New York: Guilford.

Pert, C., Ruff, M., Weber, R., & Herkenham, N. (1985). Neuropeptides and their receptors: A psychosomatic network. *The Journal of Immunology, 135(2),* 820s–826s.

Peter, B. (1994). Hypnotherapy with cancer patients: On speaking about death and dying. *Hypnos, 21,* 246–251.

Pettinati, H. M. (Ed.). (1988). *Hypnosis and memory.* New York: Guilford.

Phillips, M. (1993a). Our bodies, ourselves: Treating the somatic manifestations of trauma with ego-state therapy. *American Journal of Clinical Hypnosis, 38,* 109–121.

Phillips, M. (1993b). The use of ego-state therapy in the treatment of post-traumatic stress disorder. *American Journal of Clinical Hypnosis, 35,* 241–249.

Phillips, M. (1993c). Turning symptoms into allies: Utilization approaches with posttraumatic symptoms. *American Journal of Clinical Hypnosis, 35,* 179–189.

Phillips, M. (1997, July). *Ego-strengthening and emdr.* Workshop presented at the 1997 EMDRIA Conference, San Francisco, CA.

Phillips, M., & Frederick, C. (1992). The use of hypnotic age progressions as prognostic, ego-strengthening, and integrating technique. *American Journal of Clinical Hypnosis, 35*, 90–108.

Phillips, M., & Frederick, C. (1995). *Healing the divided self: Clinical and Ericksonian hypnotherapy for dissociative and post-traumatic conditions.* New York: Norton.

Phillips, M., & Smith, A. J., Jr. (1996, March). *Transitional states of consciousness and the hypnotherapeutic relationship.* Paper presented at the annual meeting of the American Society of Clinical Hypnosis, Orlando, FL.

Piaget, J. (1952). *The origins of intelligence in children.* New York: International Universities Press. (Original work published 1936)

Piaget, J. (1954). *Construction of reality in the child.* New York: Basic Books.

Prince, M. (1978). *The dissociation of a personality.* New York: Oxford University Press. (Original work published 1905)

Proust, M. (1970). The remembrances of things past (C. K. Scott Montcrieff, Trans.). New York: Vintage-Ransom. (*Original work published* 1913–1925)

Putnam, F. (1988). The switch process in multiple personality disorder and other state change disorders. *Dissociation, 1*, 24–31.

Putnam, F. (1989). *Diagnosis and treatment of multiple personality disorder.* New York: Guilford.

Putnam, F., Guroff, J. J., Silberman, E. K., Barban, L., & Post, R. M. (1986). The clinical phenomenology of multiple personality disorder: A review of 100 recent cases. *Journal of Clinical Psychiatry, 47*, 285–293.

Rapaport, D., & Gill, M. (1967). The points of view and assumptions of metapsychology. In M. Gill (Ed.), *The collected papers of David Rapaport* (pp. 795–811). New York: Basic Books. (Original work published 1959)

Rasmussen, S. A., Eisen, J. L., & Pato, M. T. (1993). Current issues in the pharmacological management of obsessive compulsive disorder. *The Journal of Clinical Psychiatry, 54* [suppl.], 4–9.

Reis, B. (1993). Toward a psychoanalytic understanding of multiple personality disorder. *Bulletin of the Menninger Clinic, 57*, 309–318.

Richardson, A. (1969). *Mental imagery.* London: Routledge & Kegan Paul.

Richardson, A. (1983). Imagery: Definition and types. In A. A. Sheikh (Ed.), *Imagery: current theory, research, and application* (pp. 3–42). New York: Wiley.

Ricoeur, P. (1965). *History and truth.* Evanston, IL: Northwestern University Press. (Original work published 1955)

Ristad, E. (1982). *A soprano on her head.* Moab, UT: Real People Press.

Rogers, C. (1961). *On becoming a person: A client's view of psychotherapy.* Boston: Houghton-Mifflin.

Rogers, C. (1975). Empathic: An unappreciated way of being. *Counseling Psychologist, 5*, 1–10.

Rose, D. S. (1986). "Worse than death": Psychodynamics of rape victims and the need for psychotherapy. *American Journal of Psychiatry, 43*, 817–824.

Rose, G. (1978). The creativity of everyday life. In S. Grolnick, L. Barkin, & W. Muensterberger (Eds.), *Between reality and fantasy: Transitional objects and phenomena.* Northvale, NJ: Jason Aronson.

Rosen, J. N. (1962). *Direct analytic therapy.* New York: Grune & Stratton.

Rosenbaum, J. F., Pollack, M. H., & Pollack, R. A. (1996). Clinical issues in the long term treatment of panic disorder. *Journal of Clinical Psychiatry, 57* [suppl. 10], 44–48.

Ross, C. J. (1989). *Multiple personality disorder.* New York: Wiley.

Ross, C. J. & Anderson, G. (1988). Phenomenological overlap of multiple personality disorder and obsessive-compulsive disorder. *Journal of Nervous and Mental Disease, 176,* 295–299.

Rossi, E. L. (1968). The breakout heuristic: A phenomenology of growth therapy with college students. *Journal of Humanistic Psychology, 8,* 6–28.

Rossi, E. L. (1972). *Dreams and the growth of personality: Expanding awareness in psychotherapy.* New York: Pergamon.

Rossi, E. L. (Ed.). (1980). *The collected papers of Milton H. Erickson on hypnosis.* New York: Irvington.

Rossi, E. L. (Ed.). (1989). *The collected papers of Milton H. Erickson on hypnosis* (*Vol. 4,* pp. 445–542). New York: Irvington.

Rossi, E. L. (1993). *The psychobiology of mind-body healing: New concepts of therapeutic hypnosis* (2nd ed.). New York: Norton.

Rossi, E. L., & Cheek, D. B. (1988). *Mind-body therapy: Ideodynamic healing in hypnosis.* New York: Norton.

Rossman, M. L. (1987). *Healing yourself: A step-by-step program for better health through imagery.* New York: Walker.

Ruch, J. C. (1975). Self-hypnosis: The result of hetero-hypnosis or vice versa? *International Journal of Clinical and Experimental Hypnosis, 23,* 282–304.

Saint-Exupéry, A. (1971). *The little prince* (K. Woods, Trans.). New York: Harcourt Brace Jovanovich. (Original work published 1943)

Salmon, P. G., & Meyer, R. G. (1992). *Notes from the green room: Coping with stress and anxiety in musical performance.* New York: Macmillan.

Salzman, L., & Thaler, F. H. (1981). Obsessive compulsive disorders: A review of the literature. *American Journal of Psychiatry, 138,* 286–296.

Samuels, A., Shorter, B., & Plaut, F. (1986). *A critical dictionary of Jungian analysis.* New York: Routledge & Kegan Paul.

Sanders, S. (1991). *Clinical self-hypnosis: The power of words and images.* New York: Guilford.

Satir, V. (1983). *Conjoint family therapy* (3rd ed.). Palo Alto, CA: Science and Behavior Books.

Scagnelli, J. (1976). Hypnotherapy with schizophrenic and borderline patients. *American Journal of Clinical Hypnosis, 19,* 33–38.

Scagnelli-Jobsis, J. (1982). Hypnosis with psychotic patients: A review of the literature and presentation of a theoretical framework. *American Journal of Clinical Hypnosis, 25,* 33–45.

Scharff, J. S. (1992). *Projective and introjective identification and the use of the therapist's self.* London: Aronson.

Schetky, D. H. (1992). A review of the literature on the long-term effects of childhood sexual abuse. In R. P. Kluft (Ed.), *Incest related syndromes of adult psychopathology* (pp. 35–54). Washington, DC: American Psychiatric Press.

Schneck, J. (1954). Countertransference in Freud's rejection of hypnosis. *American Journal of Psychiatry, 110,* 928–931.

Schwartz, R. C. (1995). *Internal family systems therapy*. New York: Guilford.

Schwing, G. (1940). *A way to the soul of the mentally ill*. New York: International Universities Press.

Searles, H. F. (1965). *Collected papers on schizophrenia and selected topics*. New York: International Universities Press.

Sechehaye, M. A. (1947). *Symbolic realization*. New York: International Universities Press.

Shapiro, F. (1989). Efficacy of the eye movement desensitization procedure in the treatment of traumatic memories. *Journal of Traumatic Stress Studies, 2*, 199–223.

Shapiro, F. (1995). *Eye movement desensitization and reprocessing: Basic principles, protocols, and procedures*. New York: Guilford.

Shapiro, M. K. (1991). Bandaging a "broken heart": Hypnoplay therapy in the treatment of multiple personality disorder. *American Journal of Clinical Hypnosis, 34*, 1–10.

Sheikh, A. A. (Ed.). (1983). *Imagery: Current theory, research, and application*. New York: Wiley.

Siegel, B. (1969). *Love, medicine, and miracles*. New York: Harper & Row.

Siegel, B. (1989). *Peace, love, and healing*. New York: Harper & Row.

Simmel, E. (1944). War neuroses. In S. Lorand (Ed.), *Psychoanalysis today* (pp. 227–248). New York: International Universities Press.

Simonton, O. C., Matthews-Simonton, S., & Creighton, J. (1978). *Getting well again*. Los Angeles: Tarcher.

Smith, A. (1984). Sources of efficacy in the hypnotic relationship—an object relations approach. In W. C. Wester, II, & A. H. Smith, Jr. (Eds.), *Clinical hypnosis: A multidisciplinary approach* (pp. 85–114). Philadelphia: Lippincott.

Smith, A. (1990). The hypnotic relationship and the holographic paradigm. *American Journal of Clinical Hypnosis, 32*, 183–193.

Smith, A. (1995, March). *The transitional state in hypnosis: Understanding its therapeutic potential*. Paper presented at the annual meeting of the American Society of Clinical Hypnosis, San Diego, CA.

Soskis, D. A. (1986). *Teaching self-hypnosis: An introductory guide for clinicians*. New York: Norton.

Spanos, N. P. (1982). Hypnotic behavior: A cognitive, social, psychological perspective. *Research Communications in Psychology, Psychiatry, and Behavior, 7*, 199–213.

Spanos, N. P. (1986). Hypnotic behavior: A social psychological interpretation of amnesia, analgesia, and "trance logic." *Behavioral and Brain Sciences, 9*, 489–497.

Spanos, N. P. (1991). A socio-cognitive approach to hypnosis. In S. J. Lynn & J. W. Rhue (Eds.), *Theories of hypnosis: Current modes and perspectives* (pp. 324–361). New York: Guilford.

Spanos, N. P., Weekes, J. R., & Bertrand, L. D. (1985). Multiple personality: A social psychological perspective. *Journal of Abnormal Psychology, 94*, 362–376.

Spanos, N. P., Weekes, J. R., Meanry, E., & Bertrand, L. D. (1986). Hypnotic interview and age regression procedures in elicitation of multiple personality symptoms: A simulation study. *Psychiatry, 49*, 298–311.

Spence, D. P. (1982). *Narrative truth and historical truth: Meaning and interpretation in psychoanalysis*. New York: Norton.

Spiegel, D. (1986). Dissociating damage. *American Journal of Clinical Hypnosis, 29*, 123–130.

Spiegel, D. (1991). A psychosocial intervention and survival time of patients with metastatic breast cancer. *Advances, 7,* 10–19.

Spiegel, H. (1996, March). *The low hypnotizable subject: Clinical considerations.* Paper presented at the annual meeting of the American Society of Clinical Hypnosis, Orlando, FL.

Spiegel, H., & Spiegel, D. (1978). *Trance and treatment.* Washington, DC: American Psychiatric Press.

Spitz, R. (1965). *The first year of life: A psychoanalytic study of normal and deviant development of object relations.* New York: International Universities Press.

St. Clair, M. (1986). *Object relations and self psychology: An introduction.* Monterey, CA: Brooks/Cole.

Stanton, H. E. (1977). Test anxiety and hypnosis: A different approach to an important problem. *Australian Journal of Education, 21,* 179–186.

Stanton, H. E. (1979). Increasing internal control through hypnotic ego-enhancement. *Australian Journal of Clinical and Experimental Hypnosis, 7,* 219–233.

Stanton, H. E. (1989). Ego-enhancement: A five-step approach. *American Journal of Clinical Hypnosis, 31,* 192–198.

Stanton, H. E. (1990). Ego-enhancement: A five-step approach. Enhancing esteem, self-efficacy, and confidence. In D. C. Hammond (Ed.), *Handbook of hypnotic suggestions and metaphors* (pp. 109–151). New York: Norton.

Stanton, H. E. (1993a). Ego-enhancement for positive change. *Australian Journal of Clinical and Experimental Hypnosis, 21,* 59–64.

Stanton, H. E. (1993b). Using hypnotherapy to overcome examination anxiety. *American Journal of Clinical Hypnosis, 35,* 198–204.

Stein, C. (1963). The clenched fist technique as a hypnotic procedure in clinical psychotherapy. *American Journal of Clinical Hypnosis, 6,* 113–119.

Sterba, R. F. (1934). The fate of the ego in analytic therapy. *International Journal of Psychoanalysis, 15,* 117–126.

Sterba, R. F. (1940). The dynamics of the dissolution of the transference resistance. *Psychoanalytic Quarterly, 9,* 363–379. (Original work published 1929)

Stevenson, O. (1954). The first treasured possession: A study of the part played by specially loved objects and toys in the lives of certain children. *Psychoanalytic Study of the Child, 9,* 199–217.

Stolorow, R. D., Brandchaft, B., & Atwood, G. (1983). Intersubjectivity in psychoanalytic treatment. *Bulletin of the Menninger Clinic, 47,* 117–128.

Stone, M. H. (1997). *Healing the mind: A history of psychiatry from antiquity to the present.* New York: Norton.

Strachey, J. (1934). The nature of the therapeutic action of psychoanalysis. *International Journal of Psychoanalysis, 15,* 127–159.

Stafrace, S. (1994). Hypnosis in the treatment of panic disorder with agoraphobia. *Australian Journal of Clinical and Experimental Hypnosis, 22,* 73–86.

Sugarman, A., & Jaffe, L. S. (1987). Transitional phenomena and psychological separateness in schizophrenic, borderline, and bulimic patients. In J. Bloom-Feshbach & S. Bloom-Feshbach (Eds.), *The psychology of separation and loss: Perspectives on development, life transitions, and clinical practice* (pp. 416–458). San Francisco: Jossey-Bass.

Summers, F. (1994). *Object relations theory and psychopathology.* Hillsdale, NJ: The Analytic Press.

Tan, E., Marks, I. M., & Marsett, P. (1971). Bimedial leucotomy in obsessive compulsive neurosis: A controlled serial inquiry. *British Journal of Psychiatry, 118,* 155–164.

Tart, C. T. (1975). *States of consciousness.* New York: Dutton.

Teilhard de Chardin, P. (1960). *The divine milieu.* New York: Harper & Row. (Original work published 1957)

Teilhard de Chardin, P. (1964). *The future of man.* New York: Harper & Row.

Teilhard de Chardin, P. (1969). *Human energy.* New York: Harcourt, Brace, Jovanovich.

Teilhard de Chardin, P. (1973). *On happiness.* London: Collins, St. James Place. (Original work published 1966)

Terr, L. (1991). Childhood traumas: An outline and overview. *The American Journal of Psychiatry, 148,* 10–20.

Thoren, P., Asberg, M., & Bertillson, R. (1988). Clomipramine treatment of obsessive compulsive disorders: II. Biochemical aspects. *Archives of General Psychiatry, 37,* 1289–1294.

Thorpe, G. L., & Burns, L. E. (1983). *The agoraphobic syndrome: Behavioral approaches to evaluation and treatment.* New York: Wiley.

Tillman, J. G., Nash, M. R., & Lerner, P. M. (1994). Does trauma cause dissociative pathology? In S. Lynn & J. W. Rhue (Eds.), *Dissociation: Clinical and theoretical perspectives* (pp. 395–414). New York: Guilford.

Tilton, P. (1986). Effective use of Erickson's interspersal technique. In B. Zilbergeld, G. Edelstien, & D. Aroaz (Eds.), *Hypnosis: Questions and answers* (pp. 255–260). New York: Norton.

Torem, M. (1987a). Ego state therapy for eating disorders. *American Journal of Clinical Hypnosis, 30,* 94–103.

Torem, M. (1987b). Hypnosis in the treatment of depression. In W. C. Wester (Ed.), *Clinical hypnosis: A case management approach* (pp. 288–301). Cincinnati, OH: Behavioral Science Center.

Torem, M. (1989). Recognition and management of dissociative regressions. *Hypnos, 31,* 197–213.

Torem, M. (1990). Ego-strengthening: Enhancing esteem, self-efficacy, and confidence. In D.C. Hammond (Ed.), *Handbook of hypnotic suggestions and metaphors* (pp. 109–112). New York: Norton.

Torem, M. (1992). "Back from the future": A powerful age-progression technique. *American Journal of Clinical Hypnosis, 35,* 81–88.

Torem, M., & Gainer, M. J. (1995). The center core: Imagery for experiencing the unifying self. *Hypnos, 22,* 125–131.

Torem, M., Gilbertson, A., & Kemp, K. (1990). *Future oriented guided imagery as a crisis intervention technique in the treatment of suicidal multiple personality disorder patients.* Presented at the annual meeting of the American Society of Clinical Hypnosis. Orlando, FL.

Torgersen, S. (1983). Genetic factors in anxiety disorders. *Archives of General Psychiatry, 40,* 1086–1089.

Toro, P. A. (1982). Developmental effects of child abuse: A review. *Child Abuse and Neglect, 6,* 423–431.

Tulving, E. (1972) Episodic and semantic memory. In E. Tulving & W. Donaldson (Eds.), *Organization of memory* (pp. 381–403). New York: McGraw-Hill.

Tulving, E. (1985). Memory and consciousness. *Canadian Psychology, 26,* 1–12.

Turner, S. (1985). Epidemiology of phobic and obsessive compulsive disorders among adults. *American Journal of Psychotherapy, 39*, 360–369.

Turner, S., Bidel, D., & Nathan, R. (1985). Biological factors in obsessive compulsive disorders. *Psychological Bulletin, 97*, 430–450.

Unestahl, L. E. (1983). *The mental aspect of gymnastics*. Oreboro, Sweden: Veje Publishers.

Van der Hart, O., & Brown, P. (1992). Abreaction re-evaluated. *Dissociation, 5*, 127–140.

Van der Kolk, B. A. (1989). The compulsion to repeat the trauma: Re-enactment, revictimization, and masochism. *Psychiatric Clinics of North America, 12*(2), 389–3411.

Van der Kolk, B. A. (1996a). The body keeps the score: Approaches to the psychobiology of post traumatic stress disorder. In B. A. Van der Kolk, A. C. McFarlane, & L. Weisaeth (Eds.), *Traumatic stress* (pp. 214–241). New York: Guilford.

Van der Kolk, B. A. (1996b). Trauma and memory. In B. A. Van der Kolk, A. C. McFarlane, & L. Weisaeth (Eds.), *Traumatic stress* (pp. 279–302). New York: Guilford.

Van der Kolk, B. A. (1997, July). *Current understanding of the psychobiology of trauma*. Paper presented at the 1997 EMDR National Association Conference, San Francisco.

Volkan, V. D. (1976). *Primitive internalized object relations: A clinical study of schizophrenic, borderline, and narcissistic patients*. New York: International Universities Press.

Wallace, W. A. (1974). *Causality and scientific explanation*. Ann Arbor: University of Michigan Press.

Wark, D. M. (1990a). Advanced comprehension suggestions for an alert trance. In D. C.Hammond (Ed.), *Handbook of therapeutic suggestions and metaphors* (p. 450). New York: Norton.

Wark, D. M. (1990b). Alert self-hypnosis technique to improve reading comprehension. In D. C. Hammond (Ed.), *Handbook of therapeutic suggestions and metaphors* (p. 449). New York: Norton.

Wark, D. M. (1996, March). *Alert hypnosis in education and treatment*. Paper presented at the annual meeting of the American Society of Clinical Hypnosis, Orlando, FL.

Watkins, H. H. (1980). The silent abreaction. *The International Journal of Clinical and Experimental Hypnosis, 28*, 101–113.

Watkins, H. H. (1990). Suggestions for raising self-esteem. In D. C. Hammond (Ed.), *Handbook of hypnotic suggestions and metaphors* (pp. 127–130). New York: Norton.

Watkins, H. H. (1993). Ego-state therapy: An overview. *American Journal of Clinical Hypnosis, 35*, 232–240.

Watkins, J. G. (1949). *Hypnotherapy of war neuroses*. New York: Ronald.

Watkins, J. G. (1963). Transference aspects of the hypnotic relationship. In M. V. Kline (Ed.), *Clinical correlations of experimental hypnosis* (pp. 5–24). Springfield, IL: Thomas.

Watkins, J. G. (1978). *The therapeutic self*. New York: Human Sciences Press.

Watkins, J. G. (1987). *The practice of clinical hypnosis: Vol. I. Hypnotherapeutic techniques*. New York: Irvington.

Watkins, J. G. (1992). *The practice of clinical hypnosis: Vol. II. Hypnoanalytic techniques*. New York: Irvington.

Watkins, J. G., & Watkins, H. H. (1979–1980). Ego states and hidden observers. *Journal of Altered States of Consciousness, 5*, 3–18.

Watkins, J. G., & Watkins, H. H. (1988). The management of malevolent ego states in multiple personality disorder. *Dissociation, 1*, 67–71.

Watkins, J. G., & Watkins, H. H. (1990). Ego-state transferences in the hypnoanalytic treatment of dissociative reactions. In M. L. Fass & D. Brown (Eds.), *Creative mastery in hypnosis and hypnoanalysis: A festschrift for Erika Fromm* (pp. 225–261). Hillsdale, NJ: Lawrence Erlbaum Associates.

Watkins, J. G., & Watkins, H. H. (1991) Hypnosis and ego-state therapy. In P. A. Keller & S. R. Heyman (Eds.), *Innovations in clinical practice* (pp. 23–37). Sarasota: Florida Professional Resources Exchange.

Watkins, J. G., & Watkins, H. H. (1997). *Ego states: Theory and therapy*. New York: Norton.

Watkins, P. C., Matthews, A., Williamson, D. A., & Fuller, R. D. (1982). Mood congruent memory in depression: Emotional priming or elaboration. *Journal of Abnormal Psychology, 10*, 581–586.

Weiss, E. (1960). *The structure and dynamics of the human mind*. New York: Grune & Stratton.

Weiss, E. (1966). Paul Federn: The theory of the psychosis. In F. Alexander, S. Eisenstein, & M. Grotjahn (Eds.), *Psychoanalytic pioneers* (pp. 142–168). New York: Basic Books.

Weiss, J. (1993). *How psychotherapy works: Process and technique*. New York: Guilford.

Weiss, J., Sampson, H., & the Mt. Zion Psychotherapy Research Group. (1986). *The psychoanalytic process: Theory, clinical observations, and empirical research*. New York: Guilford.

Wells, H. G. (1957). *The time machine*. New York: Berkley Publishing. (Original work published 1895)

Whitaker, C., & Malone, M. (1953). *The roots of psychotherapy*. New York: Blakiston.

Wingfield, H. E. (1920). *An introduction to the study of hypnotism*. London: Balliere Tindall.

Winnicott, D. W. (1953). Transitional objects and transitional phenomena: A study on the first not-me possession. *International Journal of Psychoanalysis, 34*, 89–97.

Winnicott, D. W. (1958). Primary maternal preoccupation. In *Collected papers* (pp. 300–305). New York: Basic Books. (Original work published 1956)

Winnicott, D. W. (1965). The theory of the parent-infant relationship. In *Maturational processes and the facilitating environment* (pp. 37–55). New York: International Universities Press. (Original work published 1960)

Winnicott, D. W. (1965). Ego integration in child development. In *Maturational processes and the facilitating environment* (pp. 140–152). New York: International Universities Press. (Original work published 1962)

Winnicott, D. W. (1971). *Playing and reality*. New York: Basic Books.

Winnicott, D. W. (1975). *Through paediatrics to psychoanalysis*. New York: Basic Books.

Winter, G. D. (1986). Hypnosis with agoraphobia. In B. Zilbergeld, M. G. Edelstien, & D. L. Aroaz (Eds.), *Hypnosis: Questions and answers* (pp. 307–1112). New York: Norton.

Wolf, E. S. (1988). *Treating the self: Elements of clinical self psychology*. New York: Guilford.

Wolff, P. H. (1959). Observations on newborn infants. *Psychosomatic Medicine, 21*, 110–118.

Wolpe, J., & Lazarus, A. A. (1966). *Behavior therapy techniques*. Oxford: Pergamon Press.

Woodworth, R. S. (1906). Imageless thought. *Journal of Philosophy, Psychology and Scientific Methods, 3*, 701–708.

Woolf, V. (1959). *The waves*. New York: Harcourt Brace. (Original work published 1931)

Yapko, M. D. (1986). What is Ericksonian hypnosis? In B. Zilbergeld, M. G. Edelstien, & D. L. Aroaz (Eds.), *Hypnosis: Questions and answers* (pp. 223–231). New York: Norton.

Yapko, M. D. (1990). *Trancework: An introduction to the practice of clinical hypnosis* (2nd ed.). New York: Brunner/Mazel.

Yapko, M. D. (1992). *Hypnosis and the treatment of depressions*. New York: Brunner/Mazel.

Yapko, M. D. (1996). A brief therapy approach to the use of hypnosis in treating depression. In S. Lynn, I. Kirsch, & J. Rhue (Eds.), *Casebook of clinical hypnosis* (pp. 75–99). Washington, DC: American Psychological Association.

Young-Eisendrath, P., & Hall, J. A. (1991). *Jung's self psychology: A constructivist perspective*. New York: Guilford Press.

Zeig, J. K. (Ed.). (1980). *A teaching seminar with Milton H. Erickson*. New York: Brunner/Mazel.

Zeig, J. K. (Ed.). (1982). *Ericksonian approaches to hypnosis and psychotherapy*. New York: Brunner/Mazel.

Zelikovsy, N., & Lynn, S. J. (1995). The aftereffects and assessment of physical and psychological abuse. In S. J. Lynn & J. W. Rhue (Eds.), *Dissociation* (pp. 190–214). New York: Guilford.

Zetzel, E. R. (1956). Current concepts of transference. *International Journal of Psychoanalysis, 37,* 369–376.

Zilbergeld, B., & Lazarus, A. (1987). *Mind power*. Boston: Little, Brown.

Author Index

Subject Index

Printed in the United States
by Baker & Taylor Publisher Services